Biotechnology

Dedication:

For our families: George and Judith-Anna; Roger, Hetty and Flora.

Commissioning Editor: Timothy Horne
Development Editor: Clive Hewat
Project Manager: Anne Dickie/Hemamalini Rajendrababu
Designer/Design Direction: Charles Gray
Illustration Manager: Bruce Hogarth
Illustrations: Robert Britton

Medical Biotechnology

Edited by

Judit Pongracz BSc PhD DrHabil
Associate Professor, Department of Immunology and Biotechnology,
Faculty of Medicine, University of Pecs,
Hungary

Mary Keen BSc PhD
Associate Professor, Department of Pharmacology
University of Birmingham,
Birmingham, UK

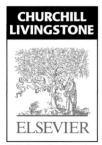

CHURCHILL
LIVINGSTONE

ELSEVIER

Edinburgh • London • New York • Oxford • Philadelphia • St Louis • Sydney • Toronto 2009

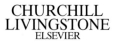

CHURCHILL
LIVINGSTONE
ELSEVIER

First published 2009

ISBN: 978-0-08-045135-0

British Library Cataloguing in Publication Data
A catalogue record for this book is available from the British Library

Library of Congress Cataloging in Publication Data
A catalog record for this book is available from the Library of Congress

Notice
Knowledge and best practice in this field are constantly changing. As new research and experience broaden our knowledge, changes in practice, treatment and drug therapy may become necessary or appropriate. Readers are advised to check the most current information provided (i) on procedures featured or (ii) by the manufacturer of each product to be administered, to verify the recommended dose or formula, the method and duration of administration, and contraindications. It is the responsibility of the practitioner, relying on their own experience and knowledge of the patient, to make diagnoses, to determine dosages and the best treatment for each individual patient, and to take all appropriate safety precautions. To the fullest extent of the law, neither the Publisher nor the Editors assumes any liability for any injury and/or damage to persons or property arising out of or related to any use of the material contained in this book.

The Publisher

ELSEVIER   your source for books,
journals and multimedia
in the health sciences

www.elsevierhealth.com

Working together to grow
libraries in developing countries

www.elsevier.com | www.bookaid.org | www.sabre.org

ELSEVIER   BOOK AID International   Sabre Foundation

The publisher's policy is to use paper manufactured from sustainable forests

Printed in China

Contents

Contributors

Andrea Bacon BSc (Hons) PhD
Institute for Biomedical Research
University of Birmingham College of Medical
and Dental Sciences
Birmingham, UK

Domokos Bartis MD PhD
Research Scientist
Department of Immunology and Biotechnology
Faculty of Medicine
University of Pecs, Hungary

Lee David Keith Buttery MSc PhD
Senior Lecturer in Cell Biology and
Tissue Engineering
School of Pharmacy
Centre for Biomolecular Sciences
University of Nottingham
Nottingham, UK

Tamas Czompoly MD PhD
Assistant Professor
Department of Immunology and Biotechnology
Faculty of Medicine
University of Pecs, Hungary

Jon Frampton
Professor of Stem Cell Biology
Institute of Biomedical Research
University of Birmingham College of Medical
and Dental Sciences
Birmingham, UK

Mary Keen BSc PhD
Associate Professor
Department of Pharmacology
Division of Neuroscience
University of Birmingham
Birmingham, UK

Krisztian Kvell MD PhD
Research Scientist
Department of Immunology and Biotechnology
Faculty of Medicine
University of Pecs, Hungary

Zsuzsanna Nagy MD DPhil
Senior Lecturer
Division of Neuroscience
University of Birmingham College of Medical
and Dental Sciences
Birmingham, UK

Karl Peter Nightingale BSc (Hons) PhD
Roberts Research Fellow
Institute of Biomedical Research
University of Birmingham College of Medical
and Dental Sciences
Birmingham, UK

Judit E. Pongracz PhD
Associate Professor
Department of Immunology and Biotechnology
Faculty of Medicine
University of Pecs, Hungary

Douglas A. Richards DPhil MIBiol
Lecturer
Department of Pharmacology
Division of Neuroscience
University of Birmingham College of Medical
and Dental Sciences
Birmingham, UK

Felicity Rosamari Rose BSc (Hons) PhD
Associate Professor in Tissue Engineering
School of Pharmacy
Centre for Biomolecular Sciences
University of Nottingham
Nottingham, UK

Kevin Shakesheff BSc (Hons) PhD
Professor in Tissue Engineering and Drug Delivery
School of Pharmacy
Centre for Biomolecular Sciences
University of Nottingham
Nottingham, UK

Acknowledgements

We thank these undergraduate medical students (University of Pecs, Pecs, Hungary) whose questions and comments helped to shape this book:

Androsics, Mónika	Novák, Zsófia
Árvai, Lilla	Pánczél, Gitta
Balasa, Tibor R.	Pere, Timea
Bernieh, Basl	Polgár, Imre
Borza, Zoltán F.	Priegl, Linda
Engel, Borbála	Prodán, Alexandra
Enyedi, Gergely	Pünkösti, Ildikó Á.
Ferenczi, Gábor	Rácz, Gábor
Fitos, Péter	Rákossy, Margaréta
Geider, Attila	Riba, János
Harta, Anikó	Sallai-Balogh, Adrienn
Jakab, Lajos	Sasvári, Kata Á.
Jakab, László	Schiller, Róbert
Józsa, Gergő	Schmeller, Bernadett
Juni, Eszter	Sirály, Enikő
Kiss, Gabriella	Stefanovits, Ágnes
Kovács, Borbála A.	Stréda, Zoltán P.
Kovács, Noémi	Szabó, Gergely
Kuperczkó, Diána	Szabó, Imre
Lengl, Orsolya	Szabó, Tímea
Lőcsei, Zoltán	Szijártó, Valéria I.
Márton, Noémi	Takács, László
Megyeri, Gábor	Turu, Dorottya
Mészáros, László	Váncsodi, József
Mózes, Réka	Varga, Diána M.
Nagy, Péter	Várnai, Lilla H.
Nagy, Tibor A.	Zalán, Petra
Nedvig, Klára	Zarka, Gyula

Our special thanks go to Lilla Árvai for reading and commenting on the sample chapters.

Preface
An introduction to medical biotechnology

Biotechnology encompasses the variety of methods available for manipulating living cells and organisms. It is having an increasing impact on all aspects of medicine, from helping in the understanding of the aetiology of disease, to its diagnosis and treatment.

The making of wine, beer and cheese and the selective breeding of plants and animals can both be viewed as biotechnology and date back to ancient times. However, it is advances in molecular biology and our ability to manipulate individual genes that really define modern biotechnology. These techniques can be used in a range of disciplines, from agriculture to medicine. It is unsurprising that the precise definition of biotechnology can vary considerably. Moreover, as it is essentially a 'tool kit' of techniques, the end result of using these techniques also varies considerably (Table P.1).

What is medical biotechnology?

Medical biotechnology can be defined as a branch of biotechnology that uses ever more specialized techniques to manipulate microorganisms, plants, animals and human tissues with the overall aim of understanding, treating and, if possible, curing human disease.

Medical biotechnology builds on our basic understanding of cell biology, genetics, molecular biology, biochemistry, microbiology, pharmacology and immunology. Fundamental to all of these is the recognition that life's basic building blocks are cells, and cells have some general similarities in addition to well-characterized differences.

The general similarities of the vast majority of cells include the fact that they are surrounded by a phospholipid plasma membrane and use the same general mechanisms of DNA replication, protein synthesis and energy metabolism.

Despite these general similarities, different cells can function in very different ways. Many organisms, such as bacteria, amoebae and yeasts, consist of single cells that are capable of independent self-replication. More complex organisms are composed of various tissue types consisting of collections of cells that function in a coordinated manner to perform particular functions. The function of some of these differentiated cells can be very specialized indeed. As an example, Table P.2 shows some of the functions of specialized cells of the human immune system.

Medical biotechnology in medical training

The growing importance of medical biotechnology means that a general understanding of this rapidly advancing field is essential for all medical graduates and medical scientists. Indeed, biotechnology courses are being established in undergraduate medical curricula in an increasing number of universities worldwide. However, as most medical graduates are unlikely to work in a basic research laboratory, the emphasis of this book is on the medical applications of biotechnology rather than the details of the experimental techniques.

Although the book is primarily intended for undergraduate students who will become medical practitioners or biomedical scientists, this summary of medical biotechnology may also be useful for current medical practitioners.

Table P.1
Examples of different uses of the same technology in different disciplines

Technique	Agriculture	Pharmacy	Medicine
Gene cloning (DNA manipulation)	Cloned crops with increased yields	Expression of human proteins into bacteria	Gene therapy
Regulation of protein expression	Muscle volume increase in cattle	Increase in the expression of medically important protein in bioreactors	Decrease of inflammatory cytokine expression by promoter inhibition
Tissue engineering		Developing novel drug test systems	Making 'transplantation-ready' human tissue

Table P.2
Specialized functions of some immune cell types

Cell type	Cell function
Dendritic cells	Antigen processing and presentation
Helper T cells	Cytokine production and antigen recognition
Cytotoxic T cells	Antigen recognition and killing of cells expressing 'non-self' antigens
Memory T cells	Retain a long-lasting 'memory' of non-self antigens
Regulatory T cells	Regulate the immune response via release of cytokines
B cells	Antibody production and antigen presentation
Memory B cells	Retain the ability to recognize a specific antigen and proliferate into antibody-producing cells in the event of reinfection
Macrophages	Phagocytosis, cytokine production, antigen presentation and elimination of pathogen
Natural killer (NK) cells	Pattern recognition and elimination of non-self cells

J. Pongracz and M. Keen

The molecular basis of disease

J. Pongracz

Recent decades have seen dramatic advances in genetics, biochemistry, biophysics, cell biology and immunology, and these have all contributed to the complex and fast-evolving field of medical biotechnology. These advances are leading to a re-evaluation of our understanding of disease, and are opening up new and sometimes unorthodox methods of diagnosis and treatment.

Clearly, human medicine deals with a highly complex multicellular organism (Fig. 1.1), and it is unsurprising that several different approaches are required to understand and potentially manipulate the regulation of the complex systems that comprise the human body. These various approaches will be considered in more detail in the chapters that follow.

Traditionally, investigation of medical problems has been confined to observations that can be made with the naked eye or reported by the patient. The wealth of knowledge accumulated by this approach is still the basis of disease nomenclature and often determines diagnosis and treatment. While technological advances, such as the invention of the microscope, have always had an impact on our understanding of disease mechanisms and have led to novel therapies, the explosion of knowledge and techniques that comprises the biotechnological revolution seems likely to change medical practice beyond recognition.

What is disease?

The *Oxford English Dictionary* defines disease as 'a condition of the body, or some part or organ of the body, in which its functions are disturbed or deranged'. This definition includes obvious diseases such as influenza, and also injuries and conditions such as depression or alcoholism, and we will stick with this broad idea of disease definition throughout the book.

What factors can cause diseases?

A number of factors can result in disease. These include:

- *infection* by bacteria (e.g. whooping cough), viruses (e.g. AIDS), fungi (e.g. candidiasis) or parasites (e.g. malaria)

- *injury* (e.g. a broken leg)
- *environmental factors* (e.g. silicosis)
- *genetic mutations*, either inherited (e.g. cystic fibrosis) or acquired (e.g. cancer).

A great many diseases seem to be caused by a combination of two or more different factors; these are the so-called 'multifactorial disorders' such as schizophrenia or heart disease.

In order to understand disease processes fully and to differentiate between diseased and healthy tissue, it is useful to understand the function of the normal human body. Often, however, it is the existence of a disease which highlights the need for further investigation and better understanding of normal tissue function.

Why is it important to understand the cause of a disease?

It is relatively easy to pinpoint the cause of some diseases. For example, mycobacterial infection is the cause of tuberculosis; mutation in the *CFT* gene is the cause of cystic fibrosis. However, in most diseases the causative agents are hard to find. Without knowing the cause, it may be impossible to effect a cure or even to alleviate the symptoms of the disease. In many cases, similar symptoms can be triggered by a variety of causes; in order to target therapy appropriately to a particular condition, it is essential to understand the cause of the disease. This can be illustrated by considering dementia as an example (Box 1.1).

The molecular basis of disease

Diseases can be categorized in a variety of ways, such as on the basis of their cause or by the time at which the symptoms appear. Box 1.2 shows some examples of how various diseases could be classified in these ways.

Figure 1.2 shows how malfunctions of various cells can lead to different conditions, depending on the time at which they occur.

However, no matter how we categorize the causes of diseases, it seems clear that precise diagnosis and

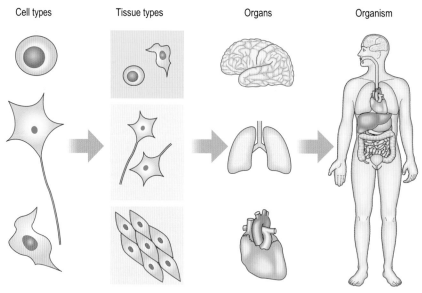

Figure 1.1
Stem cells give rise to various cell types, which differentiate into numerous tissue types that build organs and finally the organism.

 Box 1.1

Causes of dementia

Alzheimer's disease is a progressive, debilitating, degenerative condition of the central nervous system which leads to dementia. There are characteristic histological changes in the brains of patients with Alzheimer's disease, particularly amyloid plaques and neurofibrillary tangles in the cerebral cortex and hippocampus. However, these changes can only be observed upon post-mortem examination. Although Alzheimer's disease is one of the most common causes of dementia, there are numerous other conditions that can be mistaken for Alzheimer's. These include depression, thyroid dysfunction, substance abuse, nutritional deficiencies (particularly deficiencies of vitamins B_1, B_3, B_{12} and folic acid) and side-effects of prescription drugs (including drugs for Parkinson's disease, depression, allergies and migraine), all of which can mimic the decline in mental functioning associated with Alzheimer's disease. Most of the above conditions can be treated relatively easily; for example, people with dementia related to vitamin B_{12} deficiency can recover with B_{12} injections. Other less treatable disorders are also confused with Alzheimer's. These include vascular or multi-infarct dementia and progressive fronto-temporal dementia (FTD), formerly Pick's disease. While acetylcholine esterase inhibitors can slow down progression of mild to moderate Alzheimer's disease, symptoms associated with rapid shrinking of the frontal and temporal lobes cannot be treated in FTD at all. Thorough testing for alternative causes of mental deterioration is therefore essential before the final diagnosis is made. By failing to diagnose the medical condition correctly, the medical practitioner not only misses the opportunity for treatment but may also cause distress to patients and relatives alike.

Dementia with Lewy bodies is a condition associated with both dementia and parkinsonian symptoms. It is the second most common form of dementia, exceeded only by Alzheimer's disease. In this condition, the brain contains both alpha-synuclein, typical of Parkinson's disease-associated dementia, and the neurotic plaques and neurofibrillary tangles typical of Alzheimer's disease. Deficiencies are found in both acetylcholine and dopamine neurotransmission. Interestingly, treatments with cholinesterase inhibitors are more effective in patients who have dementia with Lewy bodies than in those with Alzheimer's disease. Conversely, patients who have dementia with Lewy bodies do not respond particularly well to antiparkinsonian medications. Even more importantly, anticholinergic and traditional antipsychotic medications should be avoided; they can exacerbate the symptoms of dementia or even precipitate severe reactions culminating in death.

It is likely that the ability to make more subtle distinctions amongst similar conditions will prove to be important in the future. It is a common finding that in any group of patients treated in the same way for the same condition, some individuals will respond much better than others. It may well be that differences in the underlying cause of what is outwardly the same disease may underlie these differences in response. If the precise cause of an individual's condition were known, therapy could be targeted much more accurately.

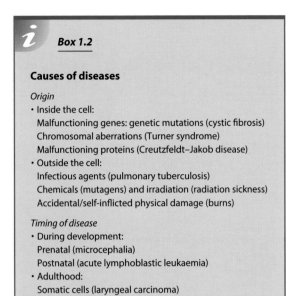

Causes of diseases

Origin
- Inside the cell:
  Malfunctioning genes: genetic mutations (cystic fibrosis)
  Chromosomal aberrations (Turner syndrome)
  Malfunctioning proteins (Creutzfeldt–Jakob disease)
- Outside the cell:
  Infectious agents (pulmonary tuberculosis)
  Chemicals (mutagens) and irradiation (radiation sickness)
  Accidental/self-inflicted physical damage (burns)

Timing of disease
- During development:
  Prenatal (microcephalia)
  Postnatal (acute lymphoblastic leukaemia)
- Adulthood:
  Somatic cells (laryngeal carcinoma)

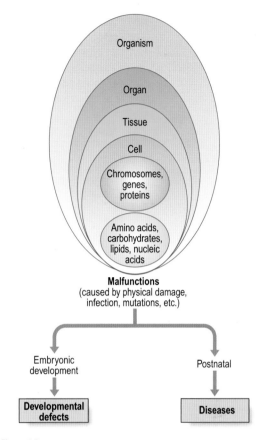

Figure 1.2
Diseases can develop at any time of life.

effective therapy require an understanding of disease processes at the molecular level. Whatever the cause of a disease, it produces an effect on the cell's physiological activity at a molecular level.

In cases like irradiation, which can cause uncontrollable cellular proliferation and malignancy, or HIV infection resulting in CD4$^+$ (helper) T cell depletion and immune deficiency, the need for understanding the molecular physiology of the cell is relatively obvious. Indeed, the use of molecular approaches in the characterization of various bacterial strains or malignant cancer types is a well-established approach. One must not forget, however, that tissue regeneration after macroscopic tissue damage, like accidental loss of limbs, burns or even idiopathic fibrosis of the lung, is basically a molecular event, orchestrated by genes and their protein products. Consequently, therapeutic approaches aimed at tissue regeneration or inhibition of tissue damage also require a thorough knowledge of the underlying molecular events.

The key molecules involved in cell function are nucleic acids and proteins, and it is these molecules that can be studied and manipulated using the techniques of biotechnology. An understanding of their roles and functional regulation is vitally important in designing new diagnostic and therapeutic techniques.

Nucleic acids and proteins

Probably the best known of the nucleic acids is deoxyribonucleic acid, or DNA. DNA is found in the chromosomes within the cell nucleus, and in smaller amounts in mitochondria (Fig. 1.3). It is the storage medium for the genetic code.

The other type of nucleic acid is ribonucleic acid, or RNA. There are a variety of different types of RNA, all

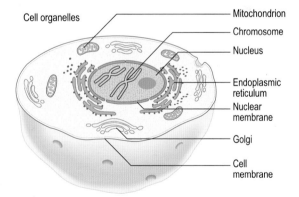

Figure 1.3
Cell organelles. All cells are built from various cell organelles, including cellular and nuclear membranes, nucleus where DNA resides, cytoplasm containing mitochondria, endoplasmic reticulum, Golgi apparatus and scaffold protein structures.

of which have different functions, and these are outlined in Figure 1.4. With the exception of the recently discovered microRNAs (miRNA) that regulate gene expression following transcription, the various types of RNA function as decoders, building the cell's proteins based on the

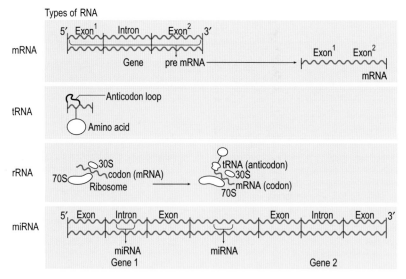

Figure 1.4
Types of RNA. Messenger or mRNA is the decoder of DNA and contains the codons for protein sequence; transfer or tRNA contains the anticodon and binds amino acids to deliver to the codon (mRNA) that is bound to ribosomal or rRNA; micro or miRNA is coded amongst regions of the DNA sequence previously believed to be 'non-coding' and regulates mRNA destruction by RNA interference.

Box 1.3

Colon cancer

A high percentage of colonic adenocarcinomas are the result of mutations in the regions of DNA encoding β-catenin, a key molecule in cell adhesion and signal transduction in the evolutionarily conserved Wnt pathway. The altered β-catenin can resist proteolytic degradation, which leads to continuous activation of genes responsible for proliferation, resulting in malignant growth of the epithelium in the colon.

---

sequence information encoded in the DNA. Consequently, any errors or changes (mutations) within the genetic material can cause errors within protein sequences, resulting in partially or completely dysfunctional proteins.

Proteins make up most of the structure of the cell, and are also the direct regulators of cell function and both intracellular and intercellular (cell-to-cell) communication. It is therefore not surprising that damaged genes and/or proteins can be underlying causes of diseases. Box 1.3 shows an example how mutation can lead to cancerous growth of tissue.

What are mutations?

Mutations are changes to the genetic material, DNA or RNA. Genetic mutations have varying effects on human health, depending on the nature of the mutation, where

the mutation occurs and whether it alters the function of essential proteins. If we understand how mutations occur, we can perhaps learn to control them and use our knowledge in order to manipulate the process or to correct the damage. Mutations can occur in all organisms, from humans to bacteria and viruses.

Each human cell contains about 2 metres of DNA. This is neatly folded and condensed into the nucleus with the help of protective and regulatory histone proteins (see Ch. 4). The genetic code seems to be more vulnerable to mutation at particular stages of the cell cycle.

During cell division, the DNA is 'unwound' to allow access to the enzymes that replicate the DNA, in order to provide each daughter cell with an identical copy. A representation of this process is shown in Figure 1.5. The replicating DNA is exposed not only to potential physical or chemical damage but also to mistakes made by the enzymes involved in the process of replication.

Similarly, during gene transcription the DNA sequence has to be exposed to enzymes in order to be transcribed into mRNA. This process is illustrated in Figure 1.6. Mistakes in transcription will lead to the production of mRNA with an aberrant sequence.

If a mutation occurs during DNA replication, the mutation occurs directly within the genetic code, and the changed sequence is likely to be transmitted to all cells produced by subsequent cell divisions. However, mistakes made by RNA polymerase during transcription only introduce errors to the mRNA, potentially resulting in a 'one-off' aberrant protein.

Mutations occur quite frequently, but the overwhelming majority have no effect, as DNA repair mechanisms have evolved which are able to reverse most changes. Mechanisms also exist to identify and eliminate

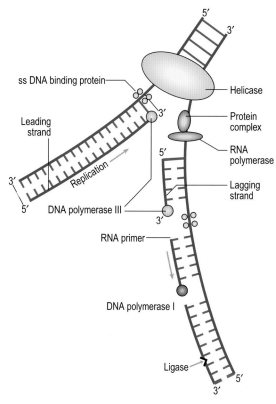

Figure 1.5
DNA replication. Several enzymes have been found to be necessary for DNA replication. As DNA polymerase cannot initiate chains de novo, primers are required. This is provided by an RNA polymerase that synthesizes a short stretch of RNA. DNA polymerase III then takes over and uses this RNA as a primer to continue the synthesis of DNA. Helicase is needed to unwind the DNA helix and to allow replication. While a single-stranded DNA-binding protein (ssDNA-binding protein) stabilizes the single-stranded regions of DNA that are transiently formed during replication. Finally, since DNA polymerase can synthesize DNA only in the (5' to 3') direction, one of the strands must be synthesized discontinuously. This leads to a series of short stretches of DNA with gaps in between. These gaps are filled by a DNA polymerase I and joined by DNA ligase.

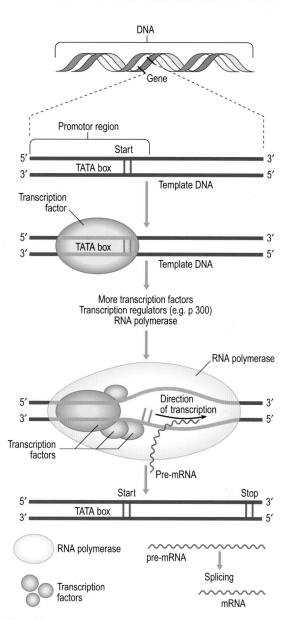

Figure 1.6
Gene transcription. A transcription factor binds to the promoter region that initiates further binding of transcription factors, RNA polymerase II and transcription regulators like p300. Following transcription from START to STOP codon, regulatory proteins and pre-mRNA leave the DNA sequence. The pre-mRNA has to go through a maturation process called splicing to become mature mRNA.

mutated somatic cells. These are outlined in more detail in Table 1.1. It is when these various repair mechanisms become faulty or are overwhelmed that problems start to occur.

Of course, mutations do not always have a detrimental effect. Mutated genes are the raw material for evolution by natural selection, generating potentially beneficial or advantageous 'new' genes.

Similarly, many mutations have rather little effect on cell function, so these altered sequences can persist in the population along with their unaltered 'parent' sequences. This gives rise to the existence of 'polymorphisms', in which somewhat different alleles of a gene exist in different members of the population. Polymorphism underlies a great deal of human genetic diversity and there is enormous interest in determining the contribution of the different alleles to various characteristics, including susceptibility to disease or to adverse drug reactions (see Ch. 9).

Types and causes of mutations

Mutations can be categorized in a variety of ways, depending, for example, on the cause of the mutation, the length of the damaged DNA, the modification of the resulting protein function, etc.

Table 1.1
Some diseases resulting from DNA repair dysfunction

Type of DNA mutation	Repair mechanism	Enzymes involved	Disease resulting from repair dysfunction
Aberrant bases (deaminated or chemically modified in other ways)	Base excision repair	DNA glycosylase, AP endonuclease, DNA polymerase I, DNA ligase	Colorectal polyposis, colorectal cancer, Alzheimer's disease; predicted to be important in all neurodegenerative disorders
Nucleotide mutation and base dimers	Nucleotide excision repair	DNA polymerase I, DNA ligase	Xeroderma pigmentosum, trichothiodystrophy, Cockayne syndrome, where patients have UV-induced DNA lesions
Inappropriately matched bases	Mismatch repair	Methylase, exonuclease, DNA helicase II, DNA polymerase III, DNA ligase	Familial colorectal cancer, folate deficiency leading to megaloblastic anaemia, developmental defects and cancer
Strand exchange from another chromosome	Recombination repair (post-replication)	Two pathways: HR (homologous recombination) and NHEJ (non-homologous end joining). DNA polymerase, DNA ligase	Ataxia telangiectasia — high frequency of spontaneous chromosome aberrations, breast cancer, leukaemia, ageing-associated disorders
Pyrimidine dimers formed by UV light	Photoreactivation	DNA photolyase, DNA ligase	Xeroderma pigmentosum — skin cancers and melanomas — defective ability to excise pyrimidine dimers

Spontaneous and induced mutations

- *Spontaneous mutations* are those which occur without any obvious external cause, such as copying errors during cell division.
- *Induced mutations* are those which are caused by exogenous factors, such as exposure to ultraviolet (UV) radiation, radioactivity, chemical mutagens or viruses.

Types of mutation by the length of DNA affected

The genetic code is preserved within the coding sequence of the DNA. The DNA is supercoiled, as shown in Figure 1.7, and stored as chromosomes. Damage to the DNA can affect anything from one or two nucleotides up to entire arms of chromosomes. When the result is a change in the number or structure of chromosomes that can be visualized under a microscope, this tends to be called a chromosomal mutation or abnormality.

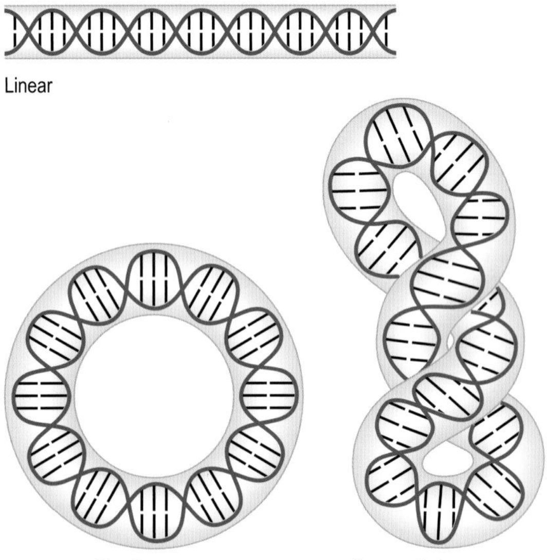

Mutations affecting short sequences
Mutations which affect only one or two nucleotides can be of the following types:

- *Point mutations* (transition, transversion: Box 1.4) take place when a single nucleotide is exchanged for another nucleotide. They are often caused by faults in DNA replication or induced by mutagens.
- *Silent mutations* code for the same amino acid.
- *Mis-sense mutations* code for a different amino acid.

Linear

Circular   Supercoiled

Figure 1.7
Supercoiled DNA. DNA loops undergo subsidiary coiling, leading to a supercoiled chromosome. The increase in coiling in the sequence is accompanied by a reduction in size.

- *Nonsense mutations* result in a premature stop codon, truncating the protein sequence.
- *Insertions* add one or more nucleotides into the DNA sequence and consequently alter the reading frame of the gene (Fig. 1.8).

Box 1.4

Types of point mutation

The most common point mutations are 'transitions', in which a purine is exchanged for a purine (A ⇌ G) or a pyrimidine exchanged for a pyrimidine (C ⇌ T). Less common is a 'transversion', which exchanges a purine for a pyrimidine or a pyrimidine for a purine (C/T ⇌ A/G). A point mutation can be reversed by another point mutation, in which the nucleotide is changed back to its original state (true reversion) or by second-site reversion (a complementary mutation elsewhere that results in regained gene functionality).

Point mutations occur fairly frequently and presumably underlie the existence of the very large number of single nucleotide polymorphisms (SNPs) which exist in the human population. The SNP Consortium Initiative is actively identifying and analysing SNPs in the human genome and the total number is estimated to be well over 10 million.

After puberty spermatocytes divide every 16 days, and by the age of 35 approximately 540 cell divisions have occurred. The risk of faults in DNA replication and in DNA repair mechanisms can accumulate over time; therefore the large number of cell divisions that occur during sperm production increases the chance of point mutations in males and naturally this also increases with paternal age. There is a positive correlation between paternal age and the occurrence of a number of conditions, including Apert syndrome, craniosynostosis, cleft lip/palate, hydrocephalus and risk of schizophrenia. However, further studies are required to identify the point mutations in spermatocytes that are responsible for these medical conditions.

- *Deletions* involve irreversible removal of one or more nucleotides from the DNA. Like insertions, these mutations can alter the reading frame of the gene.

Table 1.2 lists some short sequence mutations which result in disease.

Mutations affecting larger sequences of DNA
Mutations that affect large regions of DNA can be of the following types:

- *Gene duplication or amplification*. This leads to multiple copies of the same gene in an enlarged chromosomal region.
- *Deletions*. These lead to loss of genes within the deleted chromosomal region.
- *Gene fusions*. By juxtaposing previously well-separated DNA sequences, fusion can bring together different genes or parts of genes to form a functionally distinct entity. These can occur as a consequence of the following chromosomal rearrangements:
  - Chromosomal translocation: interchange of sequence from non-homologous chromosomes
  - Interstitial deletions: removing regions of DNA from a single chromosome, thereby apposing previously distant genes
  - Chromosomal inversions: a chromosome segment is clipped out and then reinserted into the chromosome in reverse orientation.

Some diseases produced by mutations of large sequences are shown in Table 1.3.

Chromosomal abnormalities can also arise due to mis-sorting of the chromosomes during cell division, such that daughter cells possess too many or two few copies of a particular chromosome. These abnormalities can result in disorders such as:

- Down syndrome, in which an individual possesses three copies of chromosome 21
- Turner syndrome, in which affected individuals possess only a single X chromosome.

Some more examples of this type of chromosomal abnormality are shown in Table 1.4.

Mutations categorized by their effects

Mutations may produce a spectrum of effects ranging from no effect at all, to such a dramatic effect that embryos possessing the mutation fail to survive (lethal mutations). Similarly, mutations may render a particular protein inactive (loss of function mutations) or overly active (gain of function mutations). Table 1.5 lists some of these types of mutation and the diseases with which they are associated.

Effects of mutations on descendants

The effect of a mutation on one's offspring depends on the type of cell in which the mutation occurs. Mutations in the germ cells (cells producing eggs or sperm) may well have no effect at all on the individual in whom they occur but can be passed on to descendants, who will then carry the mutation in all of his or her cells. Somatic mutations occur in other tissues and cannot be transmitted to descendants. However, they can have devastating effects on the individual in which they occur; most cancers are associated with somatic mutations (Box 1.2).

Mutations in infectious organisms

Mutations can occur in any organism that possesses genetic material. Common pathogens such as bacteria and viruses have high mutation frequencies. The

A) Addition of a base: gag gca gtg cct...

   Deletion of a base: gac agt gcc tc...

B) Parathyroid hormone receptor mutation: deletion
   of a G at position 1122

		1122			*
WT:	tgg atc atc ca	g	g tg cc c atc		
MT:	tgg atc atc cag	tgc	cca tcc		

C) The above mutation yields a truncated protein
   and a dysfunctional receptor:

```
     361
WT:  ▯ QVPILASIVLNFILFINIVRVLA       TKLR
MT:  ▯ QCPSWPPLCSTSSSSSISSGCSPPSCG

     391
WT: ETNAGRCDTRQQYRK        LLKSTVLMPLFGVH
MT: RPTPAGVTHGSSTGSCSNPRWCSCPSLAST

     421
WT: YIVFMAT  PYTEVSGTLWQVQMHYE      MLFNSF
MT: TLSSWPHHTPRSQGRSGKSRCTMRCSSTPS

     451
WT: QGFFVA I IYCFCN     GEVQAEIKKSWSRWTLA
MT: RDFLSQSYTVSAMARYKLRSRNLGAAGHWH

     481
WT: LDFKRKARSGSSSYSYGPMVSHTSVTNVGP
MT: WTSSERHAAGAAAIATAPWCPTQV       —

     511
WT: RVGLGLPLSPRLLPTATTNGHPQLPGHAKP
MT: —

     541
WT: GTPALETLETTPPAMAAPKDDGFLNGSCSG
MT: —

     571
WT: LDEEASGPERPPALLQEEWETVM
MT: —
```

Figure 1.8
Reading frame shift. (A) A frame shift mutation tends to occur as the addition or deletion of a base. (B) If the mutation affects the translated region, frame shifts can destroy the function of the encoded product. This example shows a mis-sense mutation in the parathyroid hormone receptor, which belongs to the seven-loop transmembrane receptor family. The point mutation was caused by the loss of one nucleotide (indicated in bold) at nucleotide position 1122. (C) Comparison of the amino acid sequences of the wild-type (WT) and mutant-type (MT) receptors indicates a frame shift that yielded in a diverged sequence after amino acid 364 and a truncation after amino acid 504, resulting in a dysfunctional protein.

consequence of mutation in these organisms may be the ability to evade the immune system, increased (or decreased) virulence or infectiousness, or the emergence of drug resistance. Thus genetic mutations can alter the severity of a disease and the way in which it can be treated, and can also serve as diagnostic markers for the identification of a particular strain.

Mutations in the 'non-coding' regions of genes

The spatially and temporally orchestrated expression of genes is essential for normal function of an organism. Until recently, it was a common perception that mutations are able to induce disease development only if the mutation affects a protein-encoding region of DNA or its promoter regions. Proteins are encoded by genes that in general comprise promoter sequences — to which transcription factors and transcription regulators bind — and open reading frame (ORF) coding sequences (CDS) incorporating start and stop codons. It is these sequences that are transcribed into mRNA and translated into protein at the ribosome (Fig. 1.9).

Although these sequences are undoubtedly important, they comprise only about 1–2% of the human genome and it seems very unlikely that the remaining 98–99% is entirely 'junk'. Indeed, it is now known that miRNAs, for example, are coded by 'non-coding' areas of the genome and function as important down-regulators of gene expression (Box 1.5). Mutations in these regulatory DNA sequences can be just as important as mutations in protein-encoding sequences.

Proteins in disease

For the human body to function correctly, millions of cells and extra- and intracellular proteins are required to function in the right places at the right times in a highly organized way.

Mutations in the genetic material clearly have the potential to alter protein function.

- If the mutation is in the protein-encoding region of the gene, aberrant proteins may result.
- If the mutation is in the regulatory regions of the gene, too much or too little protein may be synthesized, or it may be synthesized at the wrong time.

However, mutation is not the only way in which protein function can be altered. A large number of conditions appear to result from the inappropriate activation of the immune system, whereby normal protective mechanisms, designed to be used against infectious organisms or tumour cells, are unleashed to attack innocuous antigens (giving rise to allergies such as hay fever) or components of the human body (giving rise to autoimmune diseases such as rheumatoid arthritis). Biotechnology has a big part to play in these diseases too, as increased understanding of the molecular entities involved in the abnormal responses can open up new therapeutic possibilities.

Aberrant proteins may in themselves be infectious agents. The prion diseases, such as scrapie, BSE (bovine spongiform encephalopathy) and CJD (Creutzfeldt–Jakob disease), appear to be caused by aberrant prion

Table 1.2
Some short sequence and point mutations and resulting diseases

Short sequence and point mutations	Disease	Some symptoms
Transitions		
G (guanine) to A transition at position 6664 of the *GH-1* gene results in the substitution of Arg183 by His (R183H)	Autosomal dominant isolated GH deficiency (type II)	Dwarfism
A to G transition at position 3243 in mitochondrial DNA	Focal glomerulosclerosis	Heavy proteinuria, renal failure Focal glomerulosclerosis tends to recur in transplanted kidneys
Insertions		
Cytosine (C) insertion in exon 28, or thymidine (T) insertion in exon 14 in *VWF* gene	Von Willebrand disease type III	Bleeding disorder; homozygous form is rare, heterozygous involves easy bruising, bleeding after trauma and menorrhagia in females
C insertion in *NOD2* gene leucine-rich region in exon 11 (premature stop codon in amino acid 1007)	Crohn's disease	Chronic inflammation of the bowel with transmural inflammation and granulomas
Deletions		
4-base deletion at the 3'-boundary of exon 6 in one GR allele (delta 4)	Familial glucocorticoid resistance	Hypercortisolism, hyperandrogenism
3-base deletion in CFT leading to loss of phenylalanine in amino acid position 508	Cystic fibrosis (CF)	Recurrent bronchopulmonary infections, bronchiectasis, failure to thrive in infancy, pancreatitis
Normal: ATC ATC TTT GGT GTT **CF**: ATC AT_ __T GGT GTT		

proteins. These prions are probably identical in sequence to normal cellular proteins in the brain. The prions become dangerous when they undergo a conformational change which renders them highly stable and resistant to proteolysis. These abnormal proteins accumulate in brain cells and give rise to the characteristic spongiform encephalopathy associated with prion diseases. It seems likely that the presence of a prion is able to convert the normal cellular proteins into the prion conformation and thus lead to the spread of the disease (see also Ch. 5).

What is the role of biotechnology in medicine?

Biotechnology comprises a collection of techniques for determining nucleic acid and protein sequence, and for manipulating these sequences. Mutated genes and/or the proteins they encode can be characteristic for a specific cell type and disease and therefore can be extremely useful in diagnosis.

Biotechnology is already making an impact in therapy through the availability of recombinant human proteins for use as drugs (see Ch. 11).

Biotechnology also offers the potential to target specific sites in both the genetic material (see Ch. 10) and the resulting proteins to eliminate mutant genes or to correct mutations causing malfunctioning proteins and therefore cure disease.

Mutagenesis (the creation or formation of a mutation) can be used as a powerful genetic tool. By inducing mutations in specific ways and then observing the phenotype of the organism, the function of genes and even of individual nucleotides can be determined. This contributes enormously to our understanding of disease processes. Additionally, generating mutations in a controlled way could possibly be used to modify protein expression in a therapeutically useful manner.

Thus the importance of medical biotechnology can be summed up as contributing to:

- understanding the cause of diseases
- identifying diagnostic markers
- identifying potential targets for medical intervention
- providing new types of therapy.

To be able to fulfil these aims, diseases have to be characterized and genes and proteins manipulated. Identification of genes involves a combination of techniques, which are detailed in the next chapter.

Table 1.3
Some chromosomal abnormalities and resulting diseases

Chromosomal abnormalities	Disease	Some symptoms
Gene duplication		
A-amyloid gene duplication	Alzheimer's disease	Progressive dementia
Partial duplication of 17p11.2 (peripheral myelin protein)	Hereditary motor and sensory neuropathy (HMSN)	Increased concentration of peripheral myelin protein, hypertrophic peripheral nerves
Deletion		
46XX5p-, 46XY5p- (Ch5 short arm deletion)	Cri-du-chat syndrome (1:50 000 live births)	Severe mental retardation, characteristic miaow-like cry
Survival motor neuron (SMN) gene	Half of the patients with arthrogryposis multiplex congenita (AMC) associated with spinal muscular atrophy (SMA)	Atrophy of muscular cells resulting in progressive muscle weakness
Gene fusion		
NPM-ALK (nucleophosmin-anaplastic lymphoma kinase genes)	Anaplastic large cell lymphoma (ALCL)	Histologically wide spectrum appearance, frequent in skin, gastrointestinal tract
BCR-ABL	Chronic myelomonocytic leukaemia (CML)	Abnormal leukocytes, anaemia, massive splenomegaly
Chromosomal translocation		
T(2,5)(p23,q35)	ALCL	Same as above
Interstitial deletion		
13q (q13 q22)	Hirschsprung's disease (1:5000)	Megacolon, intestinal obstruction
Del Xq27.1 near SOX3	X-linked recessive hypoparathyroidism	Parathyroid hormone deficiency, hypocalcaemia
Chromosomal inversion		
Pericentric inversion of ChX short arm aberration involving Xp11.3	Norrie disease	Mental retardation, growth disturbances, hypogonadism, susceptibility to infections

Table 1.4
Frequency of chromosomal abnormalities

Chromosomal abnormalities	Incidence/ live births	Some symptoms
Autosomal chromosomes		
Trisomy 21 (Down syndrome)	1:1000	Mental subnormality, upward-slanting eyes, congenital heart defects
Trisomy 18 (Edward syndrome)	1:5000	Associated with ear, jaw, cardiac, renal, intestinal and skeletal abnormalities
Trisomy 13 (Patau syndrome)	1:6000	Microcephaly, small eyes, cleft palate, low-set ears
Trisomy 3, 4, 8, 9, 14 mosaicisms	Rare	E.g. trisomy 9: growth and mental retardation, abnormal hands and feet, 13 pairs of ribs

Table 1.4
Frequency of chromosomal abnormalities—cont'd

Chromosomal abnormalities	Incidence/ live births	Some symptoms
Sex chromosomes		
Klinefelter syndrome (47XXY, 48XXXY, 49XXXXY)	1: 850	Male gender with female habitus, mental retardation
Double Y males (47XYY)	1:1000	Phenotypically normal male, over 6 ft tall, aggressive, often criminal behaviour
Turner syndrome (45X)	1:3000	Female gender, underdeveloped ovaries, webbed neck, short stature
Multiple X females (47XXX, 48XXXX)	1:1200	Can be mentally retarded with menstrual disturbances, though many are normal
True hermaphrodites (46XX, 46XX/47XXY, 45XO/46XY)	1:15 000	Both testicular and ovarian tissue, depending on testosterone levels, ambiguous external genitals

Table 1.5
Types of mutation affecting protein function and some resulting diseases

Protein	Disease	Some symptoms
Loss of function mutations		
Enzyme defects	Albinism (absent melanin production due to tyrosinase deficiency)	Absence of melanin pigmentation, increased risk of skin cancer from UV light exposure
Signalling defects	Albright's hereditary osteodystrophy (GNAS1, inactive Gsα protein)	Endocrine disorder, pseudohypoparathyroidism type 1a: short stature in adulthood, brachydactyly, subcutaneous ossification, bone demineralization
Non-enzyme protein defects	Marfan syndrome (dominant negative mutation of *FBN1* (fibrillin-1) gene Ch15)	Heart conditions, aortic aneurysm, arachnodactyly, scoliosis, speech impediments, myopia
Gain of function mutations		
Signal permanently 'on'	McCune–Albright disease (*GNAS1* gene, constitutively active Gsα protein)	Somatic condition in mosaics, depending on the tissue carrying the mutation, polyostotic fibrous dysplasia, hyperfunctional endocrinopathies
Ion channel inappropriately open	Paramyotonia congenita (*SCN4A* gene)	Poor inactivation of sodium channel, rigidity developing during exercise, sensitivity to cold, uncontrollable muscle tension
Non-enzyme protein	Charcot–Marie–Tooth disease (*PMP22*)	Neuropathy affecting both motor and sensory nerves, weakness of foot and lower leg
Lethal mutations		
Mutations in collagen type 2 or diastrophic dysplasia sulphate transporter genes	Achondrogenesis	Lack of development of limbs, ribs and other major bone formations
Mis-sense mutation resulting in combined loss and gain of function	α_1-Antitrypsin deficiency (Pittsburgh variant, mutation at Met358, Met to Arg mutation)	Lethal at birth or soon after. Bleeding diathesis, from elastase inhibitor the protein becomes a constitutively active antithrombin

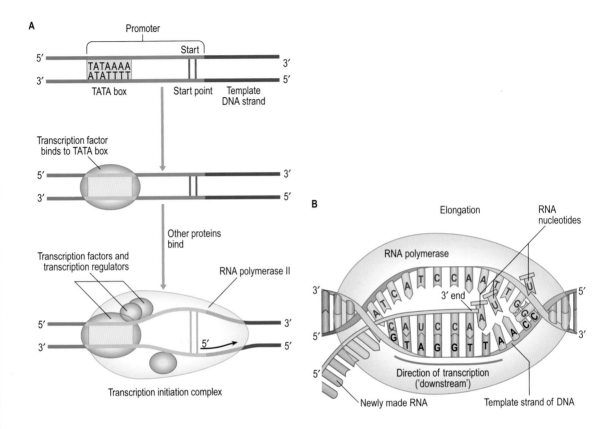

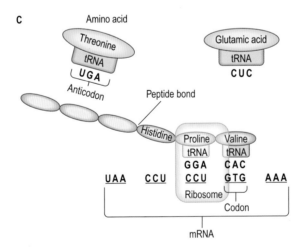

Figure 1.9

Transcription and translation. (A) Transcription factors bind to the TATA region of the promoter and initiate the binding of further transcription regulators. These lead to unwinding of the DNA and recruit RNA polymerase. (B) Transcription. RNA polymerase generates new RNA complementary to the DNA strand. (C) Following maturation of the mRNA, the smaller ribosomal subunit attaches at a specific initiation site on the mRNA molecule, forming a complex to which the larger subunit then attaches, to form the functioning ribosome. More and more ribosomal units attach, then each ribosome moves along the mRNA molecule and synthesizes the polypeptide from the amino acids delivered by tRNA. When it completes synthesis of a polypeptide, the ribosome separates from the mRNA and dissociates into 30S and 50S subunits with the aid of a specific dissociation factor.

Box 1.5

miRNA

This form of RNA was first described in *Caenorhabditis elegans* by Lee and colleagues in 1993, although the term microRNA was not introduced until 2001. The way in which regulatory or inhibitory RNA (RNAi) works is excellently illustrated in a short film that is openly accessible via the Web (http://www.nature.com/focus/rnai/animations/index.html).

RNAi molecules are all short, single-stranded, inhibitory RNAs which may be natural regulators or introduced artificially into cells for research purposes. The miRNAs are encoded by our genome, occur naturally and have a very important role in regulating normal gene expression patterns. They are transcribed from DNA to single-stranded RNA, just like messenger RNA, but are never translated into proteins. Instead, miRNAs are complementary or partially complementary to mRNA sequences. They bind to mRNA, producing a double-stranded RNA which is degraded by enzyme complexes and therefore not translated into protein.

To date, approximately 200 'genes' encoding miRNA have been discovered and methods have already been developed to use the miRNA profile of particular cells to distinguish the slow-growing or aggressive forms of chronic lymphocytic leukaemia.

FURTHER READING

Campbell AM, Heyer LJ 2003 Discovering genomics, proteomics and bioinformatics. Pearson Education, publishing as Benjamin Cummings, San Francisco, CA.

Lee RC, Feinbaum RL, Ambros V 1993 The *C. elegans* heterochronic gene lin-4 encodes small RNAs with antisense complementarity to lin-14. Cell 75(5):843–54.

Ruvkun G 2001 Molecular biology: glimpses of a tiny RNA world. Science 294(5543):797–799.

Strickberger MW 1990 Genetics, 3rd edn. Maxwell–Macmillan: New York.

Zhao Y, Ransom JF, Li A et al. 2007 Dysregulation of cardiogenesis, cardiac conduction, and cell cycle in mice lacking miRNA-1-2. Cell 129(2):303–317.

Gene hunting
J. Pongracz

The genetic basis for a number of disorders is known. For example, mutations in the *CFT* gene are the cause of cystic fibrosis, and possession of three copies of chromosome 21 gives rise to Down syndrome. However, despite our increasing knowledge about the process of mutagenesis, the root causes of many common human diseases remain unknown, although there is considerable evidence that genetics plays an important role in our susceptibility to heart disease, diabetes or depression, for example. To make matters worse, different mutations can underlie almost identical clinical symptoms. Obesity can be due to mutation in *Sirt2* that blocks fat cell formation, or mutation in the melanocortin-4 receptor (*MCR4*) that regulates food intake and energy expenditure, amongst many other factors. Moreover, most diseases appear to be multifactorial, with genetic, environmental and lifestyle factors all playing a role. This lack of knowledge regarding the precise cause of disease makes preventive measures generally inadequate and available treatments are seldom curative.

In our aim to predict, prevent and treat human diseases, we need to look for genes that are directly responsible for specific diseases and genes that increase susceptibility to diseases.

In the era of the Human Genome Project it might appear that nothing could be easier than identifying the principal genetic causes of human diseases and then using that information to find a cure for most of our medical problems. Unfortunately, simply sequencing the human genome did not take us much closer to these goals. So why is this the case?

Several issues contribute to the problem of finding the genes responsible for a particular disease. Firstly, just because we have now sequenced the full human genome, it does not mean that we now know what all that genetic information does. Secondly, it would be entirely impractical to sequence the entire genome of individuals suffering from any particular disease in order to try to detect any abnormalities. Sequencing our large genome, containing over 29 000 genes, was a lengthy and expensive project and, as such, it is not really feasible to repeat the process over and over again.

Any two humans are approximately 99.9% identical in their DNA sequences; it is the variable 0.1% of the human genome that determines disease risks and response to infectious agents, drugs and other environmental factors. These differences in sequences are the ones that need to be found and connected with specific diseases. Therefore sequencing thousands of samples without a better work plan would make a simplistic gene hunting approach more like searching for a needle in a haystack;

it would be expensive, time-consuming and probably inaccurate. Mass sequencing of individually identified and personalized human genetic samples would also raise serious ethical issues.

What is needed is a way of narrowing down the amount of sequence that needs to be determined in order to find an aberrant gene.

There are two main questions to be answered:

- What types of gene are we looking for?
- What is the most efficient way to find them?

While the answer to the first question is relatively easy (for example, we are looking for genes predisposing an individual to Parkinson's disease), the answer to the second question requires knowledge of the rules of genetics and statistics and the appropriate experimental techniques and instrumentation.

The basic set of information required for gene hunting needs to include:

- DNA sequencing data
- rules of genetic inheritance
- rules of DNA replication and mutagenesis generating genetic markers
- the principle of 'genetic linkage'
- computer-based data modelling.

DNA sequencing

Sequencing is the technique without which all our efforts to find specific disease and disease susceptibility genes would be futile. It is, as is well known, the process of determining the exact order of the bases A, T, C and G in a piece of DNA. (For an explanation of how DNA sequencing is performed, see Appendix 2.)

The most obvious application of DNA sequencing technology is the accurate sequencing of genes and genomes. The human genome contains about 3 billion base pairs (bp), arrayed in 24 chromosomes. The chromosomes themselves are 50–250 million bases long. These megabases of DNA are much too large to be deciphered in one go, even by the latest automated machines. Fragments of DNA between 400 and 800 bases long can be sequenced using currently available techniques. Larger DNA molecules, including whole genomes, must be broken into smaller fragments before sequencing and then reassembled by computer programs which search for overlaps.

Box 2.1

Sequencing the human genome

In the Human Genome Project (HGP) blood (female) or sperm (male) samples from a large number of donors were collected, but samples from only 8 males and 1 female were processed. During the design of the HGP, donor identities were carefully protected, so donor samples were anonymous.

Sperm samples were used, as it is much easier to prepare DNA cleanly from sperm than from other cell types. In sperm the DNA to protein ratio is much higher than in other cell types. It also has one other advantage, in that it provides all chromosomes for the study, including equal numbers of the

X (female) or Y (male) sex chromosomes. Thus, the reason for using mostly male samples was not sex discrimination. However, white cells from the blood of a female donor were also used, so as to include female-originated samples.

DNA samples in the Celera Genomics private sector project were collected from a variety of different individuals and then mixed before processing for sequencing. The origin of samples covers the whole human race, as donors were recruited of European, African, American (North, Central, South) and Asian ancestry.

Sequencing in gene hunting studies helps to determine not only nucleotide sequences of genes or particular DNA sequences but also the location of mutations and sequence variations in genes.

Accuracy is achieved by sequencing each template several times. Lower-fidelity, single-pass sequencing is useful for the rapid accumulation of sequence data but at the expense of some accuracy. It may, however, be necessary to resequence the same DNA molecule over and over again. This provides the level of accuracy required in order to identify single nucleotide polymorphisms, for example.

Sequencing plays an important, if not the most important, part in all gene hunting studies, as it provides the raw data for further gene hunting analysis; as such, its accuracy is of high importance. It does not matter how sophisticated the available analysis programs or computer models are, if the genetic sequence data contain errors. If there are errors in the input data, these will be amplified during analysis. For example, a 1% error in sequencing can result in a 36–58% error in the final analysis.

Under the aegis of the Human Genome Project, nucleotide sequencing of the human genome has been completed. However, we cannot consider the human genome to be fully known. Due to individual variability, the nine individual genomes that were actually sequenced in the project can only be considered as reference sequences (Box 2.1). Based on the reference database, further studies are required to reveal more about our genetic background, inheritance and function. To be able to perform all the predictive work and functional studies, an in-depth understanding of the rules of genetic inheritance is very important.

The rules of genetic inheritance

The idea that disease can run in families is not a new one. It has been widely accepted, since long before the era of genetics, that medical examination should include the patient's family history, as this information can indicate disease susceptibility and response to treatments. By now it is clear that by taking the patient's family history the doctor is assessing the patient's genetic background. The scientific basis for this assessment reaches back to Mendel's work in the late 19th century.

To be able to inherit the correct set of information for a fully functional body, gametes have to go through meiotic divisions (Fig. 2.1). In this way only one of each pair of chromosomes (haploid) gets into our gametes. When the egg is fertilized, the correct number of chromosomes is restored (diploid). As a result, we can inherit different variants of the same genes (alleles) that are localized at an identical place (locus) on each chromosome in the pair. A particular combination of alleles along a chromosome is termed a haplotype. The manifestation of genetically encoded traits is called the phenotype (Fig. 2.1). The way these alleles are inherited and influence genetic traits was recognized by Mendel and summarized in his laws of inheritance.

The laws of Mendelian inheritance

Mendelian inheritance depends on two principles:

- *the principle of segregation*, which assumes that different versions of a particular gene (alleles) account for differences in inherited characteristics, such as eye colour
- *the principle of independent assortment*, which dictates that the emergence of one trait will not affect the emergence of another encoded by a different gene.

If a disease is inherited in a Mendelian fashion, it is possible to classify the mode of transmission of a disease-causing mutation as either:

Meiosis 1
The cell divides into two but the chromososmes do not double; only the pairs separate

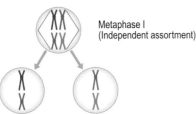

Metaphase I
(Independent assortment)

Meiosis 2
The second meiotic division is similar to mitosis. The cells divide and the chromosomes double

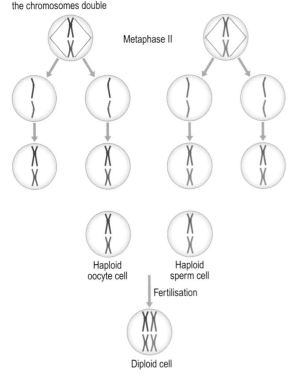

Metaphase II

Haploid
oocyte cell

Haploid
sperm cell

Fertilisation

Diploid cell

Same gene, different alleles
(e.g. chromosome 10 obesity
genes *AKR1C2*)

Chromosome terminology

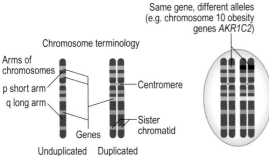

Arms of
chromosomes

p short arm

q long arm

Centromere

Sister
chromatid

Genes

Unduplicated   Duplicated

Genetic make-up
or haplotype

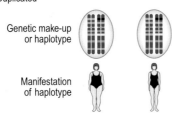

Manifestation
of haplotype

Phenotype

Figure 2.1
Meiosis. There are two divisions in meiosis: meiosis 1 and meiosis 2. The phases of cell division have the same names as those of mitosis (prophase or coiling, metaphase or alignment, anaphase or separation, telophase or uncoiling). Prophase and telophase are not shown in the figure. In the first meiotic division, the cells double without duplicating the number of chromosomes. This halves the number of chromosomes per cell. When the genetic material of the two haploid gametes merges during fertilization, the diploid set of chromosomes is restored. Depending on the manifestation of the inherited sets of genetic alleles, the phenotypic appearance can vary.

- *Dominant* — only one abnormal copy of the paired gene (allele) is necessary for expression of the disease (Fig. 2.2)

or

- *Recessive* — both copies of the paired gene are required to be mutated for expression of the disease (Fig. 2.2).

Autosomal and sex-linked inheritance

Mendelian inheritance patterns can often be seen in characteristics encoded on the autosomal chromosomes, although a number of other factors can influence inheritance and complicate Mendel's simple pattern, especially the influence of other genes.

When a characteristic is carried on one of the sex chromosomes, it still follows the pattern of segregation. However, while autosomal chromosomes come in pairs, sex chromosomes pose a difficulty for male progeny, as they inherit a single X chromosome from their mother and a single Y chromosome from their father. Thus mutations on either sex chromosome can affect males severely.

X-linked disorders

In women both maternally and paternally inherited X chromosomes would have to carry the same defective gene for a recessive abnormality to be expressed; in most instances, the normal X chromosome compensates for the genetic defect in the other X chromosome. In men there is no other X chromosome to compensate for a genetic defect.

However, both copies of the X chromosome do not remain active in females; one copy is inactivated in each cell lineage by a process known as X-inactivation. This can lead to the interesting phenomenon of genetic 'mosaicism', in which half of the cells in women express genes from the maternally derived X chromosome, while the other half of the cells express genes from the paternally derived X chromosome (Box 2.2).

Y-linked disorders

For obvious reasons, Y chromosome-linked disorders only affect men. Ninety-five per cent of the length of the human Y chromosome is inherited as a single haploid block, passed from father to son. Thus, the Y chromosome represents an invaluable record of all mutations that have occurred in the male lineage throughout evolution; variation in Y chromosome DNA can be used for

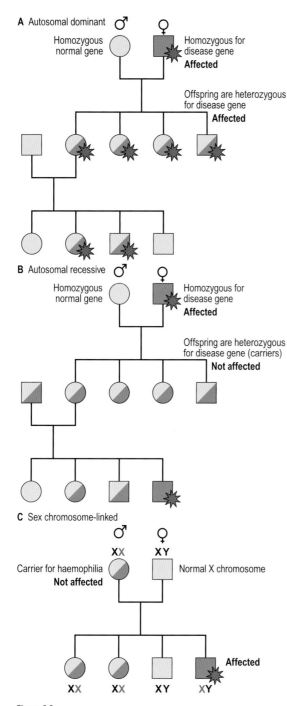

Figure 2.2
Dominant, recessive and X-linked inheritance patterns. (A) Domi-
nantly inherited genes do not skip generations; all offspring of a homozygous parent are affected by the disease. (B) Recessive disease genes
do not necessarily affect each generation. (C) X-linked inheritance patterns affect the male offspring of mothers who are carriers.

Box 2.2

Mosaicism or 'Lyonization'

Mosaicism or Lyonization was first proposed by Mary
Lyon. In X-linked skin disorders, Lyonization can give rise
to a 'mosaic pattern' in females, such that the affected
skin can appear in 'stripes', known as Blaschko lines,
separated by areas of normal skin. In the various X-linked
skin disorders, affected women can show quite dissimilar
degrees of involvement and forms of manifestation
because X-inactivation may give rise to different patterns
of functional mosaicism.

Oddly, mosaicism is not apparent for all X-linked disorders.
No such pattern is observed in women with Fabry disease,
a fat storage disorder caused by a deficiency of an enzyme
(α-galactosidase A) involved in the biodegradation of
lipids (see Ch. 11). In Fabry disease, the causative gene
seems to be inactivated in all cells. However, in another
X-linked condition, ichthyosis, the gene seems to escape
inactivation entirely, and the whole body surface is
affected by scaly skin.

Thus, while it is clear that the regulation of X-linked
gene expression is a little more complex than originally
predicted, mosaic gene expression does occur and
women can be considered functional mosaics. Analogous
X-inactivation patterns have already been documented in
human skin, bones, teeth and eyes.

investigations of human evolution, for forensic purposes
and for paternity analysis.

There are relatively few genes on the Y chromosome,
but Y-associated polymorphisms are of interest in male-
specific disorders, such as failure of sperm production and
cancer of the prostate and testes, and predominantly male-
associated disorders such as hypertension and autism.

Table 2.1 shows a number of examples of autosomal dominant, autosomal recessive and sex-linked disorders.

Non-Mendelian inheritance

Whilst the importance of Mendel's laws to the development of genetics cannot be over-estimated, the inheritance
of a large number of autosomal genetic characteristics
does not seem to follow the simple patterns of recessive
or dominant transmission. This makes it especially difficult to track down the particular genes involved.

Incomplete dominance

This is a heterozygous condition in which both alleles at
a gene locus are partially expressed, often producing an
intermediate phenotype. A good example of incomplete

Table 2.1
Some dominant, recessive and X-linked genetic disorders

Inheritance pattern	Diseases	Affected chromosome and gene	Symptoms
Autosomal dominant	Neurofibromatosis	17 Neurofibromin (*NF1*)	Multiple nerve sheath tumours, café-au-lait skin spots and tumours
	Familial adenomatous polyposis (FAP)	15 Adenomatous polyposis coli (*APC*)	Numerous benign colorectal polyps, increased risk of colorectal carcinoma
	Huntington's disease	4 Huntingtin (*HD*)	Chorea (movement incoordination), dementia
Autosomal recessive	Phenylketonuria (PKU)	12 Phenylalanine hydroxylase (*PAH*)	Neurological abnormalities, mental retardation
	Cystic fibrosis (CF)	7 Cystic fibrosis transmembrane conductance regulator (*CFTR*)	Chest infections, pancreatitis
	Albinism 1 (OCA1)	11 Tyrosinase (*TYR*)	Absence of melanin pigmentation, increased risk of skin cancer
X-linked	Duchenne muscular dystrophy (DMD)	X Dystrophyne (*DMD*)	Progressive muscular weakness
	Haemophilia A (HEMA)	X Coagulation factor VIII	Tendency to bleed
	Anaemia due to G6PD deficiency	X Glucose-6-phosphate dehydrogenase (*G6PD*)	Haemolysis, resistance to malaria

dominance is sickle cell disease; individuals homozygous for the recessive genetic mutation in the haemoglobin β-chain at amino acid position 6 have sickle cell disease, with a special haemoglobin variant which becomes crystalline at low oxygen tensions (see Ch. 5). The disease is characterized by episodes of tissue infarction and chronic haemolysis. Heterozygous individuals exhibit a mild version of the disease with normal blood count and no symptoms under normal circumstances. Sickling occurs only under severe hypoxia such as that caused by general anaesthesia. Haematuria is also an occasional feature of the heterozygous state due to renal papillary necrosis from focal sickling in the renal medulla. Homozygous-dominant individuals have normal haemoglobin (see also Box 2.5 below).

Over-dominance

This has been recognized in human leukocyte antigen (HLA) heterozygotes among individuals with favourable disease outcomes during viral infections. During the cellular immune response, T lymphocytes recognize virus antigens displayed on a host cell 'in the context of' HLA proteins and differences at the loci encoding the HLA alleles modulate the intensity and effectiveness of host response to infection. Consequently, individual combinations of HLA alleles may be especially effective, or especially ineffective, at presenting antigens from particular infections, so that carrying one or two copies of a given HLA allele can predispose an infected individual to a more or less favourable disease outcome.

Co-dominance

In the case of co-dominance, neither phenotype can be dominant over the other. Instead, the individual expresses both phenotypes. A good example of co-dominance is in human Landsteiner blood types. The gene for blood types has three alleles: A, B and i. Allele i causes O-type blood and is recessive to both A and B alleles. When a person inherits both A and B alleles, the blood type is AB, as they are co-dominantly expressed.

Multiple alleles

This is when more than two forms of the same gene are present in a population. There are three blood type alleles (A, B, O) of one blood type gene. Complexity is further enhanced by the potential increase not only by allele variations, but also by the number of genes encoding a simple trait (polygenic trait). For example, while skin

Table 2.2
mtDNA-linked disorders

Mitochondrial disorder	Mutation	Gene	Symptoms
Kerns–Sayre syndrome	Single, large deletion	Several genes	Progressive myopathy, cardiomyopathy, ophthalmoplegia
Pearson syndrome	Single, large deletion	Several genes	Pancytopenia, lactic acidosis
CPEO	Single, large deletion	Several genes	Ophthalmoplegia
MELAS	A–G, 3243; T–C, 3271	TRNL1	Myopathy, encephalopathy, lactic acidosis, stroke-like episodes
	Individual variations	ND1	
	Individual variations	ND5	
MERRF	A–G, 8344; T–C, 8356	TRNK	Myoclonic epilepsy, myopathy
NARP	T–G, 8993	ATP6	Neuropathy, ataxia, retinitis pigmentosa
MILS	T–C, 8993	ATP6	Progressive brain-stem disorder
MIDD	A–G, 3243	TRNL1	Diabetes, deafness
LHON	G–A, 3460	ND1	Optic neuropathy
	G–A, 11778	ND4	
	T–C, 14484	ND6	
Myopathy and diabetes	T–C, 14709	TRNE	Myopathy, weakness, diabetes
Sensorineural hearing loss	A–G, 1555	RNR1	Deafness
	Individual variations	TRNS1	
Exercise intolerance	Individual variations	CYB	Fatigue, muscle weakness
Fatal infantile encephalopathy (Leigh-like syndrome)	T–C, 10158; T–C, 10191	ND3	Lactic acidosis

colour is determined by three genes with six alleles, HLAs are encoded by 220 known genes and multiple numbers of potential HLA alleles. Analysis of the genetic basis for complex traits is even more difficult, as the phenotype can be the product of a range of unrelated polygenic factors and multiple alleles. Complex traits are the result of the interaction of several, potentially polygenic, multi-allele simple traits. For example, hypertension is a phenotype that is influenced by the patient's weight (obesity gene or genes), cholesterol level (genes controlling metabolism), kidney function (salt transporter genes), etc. Each one of the contributing simple traits can be polygenic and also have multiple alleles complicating genetic analysis.

Mitochondrial inheritance

While searching for genes underlying specific disease traits, it is easy to focus entirely on chromosomal DNA. However, extranuclear or cytoplasmic inheritance is also well documented in a number of species including humans. An established mechanism by which extranuclear inheritance occurs in humans is via maternally inherited mitochondrial DNA (mtDNA). However, whether mutations in mtDNA influence disease traits was, for a long time, an unanswered question.

It is now clear that mitochondrial biogenesis and function are under dual genetic control and require extensive interaction between paternally and maternally inherited nuclear genes and maternally inherited mitochondrial genes.

Mutations can occur in any nucleic acid sequence, so mutations in mtDNA can and do occur. As mtDNA is maternally inherited, the manifestation of mitochondria-linked pathologies is complex and the localization of disease genes difficult. Table 2.2 lists some mtDNA-linked disorders; mtDNA is also used in studies of human evolution and for forensic purposes.

Rules of DNA replication and mutagenesis

The main principles of DNA replication and mutagenesis were considered in Chapter 1. For the purpose of gene hunting, there are three important principles to keep in mind:

- Despite the various repair mechanisms, genetic mutations can occur in any nucleic acid sequences, either as spontaneous or induced mutations.
- Characteristic mutations can persist in a gene pool without causing disease. These are known as genetic variations or polymorphisms.
- Genes in close proximity on a chromosome can be inherited together ('linked'), even during chromosomal recombination (Fig. 2.3).

It has also been established that a single mutation in a somatic cell (see Ch. 1) rarely leads to disease; most genetic errors are attributable to inheritance through parental genes. Inherited mutations and variability are often generated during the complex, environmentally sensitive process of meiotic division during the production of haploid gametes.

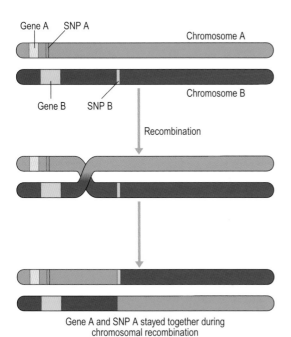

Gene A and SNP A stayed together during chromosomal recombination

Figure 2.3
Chromosomal recombination. Satellites and single nucleotide polymorphisms (SNPs) that lie near a disease gene are more likely to stay with the disease gene during chromosomal recombination and serve as markers for the disease. In the figure SNP A is near gene A; therefore during recombination these stay together. Gene B and SNP B are separated during the recombination process.

Finding disease genes

Abnormal genes may be detected either:

- *directly* from the presence of the gene itself or the defective product

or

- *indirectly* by virtue of its linkage with a detectable marker (see below).

For some of the single gene disorders, the aberrant gene is well characterized. These disorders include cystic fibrosis (CF) and glucose-6-phosphate dehydrogenase (G6PD) deficiency. Finding the genetic basis for multifactorial conditions — for example, cardiovascular diseases or cancers — is more difficult, indicating the need for complex gene hunting approaches.

Mutations in the cystic fibrosis gene

CF and congenital bilateral absence of the vas deferens (CBAVD) are 'single gene' disorders. The causative gene is *CFTR*, the cystic fibrosis transmembrane conductance regulator, which is member 7 of subfamily C of the adenosine triphosphate (ATP)-binding cassettes. However, there are several mutations within this one gene that can cause phenotypic manifestation of the disease. *CFTR* is located on chromosome 7, stretching from base pairs 116,907,252 to 117,095,950. Mutations within the sequence include deletion of F508 (the most common mutation, comprising 66% of all CF mutations), G542X, G551D, N1303K, W1282X, R553X and single nucleotide insertions and deletions. (For a more complete mutation list see www.genet.sickkids.on.ca.) Based on the recommendation of the American College of Medical Genetics in 2004, 23 different mutations are sought in genetic testing for CF.

CFTR exists in many organs, but the most prominent abnormalities are evident in airway epithelia, sweat glands, pancreas, intestine, liver and genitourinary system. Although CF is a complex multisystem disease, diagnosis is often based on acute or persistent respiratory symptoms; including chronic cough, persistent wheezing and pulmonary infiltrates. These symptoms often progress to extensive airway damage, and this is the major cause of morbidity and mortality in CF patients.

Mutations in G6PD deficiency

The relationship between genetic mutations and protein dysfunction has been extensively studied in relation to the human gene for G6PD. Mutation of this gene can cause the appearance of an enzyme variant, G6PD A⁻, which gives rise to human G6PD deficiency. The resulting protein has markedly reduced structural stability that is caused by a two-amino acid substitution. The functionally defective G6PD A⁻ shows reduced unfolding enthalpy accompanied by changes in inner spatial distances between residues in the coenzyme domain.

The loss of folding determinants leads to a protein with decreased intracellular stability.

The G6PD gene is located in a region of the X chromosome showing a high degree of genetic variability. For this particular gene, more than 100 mutations or combined mutations associated with nearly 200 variants have been detected. As over 400 million people in the world have G6PD deficiency, this medical problem is the most common human enzymopathy. G6PD deficiency is associated with acute or chronic haemolytic anaemia and neonatal jaundice. Some genetic variants have attained a high incidence in certain parts of the world, since they confer selective advantage against malaria (see also Ch. 9).

Linkage studies

While direct gene hunting has the benefit of well-identified malfunctioning proteins, indirect gene hunting approaches need to make use of circumstantial evidence for the presence of malfunctioning genes. From studies of genetic inheritance it is known that, prior to meiosis, which leads to the production of haploid germ cells from their diploid precursors, random interchange of DNA segments can occur between the homologous paternally and maternally derived chromosomes to form new recombinant chromosomes (Fig. 2.3). The process of interchange occurs over such short lengths of DNA that only those genes lying adjacent on chromosomes are likely to remain 'linked' together through successive generations. Single nucleotide mutations and nucleotide repeats persist within populations and are inherited linked to other genes. As a consequence, these characteristic variants can serve as markers that help gene hunting.

Genetic markers

There are two main types of genetic marker:

- tandem repeats (satellites)
- single nucleotide polymorphisms (SNPs).

Both satellites and SNPs can be the cause of disease. Table 2.3 lists some of the diseases associated with tandem repeats. However, both types of genetic marker can occur and persist in the genome without necessarily being an underlying cause of disease. These can be used as markers to narrow down the chromosomal location of disease genes (Fig. 2.3). Satellites have also been successfully used in forensic science for personal identification; they are the basis for 'genetic fingerprinting'.

Markers are detected and identified using either the polymerase chain reaction (PCR) or Southern blotting (see Appendix 2). Both techniques rely heavily on specific probes that are synthesized to complement specific DNA sequences.

Although SNPs are the more stable markers, currently both satellites and SNPs are used as markers in gene hunting studies. In general, both markers are used to trace genes for disease traits to specific chromosomes or even to localize a potential disease gene to a certain part of that specific chromosome. In this way a potential target sequence, much shorter than the full genome, can be sequenced repeatedly until the mutation and the disease gene are found.

Tandem repeats (satellites)

Short segments of DNA that have a repeated sequence pattern are called tandem repeats. Tandem repeats usually tend to occur among 'satellites' — a long DNA sequence of genetically inactive DNA or heterochromatin. Based on size, it is possible to distinguish:

- *minisatellites* (repeat units in the range 6–100 bp, spanning hundreds of base pairs); these are also called various number tandem repeats (VNTRs)
- *microsatellites* (repeat units in the range 1–5 bp, spanning a few tens of nucleotides); these are also called short tandem repeats (STRs).

The repeat units can vary. They can be:

- *dinucleotides*, such as CACACA, that is frequently present in the human genome
- *trinucleotides*, such as CAGCAGCAG or GCCGCCGCC
- *tetranucleotides*, such as AATGAATGAATG
- *pentanucleotides*, such as AGAAAAGAAAAGAAA
- *hexanucleotides*, such as AGTACAAGTACAAGTACA.

The efforts of the Human Genome Project have identified numerous tandem repeat sequences. So far more than 20 000 tetranucleotide STR loci have been characterized; potentially, there may be more than a million STR loci present in the human genome, depending on the way they are counted. The wide variety of tandem repeats occurring in the human genome means that they differ sufficiently among individuals and as such are useful markers not only for genetic mapping and linkage analysis of human diseases, but also in human identity testing. Box 2.3 describes an example of a genetic linkage study using STRs to find genes involved in hypertension. Table 2.3 lists several examples of human diseases which are caused by expansions of tandem repeats.

Single nucleotide polymorphisms or SNPs ('snips')

These are DNA sequence variations that occur when a single nucleotide (A, T, C or G) in the genome sequence is altered. Thus an SNP can change the DNA sequence of AACCCGTA to ATGGGCAT. For a variation to be considered an SNP, it must occur in at least 1% of the population. Two out of three SNPs involve the replacement of cytosine (C) with thymidine (T). SNPs can occur in both coding (gene) and non-coding regions of the genome. Many SNPs have no effect on cell function, but variations in DNA sequence can have a major impact on how people respond to disease, to environmental insults such as bacteria, viruses, toxins and chemicals, and to drugs and other therapies (see Ch. 9). This makes SNPs very valuable for biomedical research and for

Table 2.3
Some medical conditions caused by tandem repeats

Disease	Normal repeats	Tandem repeats	Chromosome	Protein (protein function)	Symptoms
Myotonic dystrophy type 1 (DM1)	5–35	CTG (from 35–50, up to 1000×)	19 (*DMPK* gene)	Myotonic dystrophy protein kinase (exact function unknown but has been shown to inhibit a specific subunit (PPP1R12A) of myosin phosphatase and thus regulate muscle tension)	Muscle weakness, especially of distal leg, hand, neck, and face; myotonia; posterior subcapsular cataracts
Myotonic dystrophy type 2 (DM2)	11–26	Complex (TG)n(TCTG) n(CCTG)n (from 75, up to 11 000×)	3 (*CNBP* gene)	CCHC-type zinc finger, nucleic acid-binding protein (regulates genes involved in production and use of cholesterol)	Muscle weakness; myotonia (sustained muscle contraction); posterior subcapsular cataracts; cardiac conduction defects or progressive cardiomyopathy; hypogammaglobulinaemia; insulin insensitivity; primary gonadal failure in males
Huntington's disease (HD)	6–35	CAG, 38–180 (up to 180×) with penultimate CAA interrupts	4 (*HD* or *IT15* gene)	Huntingtin (disrupts nerve signals and protein transport in brain)	Adult-onset personality changes; generalized chorea and cognitive decline
Huntington's disease 2	6–27	Pure CAG, 35–57	16 (*JPH3* gene)	Junctophilin-3 (part of junctional complexes, composed of a C-terminal hydrophobic segment spanning endoplasmic/ sarcoplasmic reticulum)	Symptoms indistinguishable from Huntington's disease; also called Huntington's disease-like 2, one of several diseases similar to HD
Friedreich's ataxia	7–22	GAA (80 or > several hundreds ×)	9	Frataxin (mitochondrial protein; its absence leads to build-up of toxic byproducts (e.g. iron) and overproduction of free radicals and oxidative stress)	First symptoms are difficulty in walking or gait ataxia; ataxia gradually worsens and slowly spreads to arms and then trunk; over time muscles begin to weaken and waste and deformities develop on limbs; also, loss of tendon reflexes, especially in knees and ankles; gradual loss of sensation in extremities, which may spread; dysarthria and fatigue; nystagmus is also common; most people with Friedreich's ataxia develop scoliosis
Fragile X syndrome (FXS)	Up to 30	CGG (from 55 to and even > 200×)	X (*FMRP* 1 gene)	Fragile X mental retardation protein (interacts with mRNA nuclear export factor NXF2)	Most common cause of inherited mental impairment; ranges from learning disabilities to more severe cognitive or intellectual disabilities; FXS is most common known cause of autism or 'autistic-like' behaviours; also features delays in speech and language development

Box 2.3

Hunting genes for hypertension

During the past decade, considerable efforts and resources have been devoted to elucidate the multiple genetic and environmental determinants responsible for multifactorial diseases. One of these diseases is hypertension. Around 900 million people worldwide suffer from hypertension and the resulting cardiovascular diseases, renal failure and cerebrovascular disease. Prevention, detection and treatment of hypertension are therefore a high priority. However, none of these aims can be efficiently achieved without the elucidation of the genetic aetiology of hypertension. So far, microsatellite association studies have been proved to be the most reliable in the search for the genetic basis of hypertension and cardiac diseases. Therefore this approach is often used in genome-wide mapping to find hypertension 'predisposition genes'.

In Japan, a study to elucidate the genetic basis of hypertension was conducted using 18 977 microsatellite markers. Blood samples were collected from 385 moderate to severe hypertensive patients and 385 normotensive control subjects. To avoid protein and RNA contamination, and also to prevent variation due to differences in DNA quality, DNA was extracted using a standard kit and DNA degradation was tested using agarose gel electrophoresis.

Using standardized pipetting of aliquoted DNA whose concentration had previously been determined, DNA templates were prepared for typing for 2 × 18 977 STR markers (first set: case subjects; second set: control subjects) and for 2 × 18 977 PCR reactions (see Ch. 3 and Appendix 2) using an automated system. The PCR reactions were performed with primer pairs designed to amplify individual sites from each of the 18 977 predetermined microsatellite sites. PCR products were visualized in agarose or capillary gel electrophoresis and product peak intensity was analysed. Standardized preparations ensured reproducibility and accuracy throughout testing, and the resulting chromatograms were analysed for peak positions and heights using computer programs.

The relatively large sample cohort increased the value of statistical analysis that was initially conducted in pooled samples in a three-stage genomic screen of three independent case-control populations, and 54 markers were extracted from the original 18 977 microsatellite markers. As a final step, each single positive marker was confirmed by individual typing, and only 19 markers passed this test. As a result, the 19 significantly different allelic loci were identified as essential hypertension markers (Yatsu et al., 2007). Clearly, gene hunting is not for the faint-hearted!

---

developing pharmaceutical products or medical diagnostics. SNPs are also evolutionarily stable, persisting in the genome, and this makes them easier to follow in population studies.

Detection of SNPs

Identification of genetic markers is a laborious task. SNPs, for example, can be located if overlapping DNA sequences are lined up and sequence analysis results are compared to find differences in the nucleotide order. False positive (change in nucleotide sequence) and false negative (no change in nucleotide sequence) results of sequence assessments are both possible. These variations result either from errors in sequencing or from the presence of paralogue sequences. Paralogues are genes related by duplication within the genome. The length of reference sequences can vary but is usually around 1 Mb; the sequences are organized for further analysis by using overlapping areas of sequence. Paralogues can be omitted from the analysis if, for example, sequences with a high number of variations are not included. All sequencing chromatograms are normally analysed using the PHRED base finder computer program. Both PHRED and PHRAP computer programs were developed by Philip Green at the University of Washington, Seattle, USA, and played a vital role in the analysis of results generated in the Human Genome Project. Further

statistical analysis can help to identify more consistently present nucleotide sequence variations. Once potential SNPs are identified, then further assessment is required to find out whether the sequence variation is anywhere near a meaningful coding sequence and whether it can be linked to a specific protein, and perhaps a specific disease. The International SNP Map Working Group has summarized human SNP distribution for each chromosome.

Statistical probability

It is not the aim of the present book to discuss the statistical requirements for genetic studies in detail; there are already some excellent books available which cover this topic (e.g. Sham, 1998). However, it is not possible to omit the main principles of statistics from this discussion of gene hunting.

We have discussed some of the basic principles of genetics used in the process of finding the genes for disease or disease susceptibility. To a superficial observer the above principles might seem sufficient to identify the appropriate coding sequences for disease genes. However, without statistics geneticists would not be able to draw

Box 2.4

The effect of diet on colorectal cancer

The connection between diet and colorectal cancer presents an excellent example of the complexity of medical issues. Changes in activation or inhibition of the protein kinase C (PKC) family of signal transduction molecules can indirectly lead to modified gene expression. Epidemiological data had strongly implicated diet as a factor in colorectal cancer. Somewhat surprisingly, various bile acids were found to influence PKC activity, which in turn affects cell proliferation, differentiation and apoptosis, and thus disease development and progression. Some clinical studies have shown increased amounts of bile acids, especially secondary bile acids, in colorectal cancer. Bile acids are normal constituents of the intestinal tract, where bile production and bile acid constitution are dependent on individual diet. The diet is dependent on geological location and also on cultural differences and individual preferences. It is not surprising, therefore, that finding the genetic background to a specific multifactorial disease like colorectal cancer is extremely difficult.

Box 2.5

Sickle cell disease

A typical and frequently cited example of the process of 'selection' is sickle cell disease. Sickle cell disease is a haemoglobin abnormality. The mutant molecule (HbS) has a valine substitution for glutamic acid at position 6 on the β-chain that makes the haemoglobin crystalline at low oxygen tensions, which results in sickle-shaped distortion of the red blood cells (see also Ch. 5). The mutation is common in West and Central Africa, the Mediterranean, Middle East and some parts of the Indian subcontinent; clinical symptoms are severe in the homozygous population, who experience chronic haemolytic anaemia and microvascular occlusion causing ischaemic tissue damage and severe pain. Despite these clinical features, the mutation persists in the population, as — similarly to G6PD deficiency — sickle cell disease creates a hostile environment for the plasmodium parasite within the red blood cells and therefore is protective against malaria.

- *Mutation*: when spontaneous or induced changes occur in the genetic sequence.
- *Migration*: when people move from one town, city or continent to another and, through reproduction, introduce novel alleles to the pre-existing gene pool. At the same time, migrating individuals also remove their alleles from the population they are moving out of, which may decrease variability in their previous population.
- *Selection*: when having or lacking a particular allele confers an advantage during evolution (Box 2.5).

Studying population genetics and hunting for disease genes are very similar in that it is exceptionally difficult in both to consider all potential factors influencing a given genetic diversity. To make specific traits easier to identify, certain assumptions have to be made. One of these is the random distribution of equally viable alleles according to the Hardy–Weinberg equilibrium.

conclusions regarding the scientific significance of the limited evidence provided by relatively small sample numbers. Furthermore, it is also important to simplify the data in order to recognize trends or relationships. In biology in general, and medical research in particular, observed relationships are rarely clear-cut. Even when the underlying relationship is simple, our picture of it is often confused by uncontrolled variations. Inherent variations are observed both within the organism and in its environment (for an example, see Box 2.4). In a genetic analysis it is often important to simplify these variations to make numerical analysis possible.

In gene hunting studies, the complexity is compounded because these studies have to be performed at a variety of levels: gene, chromosome, cell, individual, family and population. It is not unusual to identify a gene that underlies a particular disease in one family, only to find that all other sufferers from this disease do not seem to share that variant gene.

As specific traits, including disease traits, are determined in a population by the presence of alleles, it is naturally important to determine how frequently this allele is present in the gene pool.

What is genetic frequency?

Genetic frequency is the percentage or proportion of a particular allele at a genetic locus within a population. In a real population, there are several factors influencing allele frequency of disease or disease susceptibility genes. These include:

The Hardy–Weinberg equilibrium

"Under conditions of random mating in a large population where all genotypes are equally viable, gene frequencies of a particular generation depend upon the gene frequencies of the previous generation and not upon the genotype frequencies.

The frequencies of different genotypes produced through random mating depend only upon the gene frequencies".

In practice, the Hardy–Weinberg equilibrium declares that gene and genotype frequencies in future generations can be predicted if outside forces are not acting to change the frequency of the genes and if random mating occurs between all genotypes. To make some of the statistical analysis possible, it has to be assumed that the Hardy–Weinberg equilibrium applies for some of the analysis involved in looking for disease genes.

Given the assumptions necessary for the Hardy–Weinberg equilibrium to apply, it is perhaps not surprising that deviations are not uncommon. These may be due to a variety of causes. If an excess of heterozygotes is observed, this may indicate the presence of overdominant selection or the occurrence of outbreeding. Alternatively, if an excess of homozygotes is detected, it may be due to any one of four factors:

- The locus is under selection.
- 'Null alleles' (a mutant copy of a gene that completely lacks that gene's normal function) may be present.
- Inbreeding may be common in the population.
- There is a population substructure that is not immediately detectable and therefore mating is, in fact, not random — a situation that is not uncommon in human populations!

The likelihood of each of these explanations must be assessed using additional data, such as demographic information. It is understandable that, without the help of computer algorithms, it is impossible to analyse all the collected data and to take all potential variables — even in a simplified form — into consideration (see below).

Due to naturally occurring variability of the human genome, most statistical methods require nuclear families (sibling/parent studies) or extended pedigrees, where the principles of genetic inheritance can be observed, for successful implementation.

Although recognition of genetic principles and the complexity of individual genetic problems is vitally important, identification of a specific disease susceptibility gene remains hard to achieve and requires further consideration of analytical and statistical methods.

Linkage analysis

Traditionally, the search for a disease gene begins with linkage analysis.

Genetic linkage analysis is a statistical method that is used to associate potential functionality of genes with their location on chromosomes. The main idea is that markers which are found in the same vicinity on the chromosome have a tendency to stick together during chromosomal recombination when passed on to offspring, and are therefore said to be linked. Thus, if a particular disease is often passed to offspring along with specific markers, then it can be concluded that the gene (or genes) responsible for the disease is located close to these markers on the chromosome.

Searches for causative variants of disease genes in regions of a chromosome identified by linkage analysis have been highly successful for many rare single-gene disorders, especially those that follow Mendelian inheritance patterns. Health problems that appear to aggregate within families but that do not segregate like a simple Mendelian gene, such as cardiovascular disease, obesity or schizophrenia, pose additional problems for gene hunting. Linkage analysis has been less useful in finding genes that are risk factors for these multifactorial disorders. In order to improve prediction and probability studies for complex traits, linkage disequilibrium (LD) analysis has been introduced.

Linkage disequilibrium is slightly different from linkage. LD is based on the observation that common genetic variants in individuals who carry a particular polymorphism (such as an SNP) at one site, often predictably carry other specific polymorphisms at other nearby variant sites. This has led to the suggestion that chromosomal recombination may occur at particular 'hot spots' on either side of the regions of LD.

LD reflects the shared ancestry of contemporary chromosomes. When a new variant arises through mutation — whether a single nucleotide change, an insertion/deletion or a structural alteration — it is initially tethered to a unique chromosome on which it occurred, and associated with a distinct set of genetic markers. Recombination and further mutation can subsequently act to erode this association but this process occurs slowly, so that some interactions remain sufficiently stable to follow inheritance.

Linkage disequilibrium and haplotypes

High-resolution characterization of LD patterns across the genome has proved to be centrally important for association studies of disease and disease susceptibility genes, as well as the understanding of genetic processes such as recombination, mutation and selection. LD maps rely directly on marker correlation in the population and can thus guide marker selection for association studies. As regions of high LD display low haplotype diversity, common haplotypes can be efficiently tagged with only a relatively few variants or SNPs. Several parameters influence the appearance of haplotype blocks and SNP tags, including the population in which the studies are performed, the choice of markers, the density of polymorphisms and the applied computer algorithm. Nevertheless, as studies have been repeated, taking as many variables into consideration as possible, a pattern has emerged in the US population with northern and western European ancestry connecting autoimmune, inflammatory and infectious diseases with loci in the HLA gene, confirming previously identified recombination hot spots. For further details, see Centre d'Etude du Polymorphisme Humain (CEPH), which collected pedigrees with northern and western European ancestry (http://www.cephb.fr), and Ensemble Variation API (www.ensembl.org).

The correlation between causal mutations and the haplotypes in which they arise is an important tool in genetic research. Common variants of a number of individual genes have been shown to play important roles in susceptibility to specific diseases (Table 2.4).

Table 2.4
Some genetic risk factors and their chromosomal localization

Genetic risk factor abbreviation	Genetic risk factor	Gene map locus	Disease
APOE4	Apolipoprotein E4	19q13.2	Alzheimer's disease 2, late-onset
PPARG	Peroxisome proliferator-activated receptor-gamma	3p25	Type 2 diabetes
PTPN22	Protein tyrosine phosphatase non-receptor type 22	1p13	Rheumatoid arthritis and type 1 diabetes
CTLA4	Cytotoxic lymphocyte-associated antigen 4	2q33	Autoimmune thyroid disease, type 1 diabetes
NOD2	Nucleotide-binding oligomerization domain protein 2	16q12	Inflammatory bowel disease, psoriatic arthritis
NRG2	Neuregulin 1	5q23–q33	Schizophrenia, Alzheimer's disease
DTNBP1	Dysbindin 1	6p22.3	Schizophrenia
ADAM33	A disintegrin and metalloproteinase domain 33	20p13	Asthma
PDE4D	Phosphodiesterase 4D	5q12	Stroke
LTA	Lymphotoxin alpha	6p21.3	Myocardial infarction, arthritis, asthma, inflammatory bowel disease
APOAV	Apolipoprotein A-V	11q23	Hypertriglyceridaemia
ATP1A2	Na^+/K^+ transporting alpha 2	1q21–q32	Migraine
CACNA1A	Ca^{2+} channel voltage-dependent type alpha 1A subunit	19p13	Migraine (familial), spinocerebellar and episodic ataxia
BRCA1	Breast cancer type 1	17q21	Breast cancer, prostate cancer
BRCA2	Breast cancer type 2	13q12.3	Breast cancer, prostate cancer
CHEK2	Checkpoint kinase 2	22q12.1	Breast and colorectal cancer susceptibility

Computer-based data modelling

Perhaps it is obvious from the previously described genetic and statistical principles that all gene hunting studies have to be carefully constructed. It is especially important to choose the best-suited approach for the detection of the genes that may predispose an individual to a complex multifactorial phenotype.

The current literature is divided between two types of study design:

- *Model-based analysis*. It is assumed that the causative mechanisms of both the disease trait and marker phenotypes are known without error, including the number of loci involved, the mode of inheritance and allele frequencies. Thus model-based analysis makes the underlying parameters explicit. However, as our knowledge of the complexities

of the mode of inheritance and the variety of unknown and unpredictable parameters increases, the application of model-based approaches is decreasing.
- *Model-free analysis*. Here a larger data set is required. However, as the data pool increases, or becomes more heterogeneous, the number of variables is also growing and this requires some simplification of the assumptions that can be made. This is achieved in practice by repeated sampling of the same population, which allows an increase in sample size while the underlying variables remain the same.

All in all, model-based and model-free study designs are not so very different, as some assumptions have to be made in both cases in order to handle the collected data. For interested readers, there are excellent reviews providing further and more in-depth reading about the handling and analysis of genetic data (see, for example, Elston, 1998).

Currently, the most frequently used computer program for performing exact genetic linkage analysis, complete with input–output relationships, is Superlink (http://bioinfo.cs.technion.ac.il/superlink-online). The main difference between Superlink and other computer programs (see below) is that the former can run much larger files to enable analysis of general pedigrees (which may involve many individuals, inbreeding loops, many markers, etc.), two-locus traits, autosomal or sex-linked traits, and complex traits, and to perform maximum-likelihood haplotyping analysis.

Other computer programs for standard genetic linkage analysis can be found on the following websites:

- Linkage — http://linkage.rockefeller.edu/soft/linkage
- Fastlink v4.1 — http://www.ncbi.nlm.nih.gov/CBBresearch/Schaffer/fastlink.html
- Tlinkage — http://hpcio.cit.nih.gov/lserver/TLINKAGE.html
- Genehunter v2.1 — http://linkage.rockefeller.edu/soft/gh/

Hypothesis testing

The finding that a particular gene is linked to a particular disorder does not in itself tell you anything about causation. Linkage simply refers to the statistical probability that the disease-causing gene is located close to the marker gene on the chromosome; the marker gene may or may not be the causative gene itself.

The results need to be tested and manipulated at the level of protein, cell and whole animal to verify the connection between the proposed genetic mutation and the resulting pathology. For these studies transgenic animals are frequently used (see Ch. 8). These model systems allow manipulation of the suspected disease gene and detailed observation of the resulting disease phenotype. Physiological testing also helps to design and test novel pharmaceutical compounds to treat the disease, or at least to alleviate symptoms. The most immediate benefit of finding a gene for a particular disorder is usually the development of a specific diagnostic test.

Ethical considerations

To find the genetic variants of genes that cause diseases or influence disease risk and drug response, it is necessary to understand how genetic and environmental factors interact to influence health. Although the road from scientific discovery to improved health outcomes can be long, understanding these factors should eventually lead to better methods in prevention, diagnosis and treatment.

While these goals are understandable for most people, many biomedical research projects, including genetic inheritance studies, present complex ethical, social and cultural problems. Consequently, all gene hunting studies need to consider not only scientific and financial issues, but also social and ethical ones.

Investigation of disease development and inheritance is, as we have discussed earlier, population-bound. While there are some advantages to studying inheritance in isolated populations (Mendelian genetic inheritance is easier to trace and genetic mutations can be more clearly connected to specific disease patterns), other analyses require enormous sample sizes made possible only by multi-centre and multinational collaborations such as those exemplified by the HapMap project (http://www.hapmap.org).

Ethical issues before testing

Choosing populations, communities or ethnic minorities for use in the identification of a disease or disease susceptibility gene is a difficult task. First of all, to be able to generalize findings from the study, the sample cohort to be analysed needs to be large, which requires multi-centre studies. As the organization of multi-centre studies is not cheap, human genetic research often relies on financial support from worldwide organizations and funding from developed countries. This can result in ambiguity, if not downright hostility, on the part of tax-payers in the developed world.

Once the population is identified, then various genetic tests need to be performed which require human tissue samples. The use of any tissue sample for research purposes requires informed consent from the individual, so children or mentally impaired donors cannot generally be used. Researchers have to be prepared for consent to be refused on emotional or religious grounds or simply because of fear of the sampling procedure, no matter how minor that might be. Explanation of the research and its potential outcome, together with sensitivity towards people's beliefs and fears, can greatly reduce opposition to medical testing.

The next major ethical problem to be addressed is confidentiality. Samples need to be identified according to the population from which they originate and with some medical information about the donors; however, no personal identifiers are allowed. These rules were also observed during creation of the human genome reference sequence (see above).

Ethical issues after testing

The availability of genetic tests can trigger anxieties at a personal level. People worry that they may carry a specific gene that could lead to early death or chronic disease. Affected individuals need to have access to genetic counselling, and the use of genetic information by insurance companies, for example, needs to be carefully regulated. Finally, genetic studies can have ramifications for an entire community. Naming a population as a carrier for a specific disease could have important consequences for ethnic minorities or small isolated indigenous groups. Therefore, publication of test results requires careful consideration. Furthermore, issues have arisen as to who owns the results of these population studies: the population or the researchers?

FURTHER READING

Daly MJ, Rioux JD, Schaffner SF et al. 2001 High-resolution haplotype structure in the human genome. Nat Genet 29(2):229–232.

Debruyne PR, Bruyneel EA, Xuedong LI et al. 2001 The role of bile acids in carcinogenesis. Mutat Res 480–481:359–369.

Ellegren H 2004 Microsatellites: simple sequences with complex evolution. Nat Rev Genet 5(6):435–445.

Elston RC 1998 Linkage and association. Genet Epidemiol 15(6):565–576.

Krausz C, Quintana-Murci L, Forti G 2004 Y chromosome polymorphisms in medicine. Ann Med 36(8):573–583.

Kwiatkowski DP 2005 How malaria has affected the human genome and what human genetics can teach us about malaria. Am J Hum Genet 77(2):171–192.

Online Mendelian Inheritance in Man (OMIM)®, McKusick–Nathans Institute of Genetic Medicine, Johns Hopkins University (Baltimore, MD) and National Center for Biotechnology Information, National Library of Medicine (Bethesda, MD). URL: http://www.ncbi.nlm.nih.gov/omim/

Sham PC 1998 Statistics in human genetics. Arnold: London.

Sherlock R, Morrey JD (eds) 2002 Ethical issues in biotechnology. Rowman & Littlefield: Lanham, MD.

Taylor RW, Turnbull DM 2005 Mitochondrial DNA mutations in human disease. Nat Rev Genet 6(5):389–402.

Valley CM, Willard HF 2006 Genomic and epigenomic approaches to the study of X chromosome inactivation. Curr Opin Genet Dev 16(3):240–245.

Yatsu K, Mizuki N, Hirawa N et al. 2007 High-resolution mapping for essential hypertension using microsatellite markers. Hypertension 49(3):446–452.

3 Using genetic information

J. Pongracz

Now that the human genome has been sequenced and many disease genes identified, what can be done with this information?

The most immediate impact has been in the area of diagnostics, but this type of molecular genetic information is also enormously useful in medical research and in the development of new treatment strategies, such as gene therapy (see Ch. 10). It has also had a large impact on forensic medicine.

The sequencing of the genome was just the beginning of our understanding of human biology. As identification of the gene itself is seldom sufficient to understand pathology, functional genomic analysis is necessary. Regulation of gene expression and gene function is elucidated through analysis of RNA and the coded protein. Protein expression can also be regulated both at the post-transcriptional and post-translational levels. The importance of this type of regulation is well recognized and the Functional Analysis of the Genome programme (www.genome.gov) has been set up to manage and support such research. The aims of this programme include the development of improved techniques and strategies for efficient identification and functional analysis of genes, coding regions and other functional elements of the entire genomes — human and pathogens alike — on a high-throughput basis.

Medical diagnostics

Gene-based diagnostics are becoming increasingly important in medicine, to diagnose existing disease, and also as aids in disease prediction, prevention and treatment. Genome sequencing projects have generated enormous amounts of information regarding the genome of humans and a number of important human pathogens.

The mutations that are identified and associated with a specific disease or disease susceptibility trait can be introduced into high-throughput laboratory testing to aid diagnosis. Genomic testing therefore relies heavily on technical developments in nucleic acid and chromatin analysis, and development of novel technologies for taking samples, performing tests and analysing test results. With the continuous advancement of theory and technology, genomic testing has become the latest addition to a large medical diagnostic arsenal. These gene-based tests have the advantage that they are generally quicker, more specific and more reliable than more traditional diagnostic tests.

The first step for an effective medical treatment is a correct diagnosis. Thus gene-based diagnostics focuses on the characterization of reliable diagnostic markers that can identify diseases and determine potential treatment options.

Human genetics has a central place in preventive diagnosis and symptomatic screening tests.

Preventive diagnosis

The aim of preventive diagnosis is to avoid development of the disease. To this end, both pre- and postnatal tests can be used.

Prenatal diagnosis

Prenatal diagnosis requires analysis of embryonic tissue during development. Careful sampling is essential, as these procedures carry a high risk of embryo death or spontaneous abortion. Genomics has two potential applications in prenatal diagnosis:

- *Pre-implantation screening of embryos.* 'Pre-implantation genetic diagnosis' (PGD) is used prior to *in vitro* fertilization (IVF) to diagnose a genetic or chromosomal condition in an embryo before it is implanted into the mother's uterus.
- *Prenatal diagnostic screening.* Tests are performed when the baby would have an increased risk of genetic abnormality, such as spina bifida, cystic fibrosis, Duchenne muscular dystrophy, Huntington's disease, haemophilia, polycystic kidney disease, etc., or of a chromosomal abnormality such as Down syndrome.

Postnatal diagnosis

In postnatal diagnosis, newborn testing and predictive, presymptomatic and carrier screening tests are performed.

- *Newborn screening.* This is performed to detect certain genetic diseases (e.g. cystic fibrosis) for which early diagnosis and treatment are available.
- *Predictive and presymptomatic screening.* This determines the chances of a healthy individual developing a certain disease later in life. Diseases that can be screened for in this way include adult-onset conditions such as various types of cancer (e.g. breast cancer using the markers BRCA1

31

and 2), cardiovascular disease (using the ALOX5AP marker), early onset of Parkinson's disease (using the PINK1 marker), and some single gene disorders such as Huntington's disease.

- *Carrier screening*. This is performed to determine whether a person carries a copy of a particular disease-causing genetic mutation. If the inheritance pattern of the disease is autosomal recessive (see Ch. 2), then parents who both carry the same autosomal recessive gene have a 1 in 4 chance with each pregnancy of having a child with that disease (e.g. phenylketonuria or cystic fibrosis); therefore, embryonic testing of their children is particularly useful.

Symptomatic screening

Symptomatic screening tests improve the accuracy of diagnosis and can be important for deciding the best treatment strategy.

- *Obtaining diagnosis*. Genetic tests for both single-gene and multifactorial diseases, such as colonic adenocarcinomas, are becoming available. Genomic testing can also be used in infection to determine the identity of the infecting species or subspecies of microbe. As microbial infections often result in highly similar symptoms, effective treatment depends on the correct determination of the infecting pathogen.
- *Confirmation of diagnosis*. Determination of cancer markers can confirm the diagnosis or the tissue of origin of diseases.
- *Determination of treatment approaches*. Diseases with highly similar clinical symptoms, such as different types of breast cancer, may differ markedly in the way in which they respond to drug treatment, for example. Gene-based tests are being used more and more frequently to aid therapeutic decisions (see below). In cases of microbial infection, genetic tests can be used to determine drug resistance and enable selection of the most effective antimicrobial drug. Identification of drug resistance is especially important in immunocompromised patients.

Medical treatment

Genomics contributes to the effectiveness of medical treatment by allowing the monitoring of treatment efficiency and identification of novel targets for drug and/or gene therapy.

- *Monitoring the effectiveness of treatment.* Cancer-specific expression markers can be followed during the treatment of cancer to monitor how well the cells are being eradicated. Similarly, microbial markers can be monitored to assess the effectiveness of treatment of an infection.

- *Identification of drug and gene therapy targets*. Genomics aids the development of novel drugs by identifying potential new targets specific to the disease. It is hoped that it will soon be possible to treat many diseases by repairing or replacing selective genes (see Ch. 10).

Medical research

In medical research genomic studies aid the understanding of disease mechanisms at a molecular level, even in relatively inaccessible tissues like the central nervous system. These models (see Chs 8 and 12) have enabled the assessment of behavioural, pathological, cellular and molecular abnormalities, and also allow for development and evaluation of novel therapies. Medical research also aids the development of new diagnostic techniques and the improvement of existing ones.

In the rest of this chapter we will consider some of the key issues in any use of genetic information, including sample-taking, clinical categories of tested genetic markers and various techniques available in genomic testing.

Sample-taking

Specimen requirement for genomics

Genetic testing requires genetic material, so samples of DNA and RNA are required. Sampling is not without risk and the type of sample obtained determines the types of test that can be performed.

- *Pre-implantation screening*. Embryos are obtained following IVF. Screening is most important in cases where both parents are carriers of a debilitating recessive mutation and the risk of having a seriously ill child is high. Pre-implantation screening to improve the potential for disease-free embryos requires biopsy from the embryo. Procedures vary according to the developmental stage of the embryos but essentially involve removal of one cell from the embryo, often at the eight-cell stage. The embryos are kept in culture until the diagnosis is established and a mutation-free embryo can be implanted. There is a risk of the embryo being unable to survive sampling or culture, which limits the usefulness of this procedure.
- *Prenatal diagnostic sampling.* In this type of sampling taking cells from the embryo itself is not necessary; samples of the amniotic fluid, placenta or umbilical cord contain enough embryonic cellular material to be analysed with the latest highly sensitive

methodology. Nevertheless, the risk of spontaneous abortion is relatively high with all these procedures.

- *Postnatal diagnostic sampling.* This can serve several clinical purposes, including predictive, presymptomatic and carrier screening or simply obtaining diagnosis. While in predictive or presymptomatic testing a simple mouth swab, or skin or hair sample can contain a suitable number of live cells for successful analysis, a different approach might be necessary to finalize diagnosis of certain tumours or monitor efficiency of treatment. As disease-specific markers are not necessarily secreted into the blood or other body fluids, or expressed in all types of tissue, invasive sampling — for example, taking biopsies from the tumour or lymph nodes — might be necessary. Since these invasive sampling methods are often painful and not without side-effects, patients may well refuse permission for sample-taking.

Genetic material to be tested

Both DNA and RNA can be analysed. For analytical tests, nuclear and/or mitochondrial DNA samples are used, whereas the basis for functional testing is RNA; this reflects the fact that a particular gene is actually being transcribed in the cell.

- *Analytical tests.* These have been developed to identify the presence or absence of a specific disease-causing mutation (e.g. *CFTR Δ508* in cystic fibrosis) or disease susceptibility gene within chromosomes (e.g. *APOE4* in Alzheimer's disease) or mitochondrial DNA (e.g. *RNR1* in sensorineural hearing loss). Analytical testing is also suitable for distinguishing and identifying infecting microbes, including identification of human papillomavirus or *Listeria monocytogenes*, genotyping of HIV to determine viral load, and testing of HIV or *Helicobacter pylori* for drug resistance. In addition to identifying and classifying infecting microbes, genotyping can also be used to determine genetic factors that affect virulence of the pathogen. Furthermore, information concerning the antibiotic resistance of infecting pathogens and susceptibility of the host to specific infections can influence the choice of therapy.
- Functional tests are available to determine activation and inhibition patterns of gene expression that can also be characteristic for a specific disease. For example, thymidilate synthase mRNA levels are raised in various cancers (Box 3.1).

Understandably, analytical test systems for single-gene disorders like CF can be developed more easily than tests to detect an array of genes related to susceptibility to multifactorial diseases like cardiovascular disease or cancer.

However, analytical 'multi-gene' testing systems have been developed. They include a microarray to detect drug-resistant strains of *Mycobacterium tuberculosis*,

Box 3.1

Cancer prognosis based on thymidilate synthase mRNA levels

Several studies have demonstrated that the prognosis of cancer patients depends on the expression of thymidilate synthase (TS). TS is the target enzyme for 5-fluorouracil (5-FU) and catalyses the methylation of fluorodeoxyuridine monophosphate (dUMP) to deoxythymidine monophosphate (dTMP), which is an important process for DNA biosynthesis; thus high levels of TS are indicative of a rapidly advancing tumour. TS mRNA level is an accepted and clinically sensitive method for determining the prognosis of stages I and II non-small cell lung cancer (NSCLC) patients, survival in oropharyngeal cancer, or progression of colorectal carcinomas to liver metastasis. Similar effects can be seen in other cancers with different markers; in breast cancer Her2/neu mRNA levels tend to increase, while caveolin-1 and -2 mRNA and protein decrease.

or the specific species of infecting strain in *Chlamydia* infections. They are also used in forensic test laboratories.

Functional diagnostic tests involve the assessment of gene expression patterns, measured by message levels (mRNA), analysis of gene expression regulation based on miRNA (see Ch. 1) or epigenetic gene regulation patterns (see Ch. 4).

Patterns of gene expression seem to be characteristic to, and important in the understanding of, a number of phenomena, including toxic responses, distinguishing disease subsets (diagnostic gene expression microarray for type I latex allergy) or response to a pathogen. Diagnostic devices can also be used to analyse expression profiles of proteins that are the end-products of gene activity (see Ch. 6). Analysis of these complex patterns of gene expression requires advanced computer techniques which are still being developed.

Techniques

The medical application of genomics relies heavily on fast and dependable techniques that provide accurate results. A number of techniques have been developed which aid genome-based analysis of both DNA and RNA. These include:

- polymerase chain reaction (PCR)
- microarray
- fluorescence in situ hybridization (FISH)
- sequencing.

Polymerase chain reaction (PCR)

The technique of PCR is based on a single enzymic reaction, repeated over and over again until the reaction product accumulates in sufficient amounts to be analysed (see Appendix 2).

With the exception of some viruses, the genetic code is stored in double-stranded DNA and PCR exploits key features of DNA replication. The enzyme involved in the reaction is called DNA polymerase, which uses single-stranded DNA as a template for the synthesis of a complementary new strand. To be able to use PCR technology to study mRNA-based gene expression, the technique of RT-PCR was developed. In RT-PCR mRNA is transformed into cDNA, using a virally derived enzyme called reverse transcriptase. (For more details, see Appendix 2.)

DNA testing using PCR has developed into a fast-evolving field of medical diagnostics, and genetic predisposition tests are rapidly becoming available. The presence or absence of a specific gene can only be reliably tested in a PCR if sequence-specific primers are being used in the reaction. Sequence-specific primers can only be designed if the sequence of the gene of interest is available in nucleotide databases such as the National Center for Biotechnology Information (NCBI).

To perform genomic tests, only a small number of nucleated cells are required as specimens, since sequence-specific PCR can be performed from even as little as a single cell. This full DNA amplification technique has become particularly important in forensic science, where the available sample material is often limited to a single sperm or skin cell. Table 3.1 lists some diagnostic areas in which genetic tests are frequently used.

Genetic paternity tests, undertaken to confirm or exclude a person as the true biological father of a child, have become well accepted. Exclusion is essentially absolute, whilst confirmation typically provides nearly 100% certainty. Similarly, maternity and sibling analysis can also be performed. These tests are based on assessing the inheritance of highly polymorphic, independently segregating loci from across the human genome (see Table 3.2 for examples).

Both chromosomal and mitochondrial DNA can be the subject of genomic testing using PCR.

Genomic DNA analysis

Genetic testing has also given rise to dramatic improvements in the diagnosis of infectious diseases in general, and viral infections in particular. Molecular analysis is, for example, the only means of obtaining quantification of the viral load, and thus monitoring response to treatment, in HIV/AIDS and some types of hepatitis. PCR can also aid in the subtyping of bacterial pathogens and their resistance to antibiotics, or simply identifying their presence or absence in the environment.

PCR can also help in diagnosing infections caused by *Aspergillus*, *Candida* and other fungal species. It is widely known that fungal infections are associated with high mortality in cancer patients. Cultivation methods, however, fail to detect fungal infections in a large percentage of patients with invasive disease, resulting in delayed diagnoses and failure to apply appropriate antifungal therapy. Real-time quantitative PCR (qPCR) assays (see Appendix 2 for details) have been developed to detect and quantitate fungal DNA in clinical samples that facilitate the rapid and accurate diagnosis of infections. Fungal qPCR assays can be applied to blood, bronchoalveolar lavage fluid, and tissue biopsies obtained from haematopoietic cell transplant recipients at risk for invasive fungal infections. Examples of PCR-based DNA analysis in infections are shown in Table 3.3.

Mitochondrial DNA analysis

Mitochondrial DNA (mtDNA) is extremely valuable for genetic testing. As mtDNA is only passed between mother and offspring, mtDNA testing can provide evidence of maternity and sibling identity, and is also useful for determining ancestry and ethnicity.

Table 3.1
Diagnostic areas where genetic tests are used most frequently

Types of test	Disease	Tested
Genetic predisposition test	Hereditary haemochromatosis	6p21.3, *HFE* gene
	Thrombosis	Factor V Leiden, prothrombin 20210A, *MTHFR C677*
Oncology tests	Chronic myeloid leukaemia (CML)	*BCR-ABL*
	Follicular lymphoma	Translocation of t(14;18)
Human identification tests	Paternity test	See Table 3.2
	Maternity test	See Table 3.2 and mtDNA (Table 2.2)
	Sibling analysis	See Table 3.2 and mtDNA (Table 2.2)
	Forensic tests	See Table 3.2 and mtDNA (Table 2.2)

Table 3.2
Some examples of polymorphic sites of the human genome used in identity testing

Chromosome	CODIS loci	Chromosomal location
1	D1S1656	1q42
2	TPOX	2p23–2pter
3	D3S1358	3p21
4	FGA	4q28
5	D5S818	5q21–31
6	F13A1	6p25.3–p24.3
7	D7S820	7q11.21–22
8	D8S1179	8q24.1–24.2
9	D9S1122	9q21–q22
10	D10S1248	10q26.3
11	THO1	11p15–15.5
12	VWA	12p12–pter
13	D13S317	13q22–31
14	D14S1434	14q32.13
15	FES/FPS	15q25–qter
16	D16S539	16q22–24
17	D17S974	17p13.1
18	D18S51	18q21.3
19	D19S433	19q12–13.1
20	D20S482	20p13–p12
21	D21S11	21q21.1
22	D22S1045	22q12.3
X	DXS8378	X12.85
Y	DYS19	Y
mtDNA	HV1, HV2	

(CODIS = Combined DNA Index System)

Table 3.3
Detection of microbial pathogens by PCR analysis

Types of test	Microorganism	Tested
Viral infections	HIV	Viral load
	Hepatitis C	Viral load
	Hepatitis B	Viral load
Bacterial infections	*Legionella pneumophila*	Bacterial species identification and bacterial load in water supplies
	Mycobacterium tuberculosis	Antibiotic resistance
	Vibrio cholerae	Antibiotic resistance
Fungal infections	*Aspergillus* spp	Fungal species identification and fungal load
	Candida spp	Fungal species identification and fungal load

Sequence analysis of mtDNA provides an invaluable tool for forensic science too. Compared to nuclear DNA, mtDNA is more resilient, and is slower to degrade under harsh conditions. Thus, mtDNA analysis can provide important information for relationship analysis or identity testing of bodies that have been burnt or badly degraded (Box 3.2).

Microarrays

Microarrays, also known as biochips and genechips, are miniature devices, on which thousands of DNA sequences are stuck to a specific surface. They allow the simultaneous detection of thousands of different DNA or RNA sequences.

In a microarray system, known oligonucleotide sequences are arranged in a particular order (array) on a glass or silicon slide. Then both the sample DNA (from the individual to be tested) and a control DNA sample are labelled with fluorescent dyes. The labelled DNA is then allowed to hybridize with the complementary oligonucleotides in the microarray. The sample and control arrays are then placed in a special scanner which measures the brightness of each fluorescent area.

Microarray systems have also been developed to screen RNA, as activation or inhibition of gene expression can be characteristic of a specific disease and hence informative in diagnostics and therapy. Both mRNA and miRNA microarrays have been developed (see Ch. 2 and Appendix 2). In principle RNA chips are no different from DNA chips, except that in RNA arrays oligonucleotides are complementary to RNA sequences and those oligonucleotides are stuck on specific surfaces.

Because of their variability among the different human populations, two regions (hypervariable regions - HVR1 and HVR2) of mtDNA are of particular interest to test laboratories. By examining these regions in comparative mtDNA studies — usually by sequence analysis — the results can facilitate the reconstruction of maternally linked relationships.

Mitochondrial DNA can also carry mutations that can lead to complex syndromes, often exacerbated by mutations in chromosomal DNA. PCR can be used to detect these mitochondrial mutations. Some examples of currently identified mitochondria-linked syndromes are listed in Chapter 2 (Table 2.2).

Box 3.2

mtDNA in forensics

In the past decade or so, DNA typing using PCR analysis of single nucleotide polymorphisms (SNPs) or variable number tandem repeats (VNTRs) has aided the resolution of crimes, the identification of victims involved in mass disasters and missing persons understandably, reliable analysis of forensic material is of high importance. Unfortunately, the recovered tissue sample is often low on genomic DNA or the samples are badly degraded and unfit for analysis. It is not surprising that accuracy and validity of tests are frequently challenged in court. To make forensic analysis more reliable, a better source of DNA samples was needed. mtDNA has often proved to be better for forensic DNA typing methodologies, as the extranuclear mtDNA has high copy number, lacks recombination and has a distinct inheritance pattern, being maternally inherited. mtDNA also contains two hypervariable regions: HVR1 and HVR2. On average there are 8 nucleotide differences between two unrelated Caucasians, and 15 between two unrelated people of African descent, within these two HV regions. As the HV region is relatively short, it can be amplified by PCR, and the PCR product can then be sequenced for full analysis.

Box 3.3

Asthma-related gene expression studied by microarray

Microarray technology allows the analysis of many hundreds or thousands of genes that are up-regulated or down-regulated either constitutively or in response to a stimulus. One of the recent uses of microarray technology is in the identification of asthma-related gene expression patterns in childhood asthma. Microarrays have also been used to identify gene clusters specific for disease in adult asthma. Asthma is the most common chronic disease of childhood. It has a strong genetic component, and can be classified as stable asthma (asthma-S) or as exacerbation of the disease (asthma-E). Compared to healthy controls, distinct gene clusters were identified in the asthma patients. Some of these were the same in asthma-S and asthma-E, whereas others were distinctly different. This raises the possibility of better evaluation of disease status and more target-oriented and hopefully more efficient therapy. Table 3.4 summarizes asthma-S and asthma-E-related gene clusters.

Tests using microarrays have become an obvious choice for testing multifactorial disease genes (e.g. asthma; Box 3.3) and also to aid diagnosis in cases where an infectious agent could potentially be one of several different species of microorganism with a high range of antimicrobial resistance. The main requirement is that the sequence has to be precharacterized for the investigated species so it is possible to design oligonucleotides that are applicable in the array system.

Fungal infections can also be diagnosed using the microarray system. As fungal infections have become a major cause of morbidity and mortality in immunocompromised (e.g. transplantation) patients, speed and accuracy of diagnosis are of the essence. Microarrays can be particularly helpful, as conventional identification of pathogenic fungi in clinical microbiology laboratories is time-consuming and inaccurate, and consequently often imperfect for the early initiation of an adequate antifungal therapy. A diagnostic microarray for the rapid and simultaneous identification of the 12 most common pathogenic *Candida* and *Aspergillus* species has been developed by exploiting internal sequence variations. As microarray analysis is able to detect and clearly identify the fungal pathogens within 4 hours of DNA extraction from clinical specimens, this system offers a potentially valuable fungal detection system for clinical microbiology laboratories.

Some clinical uses of microarrays in diagnosis are listed in Table 3.5.

Microarrays can also be used to detect miRNA expression. These small RNA molecules specifically inhibit translation by aiding degradation of mRNAs; therefore miRNAs are regulators of gene expression at a post-transcriptional level (see Ch. 1). As a result, miRNAs affect cell differentiation, tissue development, and disease development and progression. For example, human miRNA genes are often located near cancer-associated genomic regions and fragile sites, indicating a strong connection between miRNA expression and oncogenic events. More specifically, decreased expression of some miRNAs has been found in several human cancers, including lung cancer, malignant glioma and chronic lymphocytic leukaemia (Table 3.5). Therefore detecting changes in miRNA expression patterns is of potential diagnostic value, as differences can be characteristic for a specific disease and present potential targets for gene therapy.

Comparison of PCR and microarrays

It is often the case that there is a choice between using PCR or a microarray to determine similar information. Diseases that are caused by a single gene mutation, such as Duchenne muscular dystrophy, do not require microarray analysis, as the location and sequence of the mutation are well characterized and therefore a PCR can detect the mutation efficiently. Most diseases, however, like cancers or other multifactorial disorders, develop as a result of a certain combination of pre-existing

Table 3.4
Distinct gene clusters differentially regulated in stable and acute childhood asthma

Gene cluster	Gene	Function in asthma
A (up-regulated in both asthma-S and asthma-E)	Histamine 4 receptor	Not known
B (up-regulated in asthma-S and further increased in asthma-E)	Complement 3a receptor 1	Regulation of IL-4, IgE and IgG$_1$ production
C (exclusively induced in asthma-E)	Integrin α4 (CD49d)	Eosinophil survival and recruitment
D (down-regulated in asthma-S, higher level during asthma-E)	Basic cell function genes and genes with unknown function	Not known
E (strongly increased in asthma-S)	Retinoic acid receptor α	Lung repair and remodelling
F (up-regulated in asthma-S and reduced in asthma-E)	Basic cell function genes and genes with unknown function	Not known
G (unchanged in asthma-S and down-regulated in asthma-E)	Basic cell function genes and genes with unknown function	Not known
H (reduced expression)	Interferon α/β receptor	Eosinophil survival and recruitment

Table 3.5
Available DNA and RNA microarray in diagnostics

Microarray	Nucleic acid	Disease	Microorganism
DNA		Fungal infections	*Candida albicans, C. dubliniensis, C. krusei, C. glabrata, C. tropicalis, C. parapsilosis, C. guilliermondii, C. lusitaniae, Aspergillus fumigatus, A. flavus, A. niger, A. terreus*
RNA	mRNA	Human lung, liver or kidney cancer (normal vs. tumour)	CDC2, casein kinase, etc.
	miRNA	Human lung cancer	Let-7
	miRNA	Human lymphocytic leukaemia	Mir-15a, Mir-16a
	miRNA	Human recurrent gliomas	Let-7b, Mir-125b-2, Mir-133a-1, Mir-183

genetic mutations. Therefore parallel investigation of several genes might be necessary. Microarrays can screen a vast number of genes simultaneously, while the technique of PCR (at least in its original form) would require numerous reactions to be performed repeatedly to attempt a similar screening. Additionally, specific nucleic acid sequences have to be predetermined to be able to design sequence-specific primers that are essential to PCR; often the disease-specific markers are unknown, making it impossible to find the right selection of target sequences. Obviously, a 'hit and miss' approach would be time-consuming, laborious and expensive. For these reasons, diagnostic laboratories have started to warm to the idea of using various microarrays in cases where fast and early preliminary diagnosis is necessary. Although microarrays are ideal for this type of analysis (for types of microarray and technical details, see Appendix 2), microarray testing remains less desirable in the clinical setting because of the costs involved. Microarrays have to be purchased and/or designed; sample labelling is expensive; the analysis of results requires complex computer

programs, and the initial results require further verification using custom-made microarrays and further PCR analysis. Nevertheless, microarrays have started to make their way into clinical diagnostics.

Fluorescence *in situ* hybridization (FISH)

FISH is the most commonly applied molecular cytogenetic technique used to detect chromosomal abnormalities. Sequence-specific DNA probes are fluorescently labelled and hybridized with metaphase spreads or interphase nuclei to determine chromosomal constitution (see Appendix 2).

FISH is performed when a specific numerical or structural abnormality of a chromosome, such as a microdeletion, is suspected. Interphase FISH is especially useful for studying bone marrow and cancer cells when there is poor or no growth of the specimen.

For FISH tests, sample cells are fixed on microscope slides and hybridized with specific DNA probes labelled with a variety of fluorochromes that makes possible parallel testing and simultaneous analysis with a number of probes.

Chromosomal abnormalities that can be detected by FISH include translocations, deletions, microdeletions and amplifications. The technique is also used for rapid detection of Down syndrome and other numerical chromosome abnormalities, of both autosomal and sex chromosomes (see Ch. 1).

A microdeletion is caused by the deletion of such a small region of a particular chromosome that it cannot be picked up by standard or high-resolution chromosome analysis. The FISH technique uses specific probes that were designed for a particular area of the chromosome and is able to detect the mutation. A selection of syndromes due to microdeletion is shown in Table 3.6.

The FISH technique can be used to detect common cancer-related deletions and amplifications (see Table 3.7 for examples) and to detect chromosomal translocations using dual colour translocation probes (Table 3.8).

FISH can be performed on any tissue that can be cultured for chromosome analysis, and interphase FISH can be performed on any cytogenetic sample. FISH is more sensitive and reliable than standard cytogenetic techniques, but has the disadvantage that it requires the synthesis of specific probes. However, as the human genome is known and genes have been mapped to specific chromosomes, the range of chromosomal abnormalities detectable by FISH is increasing.

Sequencing

DNA sequencing is a technique that determines the order of nucleotides (A, G, C and T) in any known or unknown DNA segments. Sequence analysis is discussed in more detail in Chapter 2 and Appendix 2.

While PCR analysis is simpler and more straightforward than sequencing, the PCR can be prone to errors, and so sequencing of DNA remains important for identifying or confirming genomic abnormalities.

Clinical genetic markers

Genetic markers were discussed in Chapter 2. However, in order for a genetic marker to qualify as a diagnostically useful disease marker, it has to fulfil some stringent criteria.

Disease markers have to produce both reliable and reproducible results in genetic tests, even when these tests are performed in different laboratories. A new diagnostic marker is useful only if it has a clear impact on the important decisions that clinicians have to make. The nature of those decisions depends on the type of disease, the stage of the disease and the range of available treatment options.

Diagnostic markers can be categorized as:

- *Preventive markers.* These indicate the need for further screening or preventative measures in populations with a high risk of a particular disease.
- *Prognostic markers.* These indicate the likely disease outcome, such as disease recurrence or patient survival, regardless of the specific treatment the patient receives.
- *Predictive markers.* These indicate the likelihood of a beneficial response to a specific therapy.
- *Tissue of origin marker.* This aids pathologists in confirming the tissue of origin of a metastatic tumour. This process is of high priority, as cancer of unknown primary (about 5% of all tumour cases) delays tissue-directed therapy and jeopardizes the chances of patient survival. Tumours of uncertain origin constitute an inconclusive diagnosis and this can add to the patient's suffering. They also result in an uncertain treatment outcome and inefficient use of healthcare resources that further increase medical costs. Understandably, finding tissue-specific markers that are easy to identify at relatively low cost is one of the aims of technological development of genomic testing.
- *Therapy response markers.* These can be used to monitor a patient's response to therapy or to detect the growth of metastases. Naturally, these markers can differ from markers in other areas of diagnostic medicine.

Some specific examples of the various types of diagnostic marker are considered in more detail below.

Preventive markers

Markers of precancerous conditions would be useful preventive markers. Early detection of various types of cancer, including colon, cervical and breast cancers, is known to improve survival. Late presentation of pancreatic cancer often renders pancreatic tumours incurable, and it has become a priority to find reliable diagnostic markers to allow detection of small precancerous and cancerous pancreatic lesions. These preventive markers are of use in populations with inheritable pancreatitis, as this frequently develops into pancreatic tumours. In this latter case, especially, understanding of characteristic genetic alterations in combination with development of high-throughput and sensitive techniques could lead to the discovery of pancreatic cancer markers that will allow early diagnosis and thus enable specific and early therapy. The National Institutes of Health-National Cancer Institute Early Detection Research Network (NIH-NCI EDRN) has been focused on the development and validation of new biomarkers for the detection of early pancreatic, lung, gynaecological, urological and other cancers (http://www.cancer.gov/EDRN).

Table 3.6
Some examples of microdeletion syndromes

Microdeletion syndromes	Chromosomal location	Genes mapped into this region	Symptoms
Wolf–Hirschhorn syndrome	4p16.3	WHSC1 and WHSC2 (Wolf–Hirschhorn syndrome candidate 1 and 2) Potential involvement in the syndrome: LRPAP1 (low-density lipoprotein-related protein-associated protein 1), A2MRAP (alpha-2-macroglobulin receptor-associated protein 1)	Midline defects, scalp defect, wide-spaced eyes, broad or beaked nose, oral facial clefts (cleft lip/palate), low simple ears, small and/or asymmetrical head; heart defects; seizures; severe to profound developmental and mental retardation
Williams syndrome	7q11.23	CYLN2 (cytoplasmic linker 2), WBSCR4, WSCR4	Dysmorphic facial features, cardiovascular disease, infantile hypercalcaemia, growth deficiency, mild or moderate mental retardation, a unique cognitive profile
Retinoblastoma	13q14	RB1	Embryonic malignant neoplasm of retinal origin with lesions in the retina. Almost always presents in early childhood and often bilateral. Spontaneous regression ('cure') occurs in some cases. (Retinoblastoma gene RB was first tumour suppressor gene cloned and is a negative regulator of cell cycle through its ability to bind transcription factor E2F and repress transcription of genes required for S phase)
Prader–Willi syndrome	15q11–q13 (inherited from father)	SNRPN (small nuclear ribonucleoprotein polypeptide N), NDN (necdin)	Affects growth and development; often weak fetal movement due to muscle weakness, evident at birth; regardless of parental inheritance: fair skin, hair, blue eyes; intellectual disability
Angelman syndrome	15q11.2–q13 (inherited from mother)	UBE3A (ubiquitin protein ligase E3A)	Microcephaly; epilepsy; severe learning difficulties (with poor communication skills and little or absent speech); unsteady or ataxic gait; characteristic facial appearance; happy disposition
Miller–Dieker syndrome (MDS)	17p13.3	YWHAE, MDCR (tyrosine 3-mono-oxygenase/tryptophan 5-mono-oxygenase activation protein, epsilon isoform)	Severe abnormalities in brain development (cerebral cortex is abnormally thick and lacks normal gyri); characteristic facial features with potential added birth defects
Smith–Magenis syndrome	17p11.2	RAI1 (retinoic acid-induced gene 1), SMCR	Short flat head, prominent forehead, broad square face, up-slanting eye slits, deep-set eyes, underdeveloped midface, broad nasal bridge, short nose, tented upper lip; mild to moderate mental retardation (including attention deficit disorders sometimes with hyperactivity, frequent temper tantrums, impulsivity, distractibility, disobedience, aggression, self-injury, toileting difficulties, self-injurious behaviours including self-hitting, self-biting and skin picking)

Continued

Table 3.6
Some examples of microdeletion syndromes—cont'd

Microdeletion syndromes	Chromosomal location	Genes mapped into this region	Symptoms
Kallman syndrome	Xp22.3	KAL1 (Kallman syndrome-1 sequence (anosmin-1)), KMS, ADMLX	Rare, X-linked, recessive disease characterized by reduced or complete absence of sense of smell (anosmia caused by absence of olfactory bulbs), underdeveloped genitalia and sterile gonads (hypothalamus produces reduced levels of gonadotrophin-releasing hormone (GnRH), resulting in low levels of LH and therefore lack of oestrogen and testosterone); greater risk for osteoporosis and brittle bone disease; primarily affects males, although there have been rare cases amongst females (autosomal recessive trait)
Placental steroid sulphatase deficiency (STS)	Xp22.3	ARSC2 (arylsulphatase C, f form)	Genetic metabolic skin disorder that affects males, caused by steroid sulphatase deficiency; insufficient cholesterol sulphate metabolism results in cholesterol sulphate accumulation in skin that prevents normal shedding of dead skin cells leading to skin scales

(p = chromosome short arm, - = deletion, q = chromosome long arm)

For a full list see OMIM Gene Map: http://www.ncbi.nlm.nih.gov/Omim/getmap.cgi

Table 3.7
Some examples of oncology-related chromosomal deletions and amplifications

Disease	Deletion	Amplification	Gene	Gene function
Tumours	7q31		*D7S486*	Tumour suppressor
Retinoblastoma	13q14		*RB1*	Tumour and growth suppressor (binds to transcription factor E2F)
Developmental delay, including cognitive abilities		13q14	*RB1*	Tumour and growth suppressor (binds to transcription factor E2F)
Malignancies (e.g. Li–Fraumeni syndrome)	17q13.1		*P53*	Regulation of cell cycle, tumour suppressor
Neurofibromatosis	17q11.2		*NF1*	Tumour suppressor

Table 3.8
Some examples of chromosomal translocations

Disease	Translocation	Gene
Chronic myeloid leukaemia (CML)	t(9;22)(q34;q11.2)	*BCR/ABL*
Mantle cell lymphoma	t(11;14)(q13;q32)	*CCND1/PRAD1*
Acute promyelocytic leukaemia (AML-M3)	t(15;17)(q22;q11.2)	*PML/RARA*
Paediatric pre-B acute lymphoblastic leukaemia (ALL)	t(12;21)(p21;q22)	*TEL (ETV6)/CBF2 (AML1)*

Prognostic markers

In most solid tumours the spread of cancer cells to lymph nodes indicates an increased likelihood of tumour recurrence, no matter which particular form of therapy the patient receives following surgery. Molecular 'staging' of malignant melanoma and of breast, colon and pancreatic cancers is therefore of high importance. Intensive research is aimed at identifying molecular markers in the sentinel lymph nodes, which would predict the recurrence of specific tumours. Despite all these efforts, useful tumour recurrence markers have remained elusive and for a long time it was believed that this approach might not prove fruitful. Recently, however, studies using animal models of breast cancer (see Ch. 8) have started to change that view.

The traditional belief is that cancer cells only start to metastasize rather late in their development. However, it appears that certain tumour cells have the ability to metastasize from the very beginning. In the case of breast cancer, tumour cells preferentially metastasize to the lung and bone marrow. A cluster of genes — *EREG*, *MMP1*, *MMP2* and *COX2* — has been determined to be vital for both aggressive growth and metastasis in breast cancer cells. Drugs targeting these genes or their products have been shown to inhibit tumour growth in an animal model, giving hope to human sufferers of disease.

Predictive markers

There is increasing interest in defining molecular targets for new therapeutic agents. The various types of breast cancer are frequently used as examples to demonstrate the importance of distinguishing specific markers to inform disease treatment. Upwards of one-quarter of all breast cancers are positive for mutations in *HER2*, the gene for the human epidermal growth factor receptor type 2, which results in fast proliferation of the cells. This mutation can also occur in other types of cancer. In breast cancer, overexpression of *HER2* indicates that the cancer is likely to be more aggressive and less responsive to treatment with anti-oestrogen drugs. The accepted treatment for *HER2*-positive breast cancers is a monoclonal antibody against *HER2*, called trastuzumab (Herceptin®; see Ch. 9). This drug can slow down the growth of the cancer, decrease its size and even reduce breast cancer recurrence by as much as 50% in many patients. Another important predictive marker in breast cancer is expression of the oestrogen receptor (*ER*) gene. Approximately 70% of patients treated for breast cancer have ER-expressing cancer cells; many of these tumours respond to hormonal therapies such as tamoxifen. Tumour cells low on ER expression cannot be expected to respond to hormone therapy. Progesterone receptors (PGR), reflecting the functional oestrogenic stimulus, have also been investigated and are believed to be at least as significant prognostic and predictive factors as the ER status. Recent trials of endocrine agents have demonstrated good levels of response among patients whose tumours are positive for both ER and PGR.

Therapy response markers

Finding markers to differentiate between highly similar tumours that can respond differently to treatment regimes is of great clinical importance. For example, gastrointestinal stromal tumours (GIST) and leiomyosarcomas (LMS) have very similar phenotypic features. As they are both of mesenchymal origin, they are difficult to distinguish and are often diagnosed as soft tissue sarcomas, although there are remarkable differences in their response to accepted treatment regimes. While patients with advanced GIST respond well to the tyrosine kinase inhibitor, imatinib (Gleevec®; see Ch. 9), patients suffering from advanced LMS respond much better to a combination of two drugs, gemcitabine and docetaxel, and do not benefit from imatinib treatment. Clearly, differentiating between the two tumours would result in far more effective therapy. Microarray analysis of samples from large populations of both GIST and LMS patients has suggested that certain genes might accurately distinguish GIST from LMS. Higher expression levels of *OBSCN*, a gene for obscurin (a cytoskeletal calmodulin and titin-interacting Rho guanine nucleotide exchange factor binding protein), have proved to be specific for GIST rather than LMS. Based on these results, an RT-PCR-based diagnostic test was developed that has proved to be 100% accurate in research laboratory tests and reliably distinguishes GIST from LMS, offering a fast and reliable diagnostic test for clinical use.

Genomics in medical research

Development of diagnostic screening methods, investigation of gene function and the use of a gene in gene therapy all require an unlimited supply of the gene or characteristic sequence in question. Fortunately, once a gene has been identified (see Ch. 2), it is possible to clone and amplify the full sequence or just part of the sequence. By using cloning primers and 'sticky ends' (Box 3.4), the gene of interest can be amplified — most frequently by PCR methods employing high-fidelity enzymes to minimize the risk of copying mistakes — and then cloned into an artificial plasmid that carries an antibiotic resistance gene as a selection marker (Fig. 3.1). A susceptible bacterial strain is then transformed with this plasmid. The bacteria are cultured in the presence of antibiotics and in the surviving ones the plasmid and the gene of interest are amplified. From these cultures the gene can be purified.

In addition, functional analysis of the gene or the encoded protein might make it necessary to amplify and also modify the genetic sequence, to be able to study the role of various exons or particular amino acid sequences in the translated protein. The techniques of site-directed mutagenesis, or the more recently developed site-saturation mutagenesis, are used most frequently to modify genetic sequences. Site-saturation mutagenesis differs from site-directed mutagenesis in one aspect only: it allows the substitution of a specific amino acid residue with all of the 20 possible amino acids at once, while site-directed mutagenesis generates these constructs individually.

Several aspects of cystic fibrosis have been discussed so far. It is not surprising that so much information has been accumulated over the years, as the *CFTR* gene mutations are direct causes of the disease. Better understanding of CF and, equally importantly, the development of gene therapy regimes with potential therapeutic value both require access to the normal *CFTR* gene and also to various mutants. The most common of all *CFTR* mutations is the phenylalanine deletion at amino acid sequence 508, leading to folding abnormalities of the protein. Genetic and functional analysis involved cloning of the *CFTR* gene, as well as site-directed mutagenesis of the gene, to make potential variations available for study.

All genetic research, be it basic or clinical, is designed to advance our understanding of the human genome and the role of individual genes or groups of genes in

---

Box 3.4

Restriction enzymes

Restriction enzymes are DNA-cutting enzymes found in and harvested from bacteria. A list of currently available restriction enzymes can be found at http://www.westburg.eu/en/site/life-sciences/enzymes-cloning/restriction-enzymes.

Restriction enzymes are endonucleases that cut DNA at a particular sequence of nucleotides. For example:

EcoRI cuts at 5′ ...GAATTC...3′
3′ ...CTTAAG...5′

If the ends of the cut have overhanging pieces of single-stranded DNA, these are called 'sticky ends', as they are able to form base pairs with any DNA molecule with complementary sticky ends. To make cloning easier, sequence-specific cloning primers are designed with complementary sticky ends to the plasmids previously cut open using restriction enzyme. When mixed together, the molecules join by base pairing and the connection is made permanent by DNA ligase. Werner Arber, Dan Nathans and Hamilton Smith won the Nobel Prize in 1978 for the discovery of restriction enzymes and their application to problems of molecular genetics.

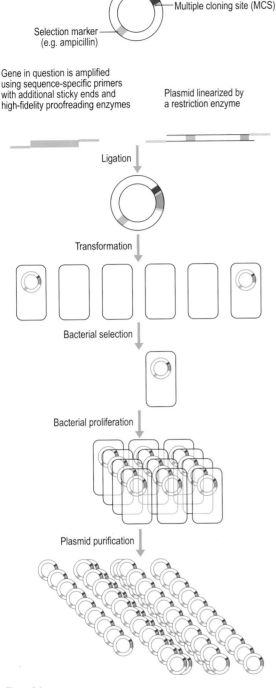

Figure 3.1
Cloning and amplification of a gene of interest. The use of primers with 'sticky ends' makes the cloning of a gene into a plasmid easier and more efficient. The gene is ligated into a plasmid which carries an antibiotic resistance gene, and a susceptible bacterium is then transformed with this plasmid. The antibiotic resistance gene allows selection of bacteria containing the plasmid. As the bacteria grow, multiple copies of the gene-containing plasmid are synthesized.

human health. Using this information, it is expected that pharmaceutical companies will develop both genetic diagnostic tests and drugs to enable fast and precise diagnosis, the identification of treatment approaches and specific and effective treatment.

Genomics in everyday medicine

Currently, more than 900 genetic tests are available from various testing laboratories, but while genomic testing has the capacity to revolutionize clinical practice, it remains very expensive. Apart from the necessary test kits and chemicals, performing and analysing the tests requires specialized equipment and trained laboratory personnel. The costs involved are rarely met by healthcare providers or healthcare insurance companies. The best genetic tests would be simple, reliable and cost-effective. Further studies of the economic benefits of genetic testing to predict, prevent and treat diseases are required to clarify the cost:benefit ratio of the various tests. However, it seems likely that the development of commercial, high-throughput test systems could lead to a dramatic decrease in cost along with an increase in reliability.

Ethical considerations

The ethical issues surrounding the use of genetic testing can be approached from two main directions: medical and public.

Medical issues

The aim of medical genomic studies is to improve human medicine by providing early diagnosis and personalized treatment of disease. Nevertheless, the availability of genomic techniques raises questions as to how the information and connected technologies affect standards of patient care.

Genetic testing has posed difficult questions in numerous areas of human medicine. For example, should patients be informed that they might be at high risk for developing an illness when there is no effective treatment or cure available? Similarly, should genetic tests be performed on an unborn fetus when the results might lead the parents to decide to terminate the pregnancy or when the sampling procedure could lead to spontaneous abortion?

The best way to conduct genetic research involving human subjects is still a matter of active investigation. Research ranges from storage of tissue specimens, through community consultation, to the issue of informed

> ## Box 3.5
>
> ### Home test kits for genetic diseases
>
> A number of companies are already offering genetic tests directly to the public. Most of these 'home' and 'mail order' test kits are for the detection of genes which predispose to diseases such as cystic fibrosis, blood clotting disorders or breast cancer. There is clearly public interest in these tests but they are not without their dangers. Some have not been clinically evaluated properly and the results can rarely be interpreted by the lay public. Commercially available genetic tests cut out the primary care physician and provide diagnostic results without the involvement of a genetic counsellor, whose role is to help the individual to deal with the psychological impact inflicted by a positive test for a life-threatening disease.

consent. Certainly, a balance needs to be achieved between the potential benefits of genetic testing and protection of the rights of the tested subjects.

Public issues

The general public is extremely interested in the idea of using genetic information for improved personal health and quality of life (Box 3.5). However, many people are also deeply concerned about the potential misuses of this sensitive and highly personal information, particularly if the uses of this genomic information extend beyond strictly medical applications. Data gained by genomic studies can potentially be made accessible to the insurance industry, the legal system, military and paramilitary organizations, educational institutions, adoption agencies and so on. While the information may well be of use to these organizations, allowing access to it may possibly not be in the best interests of the individual. For example, should a genetic predisposition to serious asthma, diabetes or even schizophrenia preclude you from adopting a child or taking up a job? Should genetic information regarding behavioural traits be admissible in court? Such uses of genomic information could jeopardize an individual's career or make health insurance prohibitively expensive.

Genomics tests are already being used by individuals who wish to trace their ethnic origins. We might see a time when genetic information could be used to define

membership of a particular race or minority group. Race is a sensitive issue and is largely a non-biological concept; a genomic definition may well not be helpful.

Members of different communities, cultures and religious traditions may have very different outlooks on the ethical issues surrounding the use of genetic information. Prenatal testing for Down syndrome leading to the abortion of an affected fetus is acceptable to many, but is considered tantamount to genocide by some people with Down's.

Research into these ethical issues is ongoing and many countries, including those in the European Union, have not yet reached any consensus on how genomic studies and genomic data should be regulated.

FURTHER READING

Barnholtz-Sloan JS, Chakraborty R, Sellers TA, Schwartz AG 2005 Examining population stratification via individual ancestry estimates versus self-reported race. Cancer Epidemiol Biomarkers Prev 14:1545–1551.

Bino J, Sander C, Marks DS 2006 MicroRNA protocols: prediction of human microRNA targets. Series: Methods in Molecular Biology, vol. 342. Humana: Totowa, NJ.

Gupta GP, Nguyen DX, Chiang AC et al. 2007 Mediators of vascular remodelling co-opted for sequential steps in lung metastasis. Nature 446:765–770.

Hillen HFP 2000 Unknown primary tumours. J Postgrad Med 76:690–693.

Joos Thomas O, Frotina P (eds) 2005 Microarrays in clinical diagnostics. Series: Methods in Molecular Medicine, vol. 114. Humana: Totowa, NJ.

Leinberger DM, Schumacher U, Autenrieth IB, Bachmann TT 2005 Development of a DNA microarray for detection and identification of fungal pathogens involved in invasive mycoses. J Clin Microbiol 43:4943–4953.

Minn AJ, Gupta GP, Siegel PM et al. 2005 Genes that mediate breast cancer metastasis to lung. Nature 436:518–524.

Price ND, Trent J, El-Naggar AK et al. 2007 Highly accurate two-gene classifier for differentiating gastrointestinal stromal tumors and leiomyosarcomas. PNAS 104: 3414–3419.

Sagara Y, Mimori K, Yoshinaga K et al. 2004 Clinical significance of caveolin-1, caveolin-2 and HER2/neu mRNA expression in human breast cancer. Br J Cancer 91:959–965.

Sambrook J, Russell DW 2001 Molecular cloning: a laboratory manual, 3rd edn. Cold Spring Harbor Laboratory Press: New York.

4

Epigenetics
K. Nightingale

Epigenetic processes control gene expression in a stable fashion, which can be passed on to daughter cells or even our children. However, these processes do not involve alteration of the genetic information encoded in the DNA; they are somehow 'apart from' or 'above' genetics. Hence the term 'epigenetics', which literally means 'above genetics'.

One of the most dramatic illustrations of epigenetic regulation is provided by the related but entirely different conditions of Prader–Willi and Angelman syndromes (Box 4.1).

How can the loss of the same region of DNA give rise to such different phenotypes as demonstrated here? It depends on whether the deletion affects the chromosome inherited from the mother or from the father, as this region of chromosome 15 is differently 'imprinted' (see below) depending on the parent from which it originated.

Imprinting results in inactivation of various genes; thus, in the region of chromosome 15 affected in Prader–Willi and Angelman syndromes, different genes will be active in the maternal and paternal chromosomes. For example, *UBE3A*, the gene for ubiquitin ligase, an enzyme important for regulation of the levels of various proteins in cells, is inactivated in the paternal chromosome. Therefore, if this gene is deleted in the maternal chromosome, Angelman syndrome will occur; loss of the gene from the paternal chromosome would have no effect.

Epigenetic gene regulation

The last two decades have seen substantial advances in our understanding of the broad mechanisms of gene regulation. The common features of promoter sequences are known, as are the components of the basal transcriptional machinery. Furthermore, the protein–protein interactions that lead to RNA polymerase recruitment have largely been characterized. This insight into the 'generic' mechanisms common to most gene promoters has been complemented by increased understanding of the roles of cell signalling pathways and individual transcription factors to the regulation of specific genes. As such, much is known about the onset of gene activation or repression, and the way transcription factors establish the coordinated patterns of gene expression that define cell identity (i.e. that make fibroblasts different from glial cells). In contrast, the epigenetic mechanisms that maintain these programmes of gene expression

and ensure that this pattern is passed to daughter cells remain far less well understood.

This epigenetic cell memory system has two primary characteristics. It must be:

- *stable*, allowing the proliferation of identical cells (i.e. in tissue growth or repair)
- *flexible*, to allow appropriate responses to extracellular signals, including the wholesale transcriptional reprogramming associated with cell differentiation, and to ensure that these changes are maintained in subsequent cell generations.

What are the basic mechanisms underlying epigenetic regulation?

Epigenetic mechanisms not only are involved in long-term phenomena, like the stable maintenance of transcription patterns, but also are integrated into short-term transcriptional control, adding a layer of regulation to processes like promoter opening or RNA polymerase II elongation. Eukaryotes have developed several distinct but interrelated regulatory systems to act over a wide range of time frames. The best understood are:

- proteins associated with chromatin structure (histones, or chromatin structural proteins), which are associated with both short- and long-term effects
- DNA methylation (primarily at CpG dinucleotides), which is associated with long-term effects.

The common thread in both of these mechanisms is that they utilize the basic elements of chromatin to influence processes that involve the DNA.

Chromatin

Chromatin is formed when DNA interacts with histone proteins. The assembly of the DNA template into chromatin has to condense the huge length of a typical eukaryotic genome (about 2 metres in humans) into the nucleus, whilst maintaining specific regions of DNA in an accessible structure to enable ongoing transcription or DNA repair. These apparently opposing functions are solved using a modular packaging approach — DNA

Prader–Willi and Angelman syndromes

These two very distinct conditions both arise from small deletions in the q11–q13 region of chromosome 15.

Prader–Willi syndrome
This is characterized by small stature, incomplete sexual maturation, muscle weakness, learning difficulties, characteristic behaviours (including temper tantrums, stubbornness and repetitive thoughts and behaviours) and, most notably, a constant and irresistible urge to eat. Unless

frustrated, this urge results in extreme obesity and early death from diabetes and the respiratory problems caused by the complications of high blood pressure.

Angelman syndrome
This is characterized by severe developmental delay, a near-absence of speech, jerky and tremulous movements, hyperactivity and frequent smiling and laughing; affected individuals give every appearance of being genuinely happy. Epileptic seizures are common and many people with this syndrome have a fascination with, and attraction to, water.

is wrapped around globular protein 'balls' or nucleosomes, which assemble on the DNA at regular (approximately 200 bp) intervals. Interactions between the nucleosomes then stabilize the subsequent folding of chromatin, which forms a helical solenoid termed the 30 nm fibre. This is then subsequently compacted via a number of poorly defined structures, ultimately allowing chromatin to adopt the level of condensation found in metaphase chromosomes.

The packaging of DNA into chromatin presents a substantial barrier to functional processes that bind to, or track along, the DNA template. This barrier arises due to several aspects of chromatin structure:

- Nucleosome-bound DNA is both highly bent and relatively inflexible, due to the multiple histone–DNA contacts needed to hold it in position on the surface of the histone octamer. This unusual DNA conformation, and steric occlusion from both the histone proteins and the adjacent turn of DNA held on the nucleosome surface (Fig. 4.1), ensure that nucleosome-bound DNA is inaccessible to most proteins that bind to specific DNA sequences.
- Processes such as transcription, replication and repair require proteins to move along the DNA. Thus they would need to displace nucleosomes at regular intervals.
- The binding of linker histones, like histone H1, and the formation of higher-order chromatin structures are associated with increased DNA inaccessibility, as DNA is 'shielded' within the core of the 30 nm chromatin fibre.

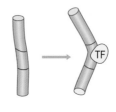

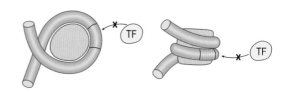

Figure 4.1
Many proteins induce DNA bending when binding to their binding site (hatched area) and cannot bind to nucleosome-bound DNA. In these examples, a transcription factor (TF) cannot recognize or bind to its site, as the DNA is highly curved by the nucleosome surface (left), and/or is prevented from binding by either the nucleosome core or the adjacent turn of DNA (right).

non-chromatinized) DNA. This ensures that transcriptional activation and silencing is the product of a highly regulated, multistep process that is targeted to specific loci. This typically involves the recruitment of histone modification enzymes and the targeting of chromatin remodelling activities, though the order in which these processes act is determined by the chromatin structure and transcription factors acting at a target locus.

Gene activation and silencing in chromatin

As well as playing a central role in packaging the DNA, the 'repressive' character of chromatin has the regulatory effect of preventing non-specific (or 'adventitious') initiation of processes that occur on 'naked' (or

Post-translational modification of the histones

The four 'core' histone proteins (histones H2A, H2B, H3 and H4) interact to form the globular protein core of nucleosomes and together generate the fundamental building block of chromatin. However, they also play a

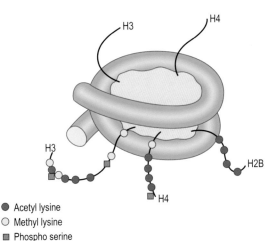

- ● Acetyl lysine
- ○ Methyl lysine
- ▪ Phospho serine

Figure 4.2

The nucleosome N-terminal tails are subject to many post-translational modifications. This diagram indicates some of the residues involved, and the range of possible modifications.

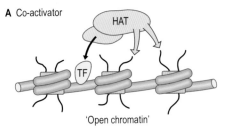

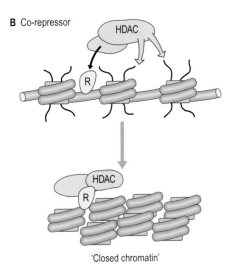

Figure 4.3

Histone-modifying enzymes are recruited to their target promoters by interactions with DNA-bound proteins. (A) In this case proteins with histone acetyl transferase (HAT) activity are recruited by interactions with activating transcription factors (TF), and subsequently acetylate residues in the adjacent nucleosomes. (B) In contrast, co-repressor complexes containing histone deacetylases (HDACs) are recruited by transcriptional repressors (R).

central role in regulating chromatin structure via their N- and C-terminal 'tails', which extend beyond the DNA and contact other components of chromatin. These are the sites of multiple post-translational modifications (Fig. 4.2), which are found at numerous residues on all four histone tails.

The regulatory effects of this bewildering array of potential modifications is a highly active area of current research, as modifications at specific histone residues are associated with different functional processes in chromatin. This has led to the concept of an 'epigenetic' or 'histone code', in which distinct histone modifications (or combinations of several associated modifications) constitute an epigenetic 'mark' that carries regulatory instructions for the adjacent DNA. Broadly, this hypothesis suggests that regulation is exerted via a number of distinct stages:

- *Recruiting modifying enzymes to target loci.*
  Histone-modifying enzymes (often in multi-enzyme complexes) are recruited to their target region of chromatin via interactions with sequence-specific DNA-binding proteins. Typically, this is a promoter-bound transcription factor, though several proteins with histone acetyl transferase (HAT) activity are associated with the RNA polymerase II. The directed targeting of enzyme activity ensures histone modifications can be restricted to a limited region of chromatin, which may be as small as around 600 bp, or 2–3 nucleosomes (Fig. 4.3A).
- *Downstream effects of histone modifications.* The histone modification can then have a direct effect on chromatin structure and/or result in the recruitment of an 'effector' protein. This can be a single protein, or a component of a multiprotein complex which recognizes and binds the specific epigenetic 'mark'. This recognition is highly specific, as both the chemical modification and the precise histone residue

are functionally relevant. For example, methylation at lysine 4 on histone H3 (short notation: H3K4me), or five residues away at lysine 9 (H3K9me), has a diametrically opposite role in transcriptional regulation; H3K4me acts as an 'activating' mark (associated with regions of active gene expression), whereas H3K9me is a 'repressive' mark, associated with silenced chromatin. Effector proteins or complexes exert their functional effects either by acting enzymatically on the adjacent chromatin (i.e. chromatin remodellers), or by assuming a structural role in stabilizing 'open' or 'closed' chromatin structures (i.e. HP1, a protein that binds H3K9me, stabilizes heterochromatin (Fig. 4.4)).

- *'Reversing' the effect of histone modifications.* The opposing processes of transcriptional activation or silencing are associated with different classes of histone modification. Thus gene silencing is initiated by the recruitment of two classes of histone-modifying enzymes: (1) enzymes which remove 'activating' histone modifications, and (2) another class which deposit 'repressive' marks. In many cases both of these enzyme activities are found in a single

A

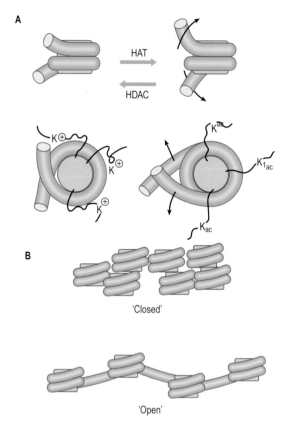

B

'Closed'

'Open'

Figure 4.4
Histone modifications exert their effects via a combination of changing chromatin structure and recruiting effector proteins.
(A) For example, histone acetylation reduces the strength of DNA binding at the level of single nucleosomes. (B) This results in a more open, decondensed chromatin structure.

multiprotein complex, such that only one targeting event is required. Repressive epigenetic complexes are recruited by similar mechanisms involved in gene activation — via interactions with gene-specific repressors, though DNA methylation also plays a central role in gene silencing (see below).

The broad concept in which enzyme-mediated deposition or removal of marks exerts its effects via effector proteins can be applied to many histone modifications, including histone acetylation, and the methylation of both lysine and arginine residues. For example, histone acetylation (an epigenetic mark associated with transcriptional activation) is targeted to promoter regions by interactions between HAT enzymes and activating transcription factors or components of the basal machinery. This results in the acetylation of histone tails in promoter-bound nucleosomes, increasing the accessibility of this chromatin (Fig. 4.4).

Specific acetylated lysine residues are also recognized by a class of chromatin remodellers, which can also lead to transcriptional activation (see below). In contrast, transcriptional silencing is often associated

with the removal of acetyl marks, typically in response to transcriptional repressor-induced recruitment of protein complexes containing histone deacetylase enzymes (HDACs) (Fig. 4.3B).

Chromatin remodelling

The assembly of nucleosomes over promoter regions prevents transcription initiation by inhibiting the binding of gene-specific transcription factors and the subsequent recruitment of the basal transcription machinery (i.e. TBP, TFIID, etc.). This inhibition largely arises due to the translational positioning of nucleosomes, or the precise 147 bp region of DNA that is associated with the nucleosome core; if this contains the relevant protein-binding site, then transcription factor-binding is effectively blocked. The use of positioned nucleosomes to generate a 'repressive promoter architecture' seems to be a widely used mechanism to maintain transcriptional silencing, as many genes contain DNA sequences which preferentially position nucleosomes over transcription factor-binding sites in their promoter and/or enhancer regions. Research on two model genes — the mouse mammary tumour virus (MMTV) and the *PHO5* gene in the yeast *Saccharomyces cerevisiae* — showed that gene activation was associated with the disruption (or 'remodelling') of a repressive pattern of nucleosomes, generating what appear to be nucleosome-free regions to which activating transcription factors could bind.

The protein complexes responsible for this chromatin remodelling activity were identified by two independent approaches:

- Genetic mutation screens in yeast identified a class of proteins necessary for the activation of two defined genes. Many of these proteins were subsequently shown to form a large multiprotein complex termed the SWI-SNF remodelling complex.
- In parallel, biochemical fractionation of *Drosophila* embryo extracts identified nucleosome remodelling factor (NURF), a multiprotein remodelling complex that could facilitate the binding of transcription factors in chromatin.

The subsequent identification and characterization of chromatin remodelling complexes from both yeast and higher eukaryotes have shown they have a number of common features.

Chromatin remodelling requires energy to disrupt nucleosomes

Chromatin remodelling requires a substantial energy input, primarily to disrupt the multiple histone–DNA interactions that constrain nucleosome-bound DNA. This is supplied by the hydrolysis of ATP, and utilized by one or more ATPase subunits in the remodelling complex.

Chromatin remodelling activities act as part of large multiprotein complexes

Chromatin remodelling complexes appear to act in a 'modular' manner, with a single subunit responsible for the enzymatic 'remodelling' activity, and other components with roles in targeting the complex to appropriate loci, or binding substrates in the correct conformation for activity. This is clearest for the *Drosophila* and human NURF and ACF complexes, where the ISWI subunit shows histone-stimulated ATPase activity, and can perform chromatin remodelling reactions in a similar manner to the intact multiprotein complex.

Recruiting chromatin remodelling complexes

Several lines of evidence, notably the use of expression microarrays to characterize the effects of remodeller mutants in yeast, suggest that chromatin remodelling is required for both gene activation and silencing. However, how these activities are recruited to their target sites, and how they are regulated once they are in place, are still areas of active research. An obvious area of focus is the role of the histone tails. These play a regulatory role with some remodelling complexes (for example, the histone H4 tail activates ISWI ATPase activity), but this is not ubiquitous as the histone tails are not absolutely required for all remodelling activities. Similarly, the histone tails act to recruit a number of remodelling activities via one or more protein domains which interact with specific histone modifications. This is a rapidly moving area, as a range of conserved protein motifs, many without clear functional roles, are found in many chromatin-binding proteins. Two of the more highly characterized motifs, 'bromodomains' and 'PHD fingers', clearly play a major role in targeting proteins to chromatin:

- *Bromodomains.* Many chromatin remodelling complexes contain multiple 'bromodomains' in one or more subunits. This is a protein fold found in HATs (Gcn5, PCAF and TAF$_{II}$250) and a family of transcriptional regulators (BET proteins), as well as in chromatin remodelling complexes, consistent with a role in acting on chromatin substrates. The domain has been shown to bind acetylated lysine, with some indications that different bromodomain sequences may have different binding specificities for defined acetylated residues on individual histone tails.
- *PHD fingers.* Histone H3 lysine 4 methylation (H3K4me) is another 'activating' modification, associated with regions of transcriptionally active chromatin. This mark is recognized by the BPTF subunit of the chromatin remodeller NURF, via a protein domain called a plant homeodomain (PHD) finger. Biochemical characterization has shown that this interaction is necessary for remodeller recruitment and activity *in vivo*.

Mechanisms of chromatin remodelling

Biochemical reconstitution experiments using purified remodelling complexes and nucleosomes show two mechanisms can disrupt nucleosome–DNA contacts and allow protein binding to DNA:

- The simplest of these is 'nucleosome eviction', or the wholesale removal of a nucleosome from the DNA sequence of interest. However, the simultaneous disruption of numerous DNA–histone interactions would generate an enormous energetic barrier without the coupled transfer of the nucleosome to another DNA molecule. This can clearly occur *in vitro* when remodelling is performed with a large excess of naked 'acceptor' DNA (Fig. 4.5A), but it is unclear whether a similar mechanism could occur in the nucleus as there are no equivalent large regions of nucleosome-free DNA.
- An alternative mechanism proposes that chromatin remodellers do not disrupt the nucleosome per se, but act to 'slide' the nucleosome into a new translational position, thus revealing protein-binding sites in the 'new' linker DNA between nucleosomes. This appears to be the means used by ISWI, which disrupts a small number of histone–DNA contacts, thereby generating a DNA 'bulge' which is stabilized and translocated around the nucleosome. Repeated cycles of this process effectively move the nucleosome to a new translational position (Fig. 4.5B). This mechanism offers a number of conceptual advantages: it minimizes the number of histone–DNA contacts disrupted at a given time, thereby reducing the energy requirement for nucleosome remodelling, and the multistep process would seem more amenable to regulation. However, the details of how the process is regulated, and how remodelling is apparently directed to specific nucleosomes, remain unclear.

Maintaining patterns of transcription: polycomb and trithorax group proteins

So far we have discussed the role histone modification plays in short-term gene regulation — where histone-modifying enzymes are integrated into the machinery of ongoing transcriptional control. However, histone modification is also involved in longer-term processes that maintain the patterns of transcriptional output that define cell identity. This 'cell memory' system is clearly important for maintaining cells in the differentiated state and is highly conserved in multicellular organisms, with similar protein complexes found in both plants and mammals; trithorax group (trxG) proteins maintain active transcription at genes, whereas polycomb group (PcG) proteins act to maintain transcriptional repression. These two families were initially

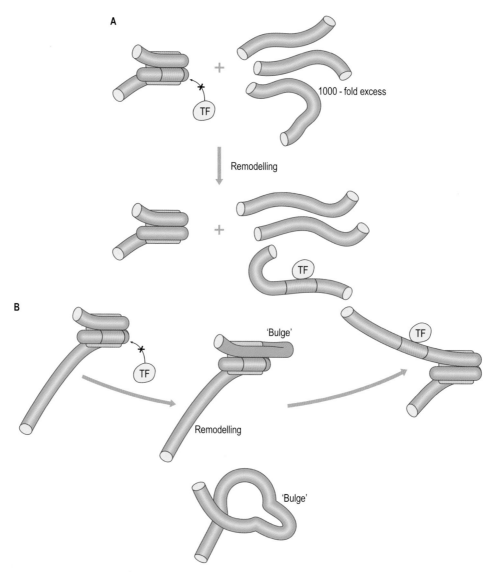

Figure 4.5

Chromatin remodelling can theoretically occur via two processes. (A) Nucleosome eviction, where it is transferred to other DNA.
(B) Translocation, where the nucleosome 'slides' along the DNA to another position. This can be accomplished by propagating a bulge of DNA
around the nucleosome. Remodelling acts to allow protein transcription factors (TF) to bind to their binding site (hatched area).

identified in homeotic mutations in *Drosophila*, in which
body sections of the fly are transformed to another, reflecting the misregulation of the *Hox* genes that establish
body patterning. Biochemical characterization shows
that the proteins act as multiprotein complexes, binding
to restricted regions of chromatin, and act via histone-
modifying activity.

Polycomb proteins act to repress transcription via two
complexes which act sequentially in chromatin: PRC1
and PRC2. PRC2 contains a histone methyl transferase
specific for a repressive mark (H3K27me), though two
subunits of the complex are required for this activity. Interestingly, an analogous complex containing different
subunits methylates a residue on histone H1 (H1K26),
confirming the fact that these complexes have distinct

substrate targeting and enzymatic subunits, similar to
chromatin remodellers. The deposition of methyl marks
by PRC2 subsequently acts to recruit the effector complex PRC1 via a chromodomain-containing subunit,
polycomb (Pc). This complex has been shown to compact chromatin and leads to transcriptional silencing,
though the mechanism used is still unclear.

In contrast the trithorax group proteins use a variety of processes to maintain transcriptional activity.
Family members show homology to components of
the yeast SWI-SNF remodelling complex (including the
BRG1/hBRM ATPases in humans), whereas others act
via histone-modifying activity, notably the mammalian MLL and hSET1 H3K4 histone methyl transferases.
Biochemical analysis of these complexes suggests that

HAT activity also contributes to their function, implying that these histone modifications either act positively to recruit activating effector proteins, or prevent the binding of negative regulators such as PRC1 (a process termed 'anti-repression'). The broad divergence in the trx family suggests that a number of the members are involved in unexplored processes.

Is histone modification only important for ongoing regulation?

Current data demonstrate that histone modification plays an integral part in both short-term transcriptional regulation (i.e. in promoter opening), and in maintaining longer-term patterns of PcG- or trxG-induced transcriptional control. This is consistent with the rapid turnover of histone modifications, many of which have half-lives measured in minutes, suggesting they are largely involved in short-term processes. However, cells also contain populations of modified histones which are highly stable, suggesting that not all histone modifications are restricted to regulating ongoing processes and may play a role in longer-term mechanisms. Similarly, 'activating' histone modifications are found in metaphase chromosomes and in highly condensed sperm chromatin. This is surprising, as both are transcriptionally silent but contain genes that will subsequently become transcriptionally active — either in the daughter cells or in the zygote. Thus we can speculate that histone modifications may act as 'epigenetic memory marks' to direct the transcriptional reactivation of chromatin. This is an active area of current research interest.

DNA methylation

The epigenetic regulation mechanisms considered so far use the deposition or removal of chromatin proteins, or their modification, to add a layer of regulatory information to the DNA to which they are bound. An alternative process uses the direct chemical modification of DNA in a similar manner, again without directly affecting the information coded by the base sequence. This is based on the methylation of the DNA bases, primarily cytosine in CpG dinucleotides. Methylation occurs at carbon 5 in the pyrimidine ring, such that the additional methyl group protrudes into the major groove of the DNA helix, but does not interfere with the cytosine hydrogen bonding to guanine on the opposite DNA strand.

Biochemical analysis of the functional activity of *in vitro* methylated templates, and the localization of CpG methylation *in vivo*, demonstrate that DNA methylation can both establish and maintain long-term transcriptional silencing. This role is consistent with the remarkable stability of this modification; global patterns of CpG methylation remain largely unchanged in somatic cells and are maintained through cell division. These are established and maintained by three enzymes termed DNA methyl transferases (Dnmt1, Dnmt3a and Dnmt3b), which contain related catalytic domains, but separate into two distinct classes with divergent regulatory domains, reflecting their different roles:

Dnmt1

This enzyme was the first cytosine-specific methylase to be identified, and acts as the 'maintenance methylase' by regenerating the pattern of DNA methylation on both DNA strands when presented with a hemi-methylated template. These are DNA sequences where cytosine residues on only one of the DNA strands are methylated; this occurs following both semi-conservative DNA replication and DNA excision repair. As such, the enzyme plays an essential role in ensuring that the information stored in the cellular pattern of DNA methylation is not lost following these processes (Fig. 4.6).

Dnmt3a/Dnmt3b

In contrast to Dnmt1, the Dnmt3a/b enzymes are responsible for generating new patterns of DNA methylation where both DNA strands are non-methylated ('de novo methylation'). In mammals this is restricted to two short developmental windows during early embryogenesis:

- The first of these developmental windows is when X chromosome inactivation occurs. The mammalian dosage compensation mechanism for balancing X chromosome-linked transcription in females (XX) and males (XY) involves the transcriptional silencing of the majority of the genes on one X chromosome in females (see also Ch. 2). This process is driven by epigenetic mechanisms in the early stages of embryogenesis, where the genes are silenced by the deposition of repressive histone modifications. This transcriptional repression is then maintained by Dnmt3a/b-deposited DNA methylation.

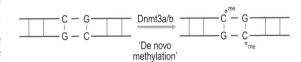

Figure 4.6
The maintenance methylase, Dnmt1, acts on 'hemi-methylated' DNA templates, whereas Dnmt3a/b generate de novo methylation at unmethylated CpG sites.

- More widespread methylation also occurs during early development. Following fertilization, the maternal and paternal pro-nuclei are subject to phases of differential demethylation. This arises due to the active demethylation of the paternal genome, leading to an apparent loss of the information stored by DNA methylation in the sperm chromatin. In contrast, DNA methylation in the maternal pro-nucleus is less substantial, reflecting the absence of the maintenance methyl transferase Dnmt1 in early embryos. Dnmt3a and 3b are involved in the subsequent remethylation of the genome that accompanies implantation of the early embryo.

DNA methylation and gene regulation

CpG methylation is an abundant epigenetic mark, and is associated with approximately 70% of the CpG dinucleotides in mammals. This ensures that the bulk of the genome is methylated and transcriptionally silenced, with the exception of 'CpG islands' — regions of DNA containing high densities of non-methylated CpG dinucleotides. These are associated with the 5′ promoter regions of genes and remain methylation-free on both transcriptionally active and silent genes, though they can become methylated in a developmentally regulated manner when the gene is to be irretrievably silenced in X-inactivation or cell differentiation. CpG islands can also become methylated in pathological processes, such as the aberrant transcriptional silencing of tumour suppressor genes in some cancers.

DNA methylation induces and maintains transcriptional silencing through two mechanisms:

- steric inhibition of transcription factor binding
- recruitment of methyl-binding proteins.

Steric inhibition of transcription factor binding

DNA methylation results in the deposition of a bulky methyl group that projects into the major groove of the DNA helix. This is where proteins form the sequence-specific interactions that determine binding site recognition; the additional methyl group effectively blocks interactions with both the modified cytosine and the adjacent residues. A number of transcription factors which have CpG within their binding site have been shown to be inhibited by DNA methylation, notably the transcriptional regulator CTCF.

DNA methylation recruits methyl-binding proteins

DNA methylation also induces transcriptional repression over larger regions via indirect, chromatin-mediated mechanisms. This is initiated by the binding of proteins

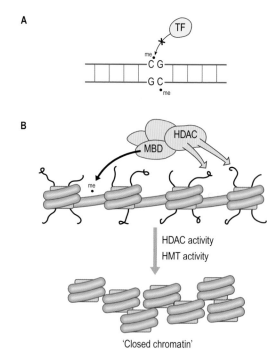

Figure 4.7
DNA methylation acts via two mechanisms. (A) Direct inhibition of the binding of a subset of transcription factors. (B) Recruitment of the methyl-binding domain (MBD) protein complexes that lead to chromatin condensation and gene silencing. For example, the protein complex containing the methyl-binding protein, MeCP2, also contains histone deacetylase (HDAC) activity. (HMT = histone methyl transferase)

containing a 'methyl-binding domain' (MBD), a protein fold that is specific for this modified residue. Biochemical fractionation and bioinformatic screening have identified five proteins that contain this conserved domain: MeCP2 and MBD1–4. Interestingly, a sixth methyl-binding protein which is also involved in transcriptional regulation, Kaiso, does not contain an MBD, suggesting that alternative modification recognition mechanisms have evolved. *In vitro* characterization suggests that the proteins recognize methyl CpG residues in different combinations or sequence environments, implying that they play distinct roles in defined regions of the genome (Fig. 4.7).

To date, several methyl-binding proteins have been characterized, and were shown to act as components of multiprotein complexes containing histone-modifying activities. These are involved in the deposition of 'repressive' modifications (i.e. MBD1 contains SETDB1, a methyl transferase) and the removal of acetyl marks (MeCP1 and 2 both contain HDAC activities), whereas MBD2 associates with the chromatin remodeller Mi2. Thus DNA methylation acts in a similar manner to histone modifications, recruiting appropriate chromatin activities to specific loci, via interactions with a specific class of effector proteins.

Genomic imprinting

Genomic imprinting, like X chromosome inactivation, is an epigenetic mechanism which uses DNA methylation to silence transcription at defined genes. The underlying basis of imprinting is highly complex, as it acts to silence genes in a parental-specific manner, using inherited patterns of DNA methylation to down-regulate either the paternal or the maternal allele.

A range of observations suggests that imprinting is essential for mammalian embryogenesis. Nuclear transfer experiments, in which nuclei can be manually transplanted into enucleated cells, show that both the maternal and paternal genomes (and the differential epigenetic information associated with them) are required for development, as neither androgenetic embryos (containing two copies of the paternal genome) nor gynogenetic embryos (containing two copies of the maternal genome) develop to term. Imprinting is largely restricted to placental mammals, although similar mechanisms are also found in a subset of plants. Only a small number of genes appear to be imprinted, and many of these are involved in embryonic or placental growth. These factors suggest that the purpose of imprinting is to balance the resources and nutrients transferred from the mother to the developing embryo. More recent data indicate that maternal imprinting tends to act to suppress, whereas parental imprinting tends to promote embryonic growth, leading to the so-called 'parental conflict hypothesis', which suggests that the mechanism reflects the different evolutionary priorities of the two parents; the father wants a large number of offspring who are likely to propagate his genes successfully, whereas the mother has to balance this against her ability to breed in the future.

Mechanistically, the establishment of an 'imprint' at a specific gene is highly complex. Imprinted genes tend to be found in clusters, in which DNA methylation at a specific locus (an 'imprint control element') regulates the expression of a number of surrounding genes. These paternally or maternally derived patterns of gene expression are dependent on interrelated mechanisms using both non-coding RNA transcripts and/or the ability of DNA sequences to block enhancer action (acting as 'insulators'), but the detail of how these processes interact is still an area of active research.

What happens when epigenetic mechanisms go wrong?

Misregulation of epigenetic mechanisms generates an 'epigenetic lesion', which can deregulate gene expression. This can be just as catastrophic for cells as a genetic mutation, leading to inappropriate differentiation or proliferation, but research in this field is still at a very early stage. This may seem surprising, given that studies on chemical-induced DNA damage and its subsequent repair are well developed and central to our understanding of cancer biology. This partially reflects the state of our knowledge about epigenetic mechanisms; we are still in the process of identifying the molecular 'players' and their role(s), whereas the basis of genetic mechanisms was largely established three decades ago.

Another factor hindering research into epigenetic lesions is that the studies are much harder to perform. Identifying an anomalous histone modification or protein–DNA interaction at a specific genetic locus requires more sophisticated experiments than PCR-based approaches. These technologies, their application to small numbers of cells, and the ability to scan regions genome-wide have only become available in the last few years, and should together enable the development of a new field of 'epigenetic toxicology'.

Examining protein (and modified proteins) binding in chromatin

One of the many practical advantages to come from genome sequencing projects is the ease of identifying DNA sequences likely to be bound by transcription factors. However, this is just the first step in experimentally demonstrating when, or indeed if, a predicted protein binds to a given site. This is particularly challenging if the protein(s) of interest do not bind a specific DNA sequence — as is the case with many epigenetic regulators. In this case analysis is usually by chromatin immunoprecipitation (ChIP), a technology based on using antibodies specific to a protein to isolate the DNA associated with it. The theory behind this approach is relatively straightforward:

- First cells are 'fixed' with formaldehyde. This cross-links proteins together and also cross-links them to DNA — essentially freezing or creating a 'snapshot' of what was happening on the chromatin at a given time.
- Chromatin is then isolated from the cells and broken into small fragments, usually by physical shearing during sonication. These are ideally 400–500 bp, roughly corresponding to the DNA associated with two nucleosomes, but the fragments also carry the proteins that were originally bound to the DNA.
- The short chromatin fragments are then incubated with an antibody specific to a protein (or protein modification) of interest, and separated into two pools: the 'bound' chromatin which should contain the protein of interest cross-linked to its binding site(s), and the 'unbound' chromatin, which should not.
- The protein–DNA cross-links are then broken by prolonged heating.

- Finally, the presence of a specific DNA sequence is probed using PCR with primers specific to it — by comparing its abundance in the 'bound' versus the 'input' chromatin (or that which originally went into the antibody-binding reaction).

This technology is remarkably powerful as it can be adapted to address many research questions. When used on cells over a time course (i.e. in response to a drug), or with multiple PCR primers which cover a large region of a gene, the approach can give detailed data on the temporal and spatial patterns of protein-binding. Similarly, immunoprecipitated 'bound' DNA can be hybridized to 'tiling' microarrays, to give an insight into the genomic distribution of a protein.

Genome-wide chromatin analysis

Epigenetic researchers are now working in a 'post-genome project' world, and this impacts on the research questions they ask and the technologies they use. On a practical level genome sequencing has given easy access to gene and promoter sequences and to the bioinformatic tools to analyse them; however, the availability of these data also prompted many to expand research questions from the detailed study of a single locus to analyse patterns of gene regulation throughout the genome.

Research questions addressing changes on a genome-wide scale are based on the use of DNA microarrays — glass slides with arrays of DNA primers spotted or printed on to them — typically covering > 10 000 distinct genes. These are targets for hybridization, so their coverage, or the sequences that they correspond to, determine the question(s) that can be addressed; for example, an 'expression' microarray containing primers derived from gene coding regions would be ideal to analyse changes in cDNA abundance. In contrast, 'genomic' microarrays contain either selected sequences from CpG islands or gene promoters, or a systematic set of primers corresponding to sequences at regular intervals over a selected chromosomal locus ('tiling arrays'), and are ideal for examining changes in transcriptional regulators. Genomic microarrays, in combination with chromatin-immunoprecipitation experiments ('ChIP-chip') are increasingly being used to analyse the distributions of epigenetic marks or regulators on a genomic scale.

How do epigenetic defects occur?

Recent developments in both the analysis of protein–DNA interactions and the use of microarrays to reveal genome-wide protein distributions have substantially increased our ability to detect and localize abnormal epigenetic processes. However, identifying the underlying cause of a lesion is more challenging, reflecting the complicated processes that generate and maintain these marks.

Some epigenetic lesions are the consequence of 'upstream' genetic defects (i.e. those that impact on transcription factor recruitment or activity). These mutations have been an important focus of cancer biology for the last decade. However, there are three mechanisms which directly impact on epigenetic regulators and could potentially generate epigenetic defects.

Genetic mutation of epigenetic regulators

Perhaps the most obvious cause of epigenetic defects results from the genetic mutation of proteins involved in epigenetic regulation, such as histone-modifying enzymes or chromatin-remodelling complexes. Mutations that result in enzyme inactivation, misregulation or mistargeting could all result in epigenetic defects and inappropriate levels of gene expression. This is indeed observed with a number of proteins (see below).

Agents which act on epigenetic regulators

The enzymes involved in epigenetic regulation have complex interaction surfaces for substrate recognition and cofactor-binding, and these are potential target sites for inhibition. A number of naturally occurring and synthetic agents act on different classes of histone-modifying enzyme, including the histone lysine demethylase, LSD1, as well as a broad class of well-characterized molecules which inhibit the class II histone deacetylases (HDACs). These agents induce genome-wide ('global') changes in the abundance of specific histone modifications. For example, HDAC inhibitors stimulate increased levels of histone acetylation ('hyperacetylation'), resulting in substantial changes in transcriptional output (both up- and down-regulation) from a large number of genes. However, the factors that determine a gene's sensitivity to HDAC inhibitors and their target enzyme(s) remain unknown. These agents, along with 5-azacytidine, which inhibits DNA methyl transferase enzymes, are currently used widely as experimental tools, but their use is also being explored clinically as epigenetic therapies (see below).

Cofactor requirement

Epigenetic regulators require cofactors, either as moiety donors/acceptors (i.e. S-adenosyl methionine for histone methylases) or as a source of energy (i.e. ATP/chromatin remodellers). This suggests that many enzymes are likely to be sensitive to cofactor concentration and, by inference, to nutrition and the metabolic status of the cell. This is a largely unexplored area of research, requiring both classical enzymology and an understanding of whether nuclear cofactor levels are within the appropriate regulatory range. The finding that most epigenetic regulators act in multiprotein complexes with multiple modifying enzymes increases both the complexity of the potential regulatory networks and the experimental hurdles to be overcome.

Epigenetic misregulation and disease

To date, several defects within the epigenetic mechanisms that contribute to 'short-term' gene regulation are known to play a role in oncogenesis and/or tumour progression; indeed, epigenetic lesions may play as important a role in these processes as genetic mutations. This section will consider:

- the broad role that epigenetic defects may play in tumour progression
- the role of defective epigenetic regulators in pathological processes
- examples of where defective imprinting is known to induce disease.

Epigenetic defects and tumour progression

Established models of cancer progression suggest that the initial event leading to tumour formation is the introduction of a key genetic mutation (or 'gatekeeper mutation') in a stem cell or partially differentiated 'progenitor' cell that leads to its deregulated proliferation. However, progression from these benign non-invasive tumours, which typically contain a single mutation, to highly invasive metastatic tumours involves the subsequent accumulation of multiple gene mutations. Thus, tumour progression involves a number of steps, in which increasingly damaged cells clonally expand, and thereby alter the tumour morphology and character. The nature of these mutations has been an active area of research, with the identification of multiple oncogenes and tumour suppressor genes involved in this process. However, both the rapid kinetics of tumour progression and DNA sequencing/mRNA expression analysis of tumour cells indicate that gene mutation is not always required. This suggests that epigenetic lesions that result in the inappropriate silencing or activation of genes also could act in a very similar manner to DNA mutation in promoting metastatic transformation.

The recognition that epigenetic mechanisms can play a key role in the cumulative process of tumorigenesis has been central to the increased interest in this field. However, several researchers have proposed that epigenetic lesions may play a larger role, in that they may precede, and thereby facilitate, subsequent gatekeeper gene mutations. This is potentially a powerful model of carcinogenesis, suggesting how apparently normal cells containing environmentally induced epigenetic errors may become predisposed to genetic mutations.

Defective epigenetic regulators and disease

Epigenetic processes play essential roles in gene regulation, often with several mechanisms interacting to regulate a single gene. This universal involvement in gene expression may explain why mutations within many classes of epigenetic regulator are linked to pathological processes. These fall into several classes of 'deregulatory' molecules:

- 'hybrid' histone-modifying enzymes, generated by chromosome rearrangements
- chromatin remodelling complexes with missing regulatory subunits
- mutations in the methyl-binding protein, MeCP2.

Deregulated histone-modifying enzymes

Acute myeloid leukaemia (AML) has long been known to associate with chromosomal abnormalities, with approximately 10% of patients showing recombination at a specific breakpoint on chromosome 11: 11q23. This cleaves the DNA sequence encoding the histone methyl transferase MLL-1, which then recombines with more than 30 genes ('fusion partners') on other chromosomes, including activating transcription factors (i.e. ETZ) and broad-specificity HATs (p300, CBP). This process generates 'hybrid' deregulated proteins containing the N-terminal of MLL, but with the transcription-activating domains of the fusion partner. This has a number of consequences, the most immediate being the loss of the MLL bromo-domain, a protein fold likely to be involved in regulating or targeting the MLL complex. However, given that MLL acts as the core of a large complex of enzymes and regulatory proteins, its truncation will also impact on the binding or activity of these proteins. These include a broad swathe of epigenetic regulators, including HATs (CBP, MOF), a chromatin remodeller (SWI/SNF), regulatory proteins (WDR5, menin) and the C-terminal MLL peptide (MLL^C), which contains the methyl transferase activity. The loss or faulty binding of many of these subunits must impact on the speed or outcome of gene expression (Fig. 4.8).

The generation of MLL fusion proteins has a profound effect on a cell's ability to regulate transcription, such that the deregulation (i.e. lack of silencing) of two key developmental MLL-driven genes, HOXA9 and MEIS1, is sufficient for the development of AML. Interestingly, three other methyl transferase enzymes (MLL2, MLL4 and MLL5) may also be associated with common chromosomal breakpoints in leukaemia and solid tumours, suggesting that these enzymes play an important role (or roles) in regulating differentiation and are potent agents of tumorigenesis when deregulated.

A similar pattern of chromosomal translocations is also involved in generating deregulated HATs. These generate fusion proteins involving two highly related HATs, MOZ (located at 8p11) and MORF (10q22), resulting in enzymes in which the N-terminal regions of the HATs are fused to C-terminal peptides derived from two further HATs (p300 or CBP). These highly active,

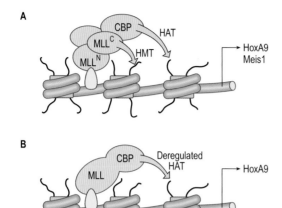

Figure 4.8
MLL-1 in gene regulation. (A) The transcriptional regulator MLL-1 forms a multiprotein complex, recruiting histone methyl transferase (HMT) and histone acetyl transferase (HAT) activities to target promoters (i.e. HoxA9 or Meis1), which contribute to gene regulation. (B) Chromosome translocations generating MLL fusion proteins (i.e. with the histone acetyl transferase, CBP) lead to constitutive gene activation, perhaps via recruiting deregulated HAT activity.

broad-specificity HATs are the likely basis of deregulation, as another MOZ fusion partner, TIF2, is a nuclear receptor co-activator which also interacts with the p300 and CBP. Interestingly, and in complete contrast to the MLL fusion proteins, MOZ-CBP and MOZ-p300 also appear to induce pathogenic processes by inhibiting transcription from key genes. This seems likely to arise due to the loss of the SM domain, a region rich in serine and methionine residues, which is involved in MOF/MORF-dependent transcriptional activation. Furthermore, both of these enzymes interact with the transcription factor Runx1, a key player in cell growth and differentiation, and also a common target of translocations in leukaemia. Thus, MOF/MORF fusion enzymes seem likely to act via inhibiting Runx1-dependent gene expression.

Absent or deregulated chromatin remodelling complexes

The deregulation of chromatin remodelling complexes is also implicated in pathological processes, reflecting their key contribution(s) to gene regulation. This is most obvious for SWI/SNF, a huge (approximately 2 Mda) remodelling complex which contains a large number of subunits and is implicated in 'promoter opening' on a broad range of genes. This broad regulatory role is consistent with roles both in embryonic development in mammals, and as a tumour suppressor via the part it plays in regulating the cell cycle.

The finding that SWI/SNF cooperates with p53 to regulate the cell cycle is key to understanding the role of the deregulated complex in tumour formation. Mutation or deletion of a single subunit, SNF5/INI1, is associated with carcinogenesis, presumably by inhibiting

remodeller tumour suppressor activity. Mutations in hSNF5 are frequently observed (in about 30% of patients) and are early events in chronic myeloid leukaemia (CML), but this protein is also mutated in a number of classes of tumour.

Defective methyl-binding proteins: MeCP2 and Rett syndrome

Differentiation and developmental processes are driven by synchronized patterns of gene expression — leading to both the activation and the silencing of networks of interlinked genes. As such, it is not a surprise that epigenetic regulators that lead to the inappropriate up- or down-regulation of key genes can have pathogenic consequences. A similar mechanism explains how mutations in the DNA methyl-binding protein, MeCP2, are catastrophic for neural development and function. This protein plays a central role in establishing transcriptional silencing over methylated genes, such that a wide range of mutations which either inactivate the protein or, more rarely, lead to increased protein levels are found in patients with Rett syndrome (RTT).

Rett syndrome is a relatively common neurological disorder found in 1 in 10 000 females. It leads to severe defects in speech and motor skills. Current hypotheses propose that the MeCP2 protein is required for the silencing of a key neuronal gene (or genes), such that faulty over-expression leads to the development of symptoms. Screens for MeCP2-dependent genes have identified *DLX5*, a gene involved in the synthesis of the neurotransmitter GABA, although whether this is central to generating the symptoms of Rett syndrome remains unclear.

Perhaps the most promising studies have come from mouse models of Rett syndrome, where genetically engineered MeCP2 mutations also induce motor and social defects. In these mice, reintroduction of normal levels of MeCP2 in postmitotic neurons at birth prevents the mice from developing Rett-like symptoms. This suggests that the brain and neural structures are developmentally normal, even in the absence of MeCP2, and that timely delivery of the protein to the correct cells could relieve the symptoms. MeCP2 mutations are also implicated in a range of other neurological diseases including autism, learning disability, schizophrenia and mental disorders.

Imprinting defects and disease

Genomic imprinting defects can occur when an individual inherits two alleles of an imprinted gene that carry the same imprint, resulting in both alleles being either transcriptionally active or silent. This typically occurs when both alleles are derived from one parent (termed a uniparental disomy, or UPD), a rare event resulting from chromosomal non-disjunction. Defects can also arise due to epigenetic mutations in the DNA methylation pattern of one allele, or due to deletion of an allele from the 'unsilenced' chromosome.

A number of disorders are linked to genomic imprinting. The best characterized are Prader–Willi and Angelman syndromes, considered previously. Genetic analysis and subsequent 'knockout' mouse experiments suggest that the underlying cause of Angelman syndrome in many patients is misregulation of the ubiquitin E3 ligase gene (*UBE3A*), though a number of patients also have mutations in the DNA methyl-binding protein, MeCP2. In contrast, the genes involved in Prader–Willi syndrome are less clear, though current research is focused on a region containing several non-coding transcripts ('snoRNAs').

Beckwith–Weidemann syndrome (BWS) is associated with a wide range of congenital abnormalities, including ear and tongue defects and a marked increase in the size of the internal organs. Patients also show an increased incidence of childhood tumours, notably Wilms' tumour, hepatoblastoma or rhabdomyosarcoma. The underlying defect that causes BWS remains unclear but various data suggest that it is linked to imprinting. Duplication of the insulin-like growth factor gene (*IGF2*) on the paternal chromosome and uniparental disomy of the chromosomal region that contains this gene (15p15.5) are both linked to the syndrome. Untangling the precise mechanism is complex, however, as the region contains a large number of co-regulated imprinted genes, in which *IGF2* is a single component.

Epigenetic therapies

So far this chapter has discussed how epigenetic mechanisms contribute to gene regulation and how the malfunctioning of these processes can lead to disease. In this final section we look to the future, to see how our knowledge of these processes can be used to develop 'epigenetic therapies': drugs that reduce or reverse abnormal gene expression by targeting epigenetic regulators. This approach holds great promise, as it aims to harness the normal nuclear processes involved in gene activation and silencing, and it should have broad application as a wide range of diseases arise due to aberrant gene regulation.

In theory, inhibitors directed at different epigenetic regulators should enable the targeted up- or down-regulation of restricted numbers of genes, but the field is currently limited to drugs targeted to histone deacetylases (HDACs) and DNA methyl transferases (DNMTs). These enzymes are largely associated with gene silencing, such that their inhibition generally leads to gene activation.

Histone deacetylase inhibitors (HDIs)

Several chemically diverse agents have been identified as HDAC inhibitors, including naturally occurring fatty acids, such as sodium butyrate, and potent synthetic agents, such as trichostatin. These drugs have a long history of use as experimental tools in the study of the effects of histone acetylation; they stimulate a rapid (approximately 15 minutes), substantial (around 5–10-fold) and genome-wide increase in histone acetylation levels ('hyperacetylation') in cultured cell lines. These HDIs have been key to identifying the sites of histone acetylation, its rapid turnover and its functional role in gene expression. Despite this insight, fundamental questions remain as to how HDIs influence gene expression in cells; for example, not all genes are affected, and the magnitude and direction of transcriptional responses are not predictable. This is largely because we do not understand the functional role of many histone deacetylase enzymes; most remain biochemically uncharacterized and their target substrates (not all of which are histones) are unknown. Despite this lack of understanding, HDIs are important clinical drugs. Sodium valproate, which is an established treatment for epilepsy, also has HDI activity.

DNMT inhibitors ('hypomethylating agents')

Two nucleoside analogues, 5-azacytidine, and a less toxic agent, 5-aza-2' deoxycytidine (Decitabine®), inhibit DNA methyl transferase (DNMT) activity and lead to reduced levels of DNA methylation ('hypomethylation') in cells. The agents act by mimicking cytosine nucleosides and are consequently incorporated into DNA, where the modified base covalently binds to methyl transferase enzymes, creating a cross-linked 5-aza-Dnmt adduct. Enzyme inactivation is a relatively slow process, as the most abundant DNMT in mammalian cells — the maintenance methylase, Dnmt1 — only acts at sites in the hemi-methylated templates created after DNA replication. This ensures that at least two cycles of DNA replication are required to reduce the levels of active Dnmt1 and DNA methylation substantially. Experiments in cultured cells demonstrate that these agents can lead to transcriptional re-activation ('derepression') of silenced genes. The observation that they frequently have a differentiation-promoting effect in many cell lines has stimulated interest in their potential clinical applications.

Clinical applications of epigenetic therapies

Current clinical studies are primarily targeted at cancers and leukaemias. These follow on from *in vitro* experiments which show that HDIs and/or hypomethylating agents promote cell differentiation or increased cell death in model tumour cell lines. Clinical trials examining the efficacy of these drugs, often in combination with differentiation-promoting agents such as retinoic acid, have been used on a variety of tumours, notably acute myeloid leukaemia. Analysis of patient samples suggests that the drugs act as predicted, increasing histone acetylation levels in target tumour cells (i.e. 'blasts') and inducing gene activation, but in an unpredictable manner. Importantly, though, a subset of patients do gain clinical benefits from these regimes. Further studies are needed to identify the gene expression changes that correlate with a positive outcome — a challenge, given the heterogeneity of tumours in individual patients.

There is an understandable concern that these epigenetic therapies may produce effects which could be inherited by the patient's offspring. For this reason, male patients taking 5-azacytidine have been warned to avoid fathering children, at least while taking the drug.

Future prospects for targeted epigenetic therapies

A number of substantial barriers need to be overcome to develop ideal epigenetic therapeutic agents — drugs that can predictably influence gene expression at defined genes. Despite real progress in our understanding, many epigenetic regulators remain essentially unexplored. For many enzymes, we know little more than their DNA sequence; their biochemical composition, substrates, target genes and control processes remain unknown.

Similarly, we are limited by the small numbers of inhibitors identified and by their broad target specificity. For example, HDIs inhibit many HDAC enzymes, though it is not clear which are therapeutically important. Thus, as with many areas of medicine, real progress is only likely to come with further basic research. As the field is expanding rapidly, with novel histone modifications and regulators being identified almost monthly, this should keep many of us busy for years to come.

FURTHER READING

Bird A 2007 Perceptions of epigenetics. Nature 447:396–398.

Oshiro MM, Kim CJ, Wozniak RJ et al. 2005 Epigenetic silencing of DSC3 is a common event in human breast cancer. Breast Cancer Res 7:R669–R680.

Strahl BD, Allis CD 2000 The language of covalent histone modifications. Nature 403:41–45.

5 Protein structure and function

M. Keen

While analysis of the genetic sequence provides a relatively simple way of determining the amino acid sequence of proteins, this is far from enough to understand protein structure and the resulting function, especially as proteins are not 'bits of wet string'. Their function depends on the three-dimensional (3D) structure that these polymers of amino acid residues assume, and this is much harder to determine experimentally than the amino acid sequence.

Understanding the structure of proteins, and the ways in which they interact, is central to our understanding of cell function and dysfunction.

As our knowledge increases, it is likely that it will bring new insights into the causes and possible treatment of disease. For example, study of the 3D structure of proteins is already having an impact on drug design. Neuraminidase inhibitors for the treatment of influenza have been developed on the basis of the way in which candidate molecules can be observed to interact with neuraminidase in X-ray crystallography. We are fast approaching the time when drugs can be expressly designed to fit the target molecule, whose structure is thoroughly understood.

It is the importance of this 3D structure, the interactions that proteins undergo with other proteins and the methods currently available to investigate these properties that are the subjects of this chapter.

Aspects of protein structure

In order to understand the role of a specific protein in human biology and disease, its structure has to be examined. Proteins have several different 'levels' of structure, referred to as primary, secondary, tertiary and quaternary (Fig. 5.1).

- *Primary structure* (Fig. 5.1A) is determined by the genetic code transcribed into mRNA and is the sequence of amino acids that makes up the polypeptide chain. The distinction between 'peptides', short sequences of amino acids, and fully-fledged proteins is largely one of size; amino acid chains of less than 40 amino acids are generally referred to as peptides.
- *Secondary structure* (Fig. 5.1B) is an area of regular structure assumed by the polypeptide chain and stabilized by hydrogen bonds. The most common types of secondary structure are α-helices and β-pleated sheets (see below). Areas of secondary structure are localized and proteins may contain many different secondary 'motifs' (see below).

- *Tertiary structure* (Fig. 5.1C) is the overall 'shape' of a single protein chain, in which the chain, with its areas of secondary structure, folds up on itself to produce the protein's active conformation. This conformation may not be fixed, as the function of a great many proteins depends on the ability of the protein to undergo conformational change.
- *Quaternary structure* occurs when several different polypeptide chains, or 'protein subunits', combine to make a large molecule which functions as a protein complex. For example, haemoglobin is tetramer consisting of two chains of α-haemoglobin and two chains of β-haemoglobin (Fig. 5.1D).

Primary structure

Primary structure describes the atoms and covalent bonds that make up the protein molecule; this is largely determined by the amino acid residues that constitute the peptide 'backbone' of the molecule. Amino acids are combined to form polypeptides at the ribosome, where amino acids corresponding to the sequence of the mRNA are combined in a condensation reaction between the carboxyl group of one amino acid and the amino group of the next, to form a peptide bond (Fig. 5.2); thus proteins are synthesized from the N-terminus towards the C-terminus. The sequence of amino acids that make up the protein is, of course, determined by the gene, and presumably this primary sequence in turn determines the final conformation of the protein. We are, however, currently quite a long way from understanding how the folding of the polypeptide into its 'proper' shape occurs, and the tertiary structure of a protein cannot yet be predicted from its amino acid sequence alone (see below).

Similarly to DNA, amino acid sequence can be determined by chemical techniques, of which the most widely used is Edman degradation (Box 5.1). However, it is now much easier and much more common to infer the primary structure of a protein from the nucleotide sequence of a gene or cDNA (see Appendix 2).

Primary structure does not depend solely upon the gene, however. Processing of RNA, post-translational modification of individual amino acid residues and proteolytic cleavage of a parent protein can all serve to modify the primary structure of a protein.

Processing of mRNA

Transcribed mRNA can be processed in two ways before translation into protein: splicing and editing.

A Primary amino acid sequence of the haemoglobin β-subunit

VHLTPEEKSAVTALWGKVNV<u>DEVGGEALGRLLVV</u>YPWTQRFFESFGDLST
PDAVMGNPKVKAHGKKVLGAFSDGLAHLDNLKGTFATLSELHCDKLHVDPE
NFRLLGNVLVCVLAHHFGKEFTPPVQAAYQKVVAGVANALAHKYH

B A region of secondary structure in the haemoglobin β-subunit.
This α helix is formed by the 13 amino acid residues underlined in A

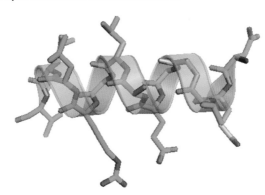

C Two views of the tertiary structure of the haemoglobin β-subunit

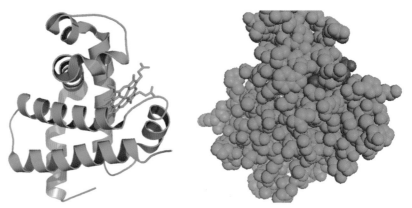

D Quaternary structure of a molecule of haemoglobin; it consists of two α- and two β-subunits

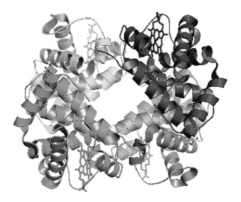

Figure 5.1
Primary, secondary, tertiary and quaternary structure of human haemoglobin. (A) The primary structure is shown as the sequence of amino acids that make up the β-subunit of haemoglobin. (B) Secondary structure shows a 'stick' model of one of the many α-helices in haemoglobin. The green 'ribbon' is the conventional way of indicating an α-helix. (C) The tertiary structure of the haemoglobin β-subunit is illustrated in two ways: a 'ribbon' diagram, which emphasizes areas of regular secondary structure, and a 'space-filling' model, in which the atoms are shown as spheres. The folding of the haemoglobin subunits involves interactions with the haem group, shown in red in the space-filling model, and as sticks in the ribbon model. (D) The quaternary structure shows the interaction of two β- (green and blue) and two α- (yellow and orange) subunits to form functional haemoglobin. Structural data is from the Protein Data Bank, accession code 2HHB, visualized using PyMOL (DeLano Scientific).

Splicing

Splicing of RNA removes introns and joins exons to form the mature mRNA. Most splicing takes place at the spliceosome: a very large macromolecular complex of RNA and proteins. A few RNA molecules are self-splicing; the intron forms a ribozyme and the spliceosome is not required. The RNA from a number of genes can be alternatively spliced, with some introns being selectively included or excluded from the mature mRNA. By this mechanism, different proteins can be encoded by a single gene.

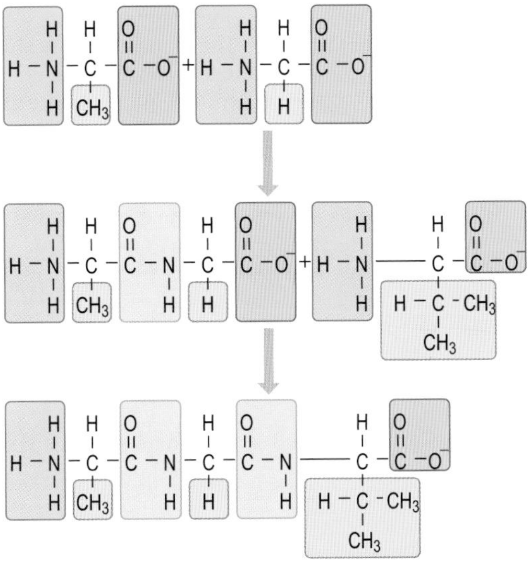

Figure 5.2

Polymerization of amino acids by peptide bonds. This diagram shows the combination of alanine (left) and glycine (right) to form a dipeptide. Valine is subsequently added to form a tripeptide. The amino and carboxyl groups of the amino acids and peptides are shown by the blue and pink boxes respectively. The green boxes highlight the peptide bonds, while the yellow boxes show the amino acid side-chains. A molecule of water is liberated during the formation of the peptide bond.

Editing

Editing of mRNA is the conversion of one base into another. In humans, the most common form of editing is the conversion of adenosine to inosine by a type of adenosine deaminase that acts specifically on RNA. Inosine is 'read' as guanosine by the ribosomes, so editing alters the protein produced. For example, in one of the subunits of a ligand-gated ion channel, the AMPA glutamate receptor, $GluR_2$, conversion of adenosine to inosine can convert a key glutamine-encoding codon (CAG) to an arginine-encoding codon (CIG). This substitution of a single amino acid has a profound effect on the functioning of the heteromeric receptor protein; the glutamine-containing form of the channel is permeable to Ca^{2+}, whereas the arginine-containing form is not. This can have profound consequences for cellular function, as Ca^{2+} is an extremely important intracellular signalling molecule.

Post-translational modifications

Amino acid residues can be modified in a number of ways: for example, by the formation of disulphide bonds between cysteine residues and by a number of post-translational modifications. Modification can be of the N-terminus — e.g. by acetylation (also known as 'N-terminal blocking'), the C-terminus — e.g. by glycosyl phosphatidylinositol (GPI) attachment (important in anchoring many proteins to the cell membrane) and/or the side-chains of the amino acid residues — e.g. by phosphorylation, glycosylation, prenylation or ADP-ribosylation. Resolution of these aspects of primary structure requires chemical analysis and it can be quite difficult to determine. Moreover, many of the modifications may be heterogeneous and/or reversible, and many of these in turn are involved in regulation of the function of the protein, phosphorylation being the best-known example.

_i_   **Box 5.1**

Edman degradation

Named after its inventor, Pehr Edman, this technique is probably the most widely used chemical method for determining the amino acid sequence of peptides.

The key step in the process is the reaction of the protein or peptide with phenylisothiocyanate. Under mildly alkaline conditions, this combines with the uncharged amino group at the N-terminus of the peptide chain to produce a phenylthiocarbamoyl derivative. The peptide bond on the C-terminal side of the modified residue becomes unstable, such that when exposed to acidic conditions the bond is cleaved. This releases the original N-terminal amino acid in the derivatized form, and leaves the next amino acid in the chain exposed as

the new N-terminus. The derivatized amino acid is extracted into an organic solvent and identified by chromatography or electrophoresis. The whole reaction is then repeated to isolate and identify each new N-terminal amino acid in turn.

The reaction can be performed with relatively small amounts of purified protein. However, it is not possible to sequence large proteins solely by this technique, as the whole process tends to grind to a halt after 50 residues or so. Moreover, it relies on the protein possessing a free amino group at the N-terminus, so it cannot be used with proteins that are N-terminal blocked (see main text). For these reasons, proteins are usually cleaved into smaller peptides and these peptide fragments are then sequenced by Edman degradation.

Proteolytic cleavage

Proteolytic cleavage may be involved in the processing of a precursor protein, translated from mRNA, to form the mature functional protein. For example, the gene for insulin is transcribed to give the 110 amino acid protein, pre-pro-insulin, which consists of a signal peptide at the N-terminus, the insulin B chain, a linker C chain and the insulin A chain at the C-terminus. The initial processing involves the removal of the signal peptide to give an 86 amino acid protein, pro-insulin. At this stage, the three disulphide bonds characteristic of mature insulin are formed, two between the A and B chains and one within the A chain. The C chain is removed and this yields active insulin, a 51 amino acid two-chain protein (Fig. 5.3).

Secondary structure

The most commonly encountered forms of regular secondary structure are the α-helix and β-pleated sheet. Both of these structures were elucidated by Linus Pauling and his colleagues in the early 1950s. Both α-helix and β-pleated sheet are formed by hydrogen bonding between the N-H and C=O groups of the peptide backbone. Both structures allow saturation of all possible hydrogen bonds in the peptide backbone, which adds stability and presumably explains why they are so commonly encountered.

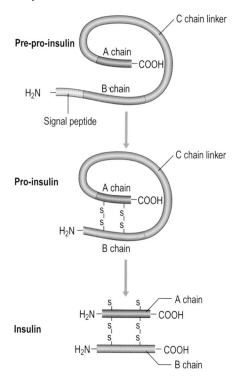

Figure 5.3
Proteolytic processing of insulin. Insulin is synthesized from pre-pro-insulin. Cleavage of the signal peptide from pre-pro-insulin yields pro-insulin; cleavage of the C-peptide linker from pro-insulin and formation of disulphide bonds yield the mature insulin protein.

- *Alpha-helix*. This is a right-handed helical structure. The N-H group of one amino acid residue forms a hydrogen bond with the C=O group from an amino acid four residues earlier in the chain (i.e. nearer the N-terminus). The side-chains point outward from the helix, as can be seen in Figure 5.4A. The α-helix is a very stable structure and occurs very commonly in proteins.
- *Beta-pleated sheet*. In this, the peptide chain is much more extended than in an α-helix. Hydrogen bonds are formed between the N-H and C=O groups in adjacent strands, and the side-chains point alternately above and below the plane of the sheet (Fig. 5.4B). The strands in a sheet can run parallel to one another (i.e. in the same direction) or antiparallel (in opposite directions). Mixed sheets, containing both parallel and antiparallel strands, do occur but are much more unusual. Antiparallel sheets are more stable than parallel. As a consequence, antiparallel sheets can occur as smaller structures (as small as two strands of only two residues each) and can be at the surface of a protein, where interactions with the aqueous environment tend to disrupt the hydrogen bonding. Parallel sheets only occur deep in the molecule and have a minimum of four strands.

Other forms of regular secondary structure are also possible, and can occasionally be observed in proteins:

- 3_{10} helix. The N-H group of one amino acid residue forms bonds with C=O from amino acid three residues earlier in the chain, and thus is more tightly wound than the α-helix.
- π-helix. The N-H group of one amino acid residue forms bonds with C=O from amino acid five residues earlier in the chain, and thus is more loosely wound than the α-helix.

Although these are energetically favourable conformations for the polypeptide, they are not found very often in proteins. They are less stable than the α-helix and packing of the side-chains is not as good. The 3_{10} helix occurs fairly frequently in proteins, but tends to be very short and usually occurs at the ends of α-helices, where these have become disrupted by the protein structure. The π-helix is very rare. A review in the year 2000 of all the structures lodged in the Protein Data Bank (Box 5.2) revealed only 10 proteins which possessed a π-helix.

Other very common aspects of secondary structure are turns and loops, stabilized by hydrogen bonds; some of these can be viewed as single residue lengths of α-helix or β-sheet. A number of combinations of secondary structure occur very commonly in proteins and these are known as structural motifs. Two examples of simple motifs are:

- the β-hairpin — two adjacent antiparallel β-strands connected by a short loop
- the β-α-β motif — in which two parallel β-strands are connected by an α-helix.

α helix

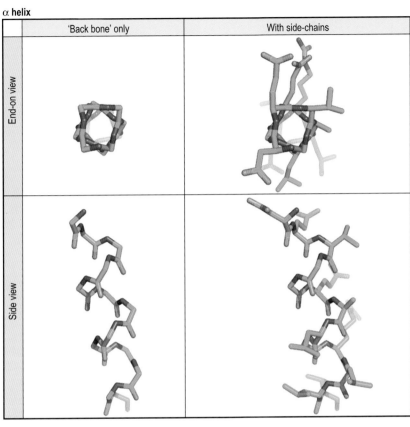

β sheet

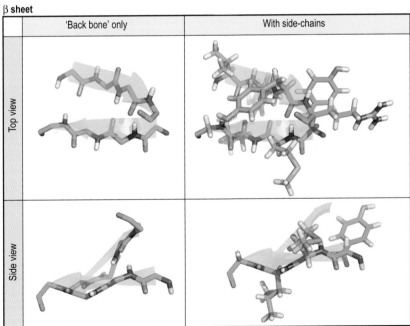

Figure 5.4

The structure of an α-helix and a β-sheet. The α-helix shown in the top panel is formed from 13 amino acid residues of the α-helix from the hae-moglobin β-subunit, also shown in Figure 5.1 (Protein Data Bank accession code 2HHB). The β-sheet shown in the bottom panel is of two antiparallel strands of four amino acid residues each, from a prion protein (Protein Data Bank accession code 1E1G). In the side view of the β-sheet, the side-chains of the front strand only are illustrated to improve clarity. It is fairly clear that side-chain geometry has a large impact on secondary structure.

Box 5.2

The Protein Data Bank

The Protein Data Bank (PDB) is the key resource in structural biology. It is an online repository for 3D structural data on proteins and nucleic acids. It provides free access for everyone to all of these structures. With the exception of some commercially sensitive molecules, such as biopharmaceuticals, all structural information obtained is deposited with PDB.

PDB was founded in 1971 with the structures of only seven proteins. Since that time, the database has grown more or less exponentially and now contains well over 40 000 structures.

PDB is run by a variety of organizations who all contribute to the deposition of structural data, data processing and distribution. The various sites all provide access to the structural information, with links to (much larger) databases, such as Swiss-Prot, which contains amino acid sequences, and the International Sequence Database Collaboration, which houses information on mRNA and gene sequences.

Since 2007, structural data have been remediated and are now stored as part of the World Wide Protein Data Bank (wwPDB). While this resource is continually updated it is, sadly, much less user-friendly than the old PDB. Fortunately, PDB remains available, although it is no longer updated.

Not all of the protein adopts secondary structure and some stretches of amino acid residues appear to exist as rather disordered conformations.

X-ray crystallography (Box 5.3) and NMR (see Box 5.4 below) are the most accurate ways of determining secondary structure. Spectrographic techniques, such as circular dichroism and infra-red spectroscopy, are also used. However, these require rather large amounts of pure protein and can only provide information regarding the proportion of secondary structures in a molecule, e.g. 20% α-helix and 15% β-sheet.

Tertiary structure

Tertiary structure describes the overall 3D arrangement of the protein chain. As the chain folds, it allows amino acid residues that are rather distant from one another in the primary sequence to come into close proximity and interact. The tertiary structure is stabilized by a variety of bonds, including hydrogen bonds, salt bridges between ionized side-chains and hydrophobic bonds. In a globular protein, hydrophobic residues tend to be clustered in the middle of the protein, where water does not penetrate, whilst hydrophilic residues are more concentrated on the outer parts of the molecule. In integral membrane proteins, hydrophobic residues tend to be clustered in the parts of the molecule that interact with the lipid bilayer of the plasma membrane, and these protein–lipid interactions can be very important for maintaining tertiary structure.

A number of similar tertiary structure 'domains' appear again and again in unrelated proteins. A structural domain is a region of the protein that seems to be self-stabilizing and therefore folds independently of the rest of the protein. Different domains can often be identified as being involved with different aspects of the protein's function, e.g. ligand-binding, tyrosine kinase activity, etc. Because they fold independently, these domains can be combined to produce multidomain proteins and 'shuffled' among different proteins, either spontaneously during evolution or as the result of protein engineering. Tissue plasminogen activator (alteplase;

see Fig. 5.6 below and Ch. 11) is an example of the very many multidomain proteins that exist in eukaryotes. It contains four distinct types of domain:

- a fibronectin finger
- an epidermal growth factor-like domain
- two kringle domains
- a protease domain.

The domaMin structure of tissue plasminogen activator (alteplase)

The domain structure of alteplase is shown schematically in Figure 5.6. Each domain has a distinctive structure and function:

- *The fibronectin finger* is made up of two antiparallel β-sheets, cross-linked by a disulphide bond.
- *The epidermal growth factor (EGF)-like domain* is made up of two two-stranded β-sheets linked by a loop. Both the fibronectin finger and the EGF-like region of alteplase are involved in binding to fibrin and also binding to a clearance receptor in hepatocytes. It has been suggested that these two domains function as a single domain in this protein.
- *The kringle domains* are triple-looped structures, stabilized by three disulphide bonds. Kringle domains are found in all of the blood clotting factors and fibrinolytic proteins. They seem to be important in regulating activity of the protease domain, via the binding of a variety of mediators. In alteplase, kringle 1 seems to be particularly associated with clearance of the molecule by hepatic endothelial cells, whereas kringle 2 is important for binding to fibrin.
- *The protease domain* is itself made up of two β-barrel domains, which presumably arose as the result of gene duplication; however, these have since diverged such that there is no obvious sequence homology between them. The active proteolytic site is in the cleft between the two barrels, with key residues contributed by both.

Box 5.3

X-ray crystallography

In X-ray crystallography, a beam of X-rays is passed through a crystal of the molecule of interest, and the resulting diffraction pattern is used to determine the precise location of the atoms within the crystal.

Diffraction is the process by which a wave is distorted as it passes a barrier or through a gap. Look at Figure 5.5 for a very simple example. It is this simple phenomenon that is exploited in X-ray crystallography.

Diffraction is most marked when the width of the gap is close to the wavelength of the wave. The wavelength of X-rays is similar to the size of the gaps between the outer electrons of the various atoms in a molecule. Crystals are required because a single molecule just would not produce sufficient diffraction of the X-rays. A crystal provides a repeated array of the same molecule, in the same orientation, which allows the diffraction effect to be multiplied many times over. During X-ray irradiation, the crystal is usually cooled using liquid nitrogen. This serves two purposes; it reduces the thermal motion of the atoms and also reduces the heating, and therefore damage to the crystal lattice, which occur as a result of the X-ray bombardment.

The X-ray diffraction pattern obtained is essentially the interference pattern between the diffracted waves, where waves that are in phase reinforce each other and waves that are out of phase cancel each other out.

It is at least reasonably obvious intuitively that there must be a relationship between the spatial arrangement of atoms in the crystal and the diffraction pattern produced. However, the actual determination of the atomic arrangement from the diffraction data is much more difficult. In essence, the diffraction pattern is used to produce an estimate of the electron density map of the molecule; this is then used to create an initial model of the structure, which undergoes several rounds of refinement until the best fit between the model and the observed diffraction data is achieved.

Undoubtedly, the most difficult part of the whole process is obtaining a good crystal. Clearly, the crystal needs to be very regular; the protein molecules should be stacked in identical conformations (something which is quite difficult to achieve for proteins, which are generally very flexible) and the crystal should be free of contaminants and impurities. Temperature changes during crystallization can lead to convection currents that damage the crystal. For this reason, there is considerable interest in growing crystals in zero gravity, where convection does not occur.

It is perhaps surprising that proteins can ever be induced to crystallize at all. The first protein structure to be determined by X-ray crystallography was sperm whale myoglobin. Why was this chosen? Because crystals of myoglobin had been observed to form spontaneously in pools of drying blood on whaling ships. Nowadays, however, crystallographers may have to try thousands of different conditions before obtaining a usable protein crystal, and a great many proteins have yet to be successfully crystallized.

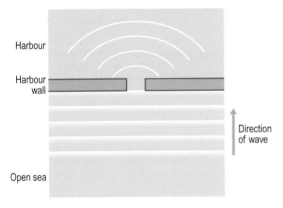

Figure 5.5
Diffraction. In this very simple example, the linear waves on the sea are diffracted into curves as they pass through the gap in the harbour wall.

conformational change. Furthermore, not all polypeptide chains adopt a well-ordered tertiary structure. Some small proteins, and the terminal and loop regions of some larger ones, seem to exist in a rather disordered state.

The most widely used method of determining tertiary structure is X-ray crystallography (see Box 5.3 above) and currently around 90% of the protein structures lodged in the Protein Data Bank (see Box 5.2 above) have been determined using this technique. The vast majority of other structures (9%) were determined by NMR spectroscopic techniques (Box 5.4). Other techniques, such as cryoelectron microscopy, tend to be of a much lower resolution and are much more rarely used. It is worth noting, however, that these structural methods all work much better for small globular proteins than they do for integral membrane proteins, for example.

Many proteins cannot be said to have a single tertiary structure. Conformational change can be extremely important in protein function and the activity of enzymes and receptors, for example, is regulated by

Quaternary structure

Quaternary structure occurs when two or more proteins interact to form a multimeric complex. For many proteins, the formation of a quaternary complex is vital to

65

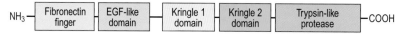

Figure 5.6
The various domains that make up tissue plasminogen activator (alteplase). (EGF = epidermal growth factor)

Box 5.4

Nuclear magnetic resonance (NMR) spectroscopy

While X-ray crystallography detects the gaps between electron shells (see Box 5.3), NMR is, unsurprisingly, concerned with the nucleus. It makes use of one of the fundamental properties of subatomic particles: that of 'spin'. Like most science that involves subatomic particles, it is inherently very complex!

Electrons, protons and neutrons all possess spin of either + or − ½. Nuclei in which the sum of the spin values for all the protons and neutrons is not equal to zero are said to be 'unpaired'; it is these nuclei that are important in NMR. The nuclei used most often in the study of protein structure are those of hydrogen, carbon-13 and nitrogen-15.

The unpaired nuclei behave as tiny magnetic dipoles and can be aligned in a strong magnetic field. During NMR spectroscopy, radio waves of the correct frequency are used to 'knock' the nuclei out of alignment with the field. Following the radio pulse, the nuclei 'relax' back into alignment with the field. As they do, the movement of the minute magnetic dipole in the magnetic field sets up a current that can be detected as the NMR signal.

The precise behaviour of each nucleus is affected by its environment; the different hydrogen nuclei in a molecule will experience slightly different magnetic fields due to differences

in the local electron density, bonding and the nature of the surrounding nuclei. Sophisticated tricks involving sequences of radio pulses (known as 2D and even 3D NMR spectroscopy) can be used to determine the precise behaviour of each nucleus and thus its spatial relationship to other nuclei in the molecule. Correlated spectra look at interactions between nuclei along the peptide backbone and thus reveal information about primary structure. NOESY (nuclear Overhauser effect spectroscopy) spectra detect interactions between nuclei through space and thus provide information regarding the folding of the peptide chain. NOESY spectra make use of the nuclear Overhauser effect, predicted by Overhauser in the 1950s, when he was still a PhD student. The effect is so counterintuitive that even most NMR specialists did not believe that it could occur until it was actually demonstrated!

NMR techniques have some advantages over X-ray crystallography for examining protein structure, the main one being that the structure can be examined in solution, avoiding the need to crystallize the protein. This makes it much easier to examine the conformation of molecules under a variety of different conditions, such as in the presence or absence of a ligand, for example. NMR is becoming increasingly important as a structural tool. However, it requires rather large amounts of purified protein and is best suited to small proteins, as the spectra of large molecules are simply too complex to analyse at present.

---

their function. For example, microtubules have essential roles in:

- maintaining the cytoskeleton
- mitosis
- cell movement
- vesicular transport.

They are made up of assemblies of tubulin monomers. Reorganization of the microtubular structure is achieved by depolymerization and repolymerization of these tubulin subunits.

Haemoglobin is a complex of four protein subunits: two α- and two β-subunits (see Figure 5.1D). Interaction between these subunits is essential in mediating the co-operative binding and disassociation of O_2; the mechanism which allows O_2 to be bound in the lungs and released in the tissues so effectively.

How can it be determined whether a protein has quaternary structure? Usually the evidence is that the native protein appears larger than its isolated subunit.

Methods for determining the size of native proteins include sedimentation rate in centrifugation, size exclusion chromatography and radiation inactivation. Even when it is clear that a particular protein exists as part of an oligomeric complex, it is far from straightforward to determine precisely with which other proteins, and in what stoichiometry, it is complexed. To add further to the problems, most proteins interact with other proteins as a critical part of their function. Transient interactions are not really considered as quaternary structure but many of the same considerations apply, and this information could provide enormously useful information about protein and cell function. These more transitory protein–protein interactions are considered in more detail below.

Some quaternary structures are stabilized by the formation of disulphide bonds between the different subunits. Others are stabilized by a phenomenon known as 'domain swapping', by which the protein subunits intertwine so that one domain of a subunit interacts with the bulk of the protein of another subunit.

Is it possible to predict structure from amino acid sequence?

As noted before, the amino acid sequence of a protein can be determined very easily from genetic sequence data, whilst the experimental methods required to determine secondary, tertiary and quaternary structure are much more complex. Nevertheless, it is these higher levels of protein structure that tell us most about function. It would greatly facilitate our understanding of cell function if it were possible to predict the final structure of a protein from its amino acid sequence.

It seems a reasonable assumption that the secondary structure of a protein must be determined by its primary amino acid sequence, and a number of strategies are used in an attempt to predict secondary structure from sequence data, particularly in order to identify potential antigenic sites for antibody production (Box 5.5).

It is clear that some amino acid residues have a particular 'preference' for different types of secondary structure. Some amino acid residues (alanine, glutamate, leucine, lysine and methionine) are commonly found in α-helices, whereas amino acid residues with bulky side-chains, such as phenylalanine, valine and tryptophan, tend to occur in strands of β-sheet. Proline and glycine have unusual geometry and tend to introduce kinks in the polypeptide backbone. Thus these amino acids are often seen as 'helix-breakers', disrupting the orderly arrangement of a helix. However, they are commonly found in turns of the polypeptide chain.

Unfortunately, the influence of individual amino acid residues on secondary structure is not sufficiently strong to allow this information alone to be a good predictor of secondary structure. Better accuracy can be obtained by looking at the nature of the amino acids in a region of the chain (e.g. seven residues on either side of a particular amino acid), both in an individual protein and in a variety of similar proteins. The various structural prediction methods are continually being tested and refined; PSIPRED is among the best at present (McGuffin et al., 2000).

Predicting tertiary structure is even harder. It is thought that the tertiary structure does depend largely upon primary sequence and methods are being developed to predict tertiary sequence. Most methods rely on comparison with published structures. Homology techniques look at similarities to proteins of known structure; by using this method it is possible to identify protein sequences with seven hydrophobic domains tentatively as members of the superfamily of G protein-coupled receptors, for example. Threading is a more sophisticated technique, where the sequence of the protein of interest is 'threaded' on to the 3D structure of a known protein; a scoring function is then generated to determine how compatible the sequence is with the structure. *Ab initio* techniques start with only the amino acid sequence and attempt to compute an energetically favourable conformation; some of these have been reasonably successful for small proteins with well-defined secondary structure.

However, whilst sequence is undoubtedly important in determining tertiary structure, protein folding also depends upon the environment in which the protein is made, and a number of molecules are known to have a role in mediating the correct folding of a number of proteins. These are generally known as 'chaperones'.

Protein chaperones

Examples of chaperones are calnexin, calreticulin and Erp57. These assist with the folding process of the major histocompatibility complex-I (MHC-I) molecule inside the endoplasmic reticulum.

MHC-I molecules consist of three protein chains and these are unstable until the correct peptide is locked into the 'peptide-presenting groove'; these peptides are provided as the result of proteosomal degradation of cytoplasmic proteins. Chaperones stabilize the MHC-I protein chains until a suitable peptide is available. Once the peptide binds to its MHC-I molecule, the now stable MHC-I–peptide complex can leave the endoplasmic reticulum and enter the Golgi apparatus before reaching the cell surface to be sampled by the adaptive immune system.

Some viruses interfere with this process to avoid recognition and elimination by the immune system. These include the cytomegaloviruses which accelerate the process by which MHC-I molecules leave the endoplasmic reticulum. As the MHC-I molecules are still not properly folded at that stage, they are degraded by the proteosome and therefore unable to present viral peptides to the immune system.

Research is ongoing to predict quaternary structure from tertiary structure. As part of the Macromolecular

Box 5.5

Prediction of antigenic sequences

There are currently attempts to predict secondary structures of proteins based on their primary sequences to identify potential antigenic sites of the protein. As any given protein can carry more then one antigenic site (epitope), which can trigger immune reactions of different strengths, determination of protein folding is important, as in reality not all of these epitopes are 'visible' to the immune system. Selection of the best epitopes is important, as during the production of diagnostic antibodies the animals are rarely immunized with the whole antigenic protein, but rather with a peptide corresponding to a particular specific epitope. Similarly, in vaccination it is useful to be able to vaccinate with a particular epitope sequence (e.g. part of a viral coat protein) rather than the entire pathogen, as this makes the process much safer (see Ch. 7).

Structure Database, the European Bioinformatics Institute routinely applies an algorithm to all protein structures lodged in PDB to try to predict their likely quaternary structure; the results form the Protein Quaternary Structure (PQS) database (http://pqs.ebi.ac.uk/).

When protein conformation goes wrong

The importance of the 3D structure of proteins can perhaps best be illustrated using examples of what happens when this structure goes wrong. We will look at two examples of aberrant protein structure:

- the abnormal haemoglobin (haemoglobin S) that occurs in sickle cell anaemia
- the aberrant conformation of the prion protein that seems to underlie diseases such as scrapie, bovine spongiform encephalopathy (BSE) and Creutzfeldt–Jakob disease (CJD).

Haemoglobin S

Sickle cell anaemia is an autosomal recessive condition that occurs as a result of a point mutation in the gene for the haemoglobin β-subunit (see also previous chapters). The mutation results in the substitution of a hydrophobic residue, valine, for the normal hydrophilic residue, glutamate, as the sixth amino acid in the β-subunit.

Haemoglobin S functions normally. Binding of O_2 to the haem groups in the molecule induces a conformational change in the molecule, increasing its affinity for O_2; upon dissociation of the O_2 molecules, the quaternary structure of haemoglobin S reverts back to its original lower-affinity conformation. Unfortunately, however, when haemoglobin S (or normal haemoglobin) is in this deoxygenated condition, it reveals two hydrophobic amino acids at the surface of the β-subunit: phenylalanine in position 85 and leucine in position 88. These amino acids are buried in the molecule when haemoglobin is in its oxygenated conformation. Figure 5.7 compares the 3D structure of normal haemoglobin and haemoglobin S in their deoxygenated conformations.

The exposed hydrophobic residues provide partners with which the mutant valine residue can form a hydrophobic bond. This can lead to the formation of abnormal chains of haemoglobin S molecules, joined by the hydrophobic interaction. These chains can form such long fibres that they distort the red blood cells into the characteristic sickle shape that gives sickle cell anaemia its name.

Prions

Prion proteins seem to be the causative agents of a number of mammalian diseases, including CJD, BSE and scrapie. These diseases are characterized by neurodegeneration with an accumulation of fibrils and plaques of a highly insoluble protein known as prion protein-scrapie, or PrP^{sc}.

The amino acid sequence of PrP^{sc} seems to be identical to that of the normal prion protein, PrP. It seems that PrP^{sc} is in fact PrP in an abnormal conformation. Moreover, inoculation of the brain with PrP^{sc} does not produce disease in animals that do not express PrP. It seems that PrP^{sc} is able to transmit its abnormal conformation to other PrP molecules, forming new PrP^{sc} molecules,

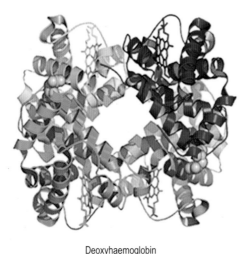

Deoxyhaemoglobin

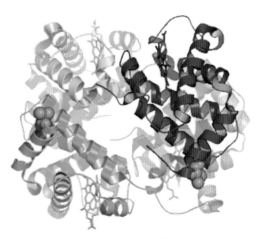

Deoxyhaemoglobin S

Figure 5.7

Comparison of the 3D structure of deoxygenated haemoglobin and haemoglobin S. The normal glutamate in the haemoglobin β-subunit is shown in pale pink; the mutant valine at the same position in the haemoglobin S β-subunit is shown in bright pink. Structural data are from the Protein Data Bank, accession codes 2HHB and 2HBS, visualized using PyMOL (DeLano Scientific).

which can in turn convert more PrP molecules to PrP^{sc} in a process that is not yet fully understood. Thus the prion diseases seem to be diseases caused by an abnormal protein conformation.

The structure of human PrP has been determined by NMR spectroscopy and is shown in diagrammatic form in Figure 5.8. This figure also shows a putative conformation for the PrP^{sc} form of the protein; PrP^{sc} is so insoluble that it has so far proved impossible to determine its structure directly.

A minority of cases (15%) of CJD appear to be inherited and these familial forms are associated with mutations in PrP. A particularly common mutation is the conversion of glutamate at position 200 to lysine. Perhaps surprisingly, however, the tertiary structure of the E200K variant of PrP is virtually identical to 'normal' PrP; clearly, this mutation alone is not sufficient to trigger the conversion of PrP to PrP^{sc}.

Normal conformation of the prion protein, PrP

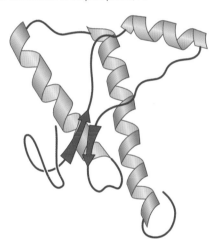

Putative conformation of the pathogenic prion protein, PrP^{sc}

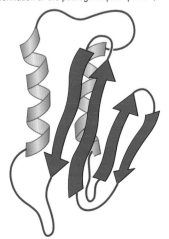

Figure 5.8
Comparison of the 3D structure of the normal prion protein, PrP, and its probable pathological conformation, PrP^{sc}. Adapted from Cohen and Prusiner (1998).

Protein–protein interactions

The function of proteins depends on their interactions with other proteins, and other molecules such as DNA, RNA and small molecule ligands. Thus in order to have a full understanding of cell function and to understand the pathologies underlying protein malfunction, we need to be able to determine all the ways in which cellular proteins interact with other molecules. This area of biology has become known, somewhat inevitably, as 'interactomics'.

The interactome

Work is underway to determine the interactome of a number of species, including *C. elegans* and human. This is a huge task. As an example, take one (any) protein — a member of the G protein receptor family — Frizzled. With how many other proteins does it interact? More than one, certainly: its ligands (a combination of the 19 known Wnts), co-receptors LRP6, Kremen, regulatory proteins (WIF, Dkks, etc.) and signal transducing proteins (G proteins, Dsh, etc.), to name only the interactions we already know about. In addition, we can multiply that number by the number of protein-encoding genes, add in a factor for interactions that we have yet to discover, and include interactions with other molecules (RNA, DNA, ligands, Ca^{2+}, etc.) and you will have some idea of the scale of the problem. Furthermore, early work in this field suggests that there is surprisingly little overlap between the interactome of different species.

The challenges of the interactome do not simply lie in finding out which proteins interact; presenting the data in a usable form is also far from straightforward.

Methods for detecting protein–protein interactions

A number of methods are available to determine whether two proteins interact. The 'gold standard' is co-immunoprecipitation (see Appendix 2). In this technique an antibody specific for one protein will precipitate that protein from a cell extract, along with another protein with which it can be assumed that the first protein was interacting. This technique is very reliable and does not yield many 'false positive' results (suggesting that two proteins interact when, in fact, they do not). However, it relies on having a good precipitating antibody for one of the proteins of interest, and it is also best used when we already know the nature of the second protein with which we are hoping to prove an interaction, as identification of an unknown protein from an immunoprecipitate can be difficult and time-consuming. Clearly, a more 'high-throughput' screening technique is needed if the aim is to systematically identify all the interactions of all the proteins in a cell.

Medical biotechnology

The most widely used high-throughput technique for detecting protein–protein interactions is currently the yeast two-hybrid system (see Appendix 2). The yeast two-hybrid system makes use of the Gal4 transcriptional activator. 'Normal' Gal4 is a protein with two distinct functional domains: a DNA-binding domain, which interacts with the promoter sequence, and an activating domain, which interacts with RNA polymerase. The two domains have to be close together in order for the downstream gene to be expressed.

In the two-hybrid system the Gal4 gene is split into two parts: one encoding the binding domain and the other encoding the activating domain. Each part is then fused to cDNA (see Ch. 4 and Appendix 2) encoding another protein, so that translation results in the production of fusion proteins. These constructs are expressed in different yeast plasmids. One plasmid will contain the 'bait' gene: part of the Gal4 gene fused to the gene for your protein of interest. The other type will contain the 'prey' genes: the other half of the Gal4 gene fused to a variety of genes with which your protein may interact — often an entire cDNA library.

To detect protein interactions, the yeast strains possessing each of the plasmids are mated, resulting in yeast expressing both of the fusion proteins encoded in the plasmids. If the two proteins interact, it will bring the binding domains and the activation domains sufficiently close together to activate the Gal4 promoter and lead to the expression of a reporter gene, which has been cunningly engineered to be downstream of the promoter, so that the colonies expressing interacting proteins can easily be identified. Figure 5.9 shows this in diagrammatic form.

The advantage of the yeast two-hybrid system is that it is relatively quick and easy to use. Its big disadvantage is that it throws up lots of false positives: proteins that clearly can interact (in the nucleus of a yeast and when fused to components of Gal4) but do not actually interact when expressed endogenously in a real cell. Thus this system is often used as a preliminary screen, with promising interactions being further investigated using co-immunoprecipitation, for example.

A number of other techniques are also available for detecting protein–protein interactions, including tandem-affinity purification, phage display libraries, protein microarrays and flow cytometry (see Appendix 2). The number of techniques available seems likely to increase as the effort to determine the entire human interactome gains momentum.

Can protein–protein interactions be predicted from sequence?

This is clearly even more of a gargantuan task than trying to predict just structure from sequence. Nevertheless, computational methods to predict protein–protein

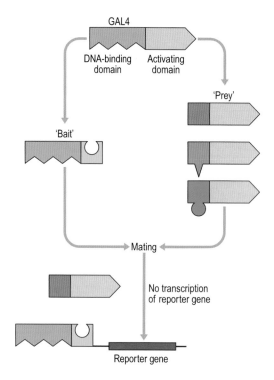

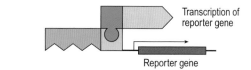

Figure 5.9
The yeast two-hybrid system. The protein of interest is expressed in yeast as a fusion protein with the DNA-binding domain of Gal4; this forms the 'bait'. The activation domain of Gal4 is expressed in another yeast strain, fused with a whole range of proteins which might potentially interact with the 'bait'; these are the 'prey'. The two yeast strains are then mated, bringing the bait and the prey together. If a particular cell possesses a bait and a prey molecule that do not interact, the reporter gene is not expressed. However, if the bait and prey molecules do interact, the reporter gene is expressed, allowing detection of the interaction.

interactions are being developed alongside the experimental approaches to determine the interactome.

It some cases it is reasonably easy to make an informed guess as to the likelihood of two proteins interacting. Proteins have evolved a number of key domains involved in protein–protein interactions and a number of these can be identified from the amino acid sequence. Thus, proteins which possess an SH2 (src homology type 2) domain are likely to interact with phosphorylated tyrosine residues; those with an SH3 (src homology type 3) domain are likely to interact with polyproline sequences.

However, for some proteins that are known to interact, it can be remarkably difficult to identify any components of the amino acid sequence which underlie this interaction. Proteins in the superfamily of G protein-coupled receptors interact — unsurprisingly — with G proteins. Moreover, different receptors interact reliably and reproducibly with different subtypes of G protein. However, despite extensive examination of the amino acid sequences of a range of receptors and G proteins, no sequence similarities can be detected between any regions of those receptors that bind G_s, for example, or distinguish those receptors from those that bind G_i. In this case it would seem that the interaction between receptor and G protein involves several regions of the molecule, so that overall shape is more important than regions of sequence and/or that other factors are involved in regulating the receptor–G protein interaction.

More sophisticated computational methods for predicting protein–protein interactions use a combination of techniques, including phylogenetic approaches (on the assumption that interacting proteins are likely to have evolved together) and comparison of regions of protein with regions known to interact in other proteins. A closely related field is that of protein–protein docking, which attempts to model the nature of the interaction of two proteins using information regarding their 3D structure.

difficult endeavour, which uses an enormous amount of computing power. Nevertheless, if successful methods could be developed, we would at last be in a position where knowing the genetic sequence of an organism would mean great progress towards decoding the ways in which that organism functions.

FURTHER READING

Cohen FE, Prusiner SB 1998 Pathologic conformations of prion proteins. Annu Rev Biochem 67:793–819.

McGuffin LJ, Bryson K, Jones DT 2000 The PSIPRED protein structure prediction server. Bioinformatics 16:404–405. http://bioinformatics.oxfordjournals.org/cgi/reprint/16/4/404.

Protein Data Bank: http://www.pdb.org. This is the old but more user-friendly version. Remediated and updated structural information is available via the Worldwide Protein Data Bank: http://www.wwpdb.org/

The importance of understanding protein structure

The potential of being able to predict the 3D structure and function of a protein from its amino acid sequence is enormous. As considered in this chapter, this is a very

Proteomics and metabolomics
Z. Nagy and D. Richards

In the wake of the Human Genome Project and the interest in 'genomics', other '-omics' have been coined to describe some of the scientific disciplines aimed at the study of distinct subpopulations of molecules in the cell. Descriptions of some of these '-omics' can be found in Box 6.1.

Proteomics

Based on the definitions in Box 6.1, proteomics involves the study of the expression, localization, function and interaction of all proteins produced by an organism — the proteome.

So how is this 'stamp collecting' exercise useful to medicine? Medical proteomics usually starts with a comparison of the proteins expressed by a diseased cell or tissue, with the proteins expressed by its healthy counterpart. Changes in the nature of the proteins expressed — their levels or their degree of phosphorylation, for example — can be detected. This can give important insights into the disease process, while also identifying possible new biomarkers for use in diagnosis or drug targets for the development of novel treatments (Box 6.2).

Studying the proteome

A variety of techniques can be used to investigate the proteins expressed in a particular cell or tissue. These include:

- 2D gel electrophoresis in combination with microsequencing techniques
- Western blotting, in which antibodies are used to label proteins that have been separated by electrophoresis
- immunohistochemistry and immunocytochemistry, in which antibodies are used to label proteins in situ in a tissue or cell, respectively
- enzyme-linked immunosorbent assay (ELISA), which is mainly used for the detection of secreted proteins, such as inflammatory cytokines
- more sophisticated techniques, such as protein microarrays and SELDI-TOF.

These techniques are considered in more detail below.

2D gel electrophoresis

This is actually rather an old technique, in which proteins extracted from a cell or tissue are first separated according to their isoelectric point using an isoelectric focusing gel. This separates the proteins in a single dimension. The 'lane' of separated proteins from this first gel is then excised and laid across the top of a second gel, in which the proteins are then separated under denaturing conditions according to their molecular weight (Fig. 6.1). Thus the proteins are separated in two dimensions, according to both isoelectric point and molecular weight; this gives a much better separation than can be achieved using one-dimensional techniques. Stained 2D gels reveal a constellation of a myriad protein 'spots'; the problem is then to identify what each of these 'spots' is.

This technique has been around for a long time but has recently undergone something of a revival, due to improvements in techniques for analysing the data. Pattern recognition software, such as Delta2D and PDQuest, enables the size and position of individual protein spots to be compared between healthy and disease samples, for example, and readily identifies any that have changed. Advances in protein sequencing techniques mean that it is now possible to excise these changed proteins and sequence them, allowing them to be identified using the wealth of protein sequence data available online (see Ch. 5).

Antibodies

Antibodies were first used for the detection of proteins as early as 1948, and they have been a standard research and diagnostic tool since the 1970s. The usefulness of antibodies rests on the fact that they provide a specific and versatile way of identifying particular proteins. They can be used in a variety of techniques for the detection, quantification and purification of proteins. For a consideration of how antibodies specific for a particular protein can be produced, see Appendix 2.

The advent of relatively cheap commercial antibodies (typically either mouse or rabbit IgGs) and antibody production services has made the production of home-made primary antibodies a practice of the past.

Western blotting

Western blotting provides both qualitative and quantitative information about particular proteins in cell or tissue extracts.

73

Box 6.1

The '-omics'

- *Genomics* is concerned with the all the genetic material of an organism.
- *Transcriptomics* is concerned with mRNAs, or transcripts in a particular tissue. It encompasses the entire set of mRNA expressed while 'building, running and maintaining an organism'. Unlike the genome (which is fixed for a given organism), the transcriptome varies, depending upon the environmental context or developmental stage of the organism.
- *Proteomics* is the study of the complete set of proteins produced from the information encoded within the genome and is thus the complete set of proteins expressed by a cell, tissue or organism. The proteome can be defined as the proteins expressed at a specific time and under specific conditions, or the complete complement of proteins made by a given species in all its tissues and stages. It is estimated that there are 250 000–300 000 proteins in human cells, of which only around 10 000 have been fully characterized.
- *Metabolomics* is the study of all the small molecules within a particular biofluid, cell, tissue or organism. Of particular interest are the small molecules that are involved in the metabolic processes of the cell; hence the name.

Box 6.2

The HER2 antigen and breast cancer

In many breast cancers, the HER2 protein is found to be over-expressed compared with healthy breast tissue and less aggressive forms of breast cancer. HER2 is still routinely detected in diagnostic laboratories using immunohistochemistry, in which a labelled antibody specific for the protein (in this case, Herceptin®) is used to visualize the protein.

HER2 expression has become established as a marker for more aggressive forms of breast cancer. Moreover, the over-expression of HER2 appears to cause the increase in cell growth, and inhibiting the action of the HER2 protein with the antibody is an effective treatment in HER2 positive breast cancers (see Chs 3 and 9 for more information).

The procedure is very simple and involves the size-dependent separation of proteins on a polyacrylamide gel, followed by transfer to a membrane and then immunolabelling. The principle of immunolabelling is identical to that of immunohistochemistry (Fig. 6.2). The difference is that the target protein is attached to a membrane.

The assay has the advantage that non-specific labelling is fairly easy to distinguish from specific labelling on the basis of molecular weight. It is also more readily quantifiable — albeit with caution. Some post-translational modifications can also be detected using Western blotting, including glycosylation and phosphorylation.

The major drawback of Western blotting is its sensitivity to proteolytic fragmentation of proteins in post-mortem tissues. It also requires a relatively large amount of protein extract from frozen tissues or cell culture samples, and only allows the analysis of a single protein at the time.

Immunohistochemistry and immunocytochemistry

These techniques are widely used both in diagnostics and basic research (Box 6.3).

The process begins with the preparation of tissue sections or cells, e.g. from clinical biopsies. This is followed by 'antigen retrieval' to improve access of the antibody to the antigen. This may involve many different procedures, such as microwave heating, enzymatic digestion and chemical treatments. The choice of retrieval technique depends on the nature of the sample, the length of fixation time and the antigen of interest.

The choice of detection technique is most often dictated by the abundance of the antigen in the tissues or cells to be analysed. Nowadays, many different amplification systems are commercially available which allow the study of proteins present in very small quantities. While most detection techniques (using coloured or fluorescent labels) do not allow more than a qualitative assessment, the use of radioactively labelled antibodies followed by autoradiography allows the quantification of proteins in tissue sections or cells.

ELISA

In ELISA, either the antigen or the 'capturing' antibody is attached to a plastic plate. The ELISA technique is less sensitive to proteolytic degradation than Western blotting and can provide very accurate measurements of specific proteins.

Since the technique allows the analysis of tissue and cell extracts, it requires accurate controls to diminish artefacts due to changes in cell numbers and variations in the relative ratio of different cell types in the samples. It does not provide information on post-translational modification of proteins, nor on possible protein isoforms, unless isoform-specific antibodies are available. The analysis of subcellular localization of proteins by ELISA is only possible if the tissue samples are very carefully fractionated to allow the separation of different cellular components.

One major advantage of ELISA is that it can be automated, allowing the routine quantitative assessment

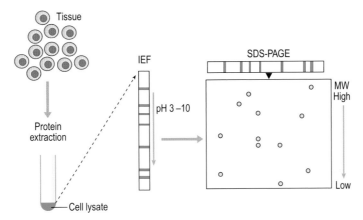

Figure 6.1
The main principles of 2D gel electrophoresis. Protein is extracted from sample tissue and loaded on an isoelectric focusing (IEF) gel which separates proteins according to their isoelectric point. This gel is then turned through 90° and placed on top of an SDS polyacrylamide gel, where proteins are separated according to their molecular weight.

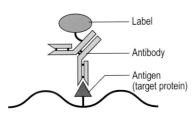

Figure 6.2
Detection of a protein by a labelled antibody.

of proteins in tissue extracts or body fluids. High-throughput (96 well format) ELISA kits are commercially available and are used by clinical diagnostic laboratories. For example, ELISA has been used for a long time to detect antibodies against cytomegalovirus, rubella and *Toxoplasma* in the serum of pregnant women; these pathogens have the potential to cause serious damage to the developing fetus and so the mother's immune status is of prime importance.

Similar ELISA-based assays are used for the detection of auto-antibodies in autoimmune diseases, and for disease biomarker assessment in situations such as inflammatory conditions, cardiomyopathy and different types of tumour. The sensitivity and specificity of these tests are good and clinical studies indicate that their use in everyday clinical diagnostics adds greatly to the accuracy of diagnosis.

As with most of the antibody-based techniques, a limitation of ELISA-based diagnostic assays is that they can test for a single or at most only a few biomarkers at a time.

Protein microarrays

Protein microarrays have been developed using similar principles to those used in the gene-based microarrays considered in Chapter 3. There are various types

> **Box 6.3**
>
> **Expression of CXCR4 in non-small cell lung cancer**
>
> CXCR4 is a chemokine receptor implicated in the metastasis of a number of different types of cancer. Immunohistochemical analysis of CXCR4 expression in samples from patients with early-stage non-small cell lung cancer suggested that, in these patients, strong nuclear staining for CXCR4 was associated with significantly better disease outcome and longer survival than in patients without nuclear staining for this protein.

of protein microarray which can be used to detect and quantify proteins. The ones most widely used at present are antibody microarrays.

Antibody microarrays

In an antibody microarray up to 1000 capturing antibodies (often monoclonal) are immobilized on to a plate or slide. The array is incubated with the protein sample, and interactions of the proteins with the antibodies are detected:

- directly by fluorescence (a label-based assay), or
- using a second antibody to detect the bound proteins (a sandwich assay; see Fig. 6.3).

The development of antibody arrays overcomes the limitations of ELISA assays by allowing testing for multiple markers simultaneously. The clinical applications include:

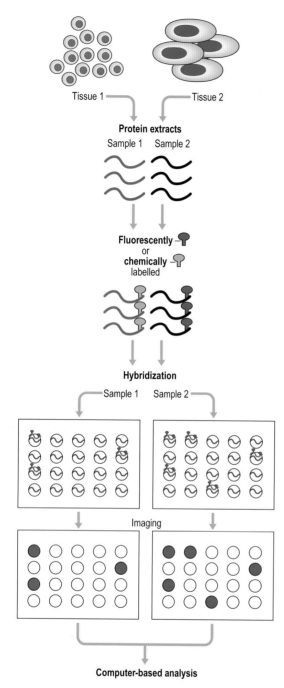

Figure 6.3
Comparison of protein expression patterns from different tissue samples using an antibody microarray (see text).

- measurement of cytokine expression levels
- detection of multiple bacteria and viruses
- diagnosis of allergies
- detection of protein–protein interactions
- protein modifications.

Furthermore, the expression pattern of different proteins may determine the choice of therapy given to individual patients (see Ch. 9).

At present, very limited numbers of commercial antibody arrays are available, so most antibody arrays have to be 'home-made', which is expensive and time-consuming. The few antibody arrays that are commercially available (from Novagen and Whatman Schleicher & Schuell) do not yet have the necessary regulatory approval for use in clinical diagnostics. However, with growing numbers of approved disease biomarkers it seems only a matter of time before relatively cheap antibody arrays will become available.

Tissue microarrays

Tissue microarrays have been developed as a way of dramatically improving the efficiency of immunohistological testing and in situ hybridization studies (see Ch. 3). Tiny tissue samples (0.6 mm in diameter) are obtained using hollow needles and embedded into a paraffin block in a precise pattern (the array). Each block can contain several hundred samples, from different patients and/or different tissues. Each paraffin block is then sliced on a microtome into 100–500 sections; each of these thin sections can then be mounted on to a slide and probed with a different antibody or oligonucleotide. Thus multiple samples can be tested with multiple antibodies simultaneously. Tissue microarrays have proved especially useful in the analysis of cancer samples.

Chemical compound microarrays

In chemical compound microarrays, various chemicals are immobilized on a glass or plastic surface. These are then used to 'trap' proteins or other molecules that interact with them. This kind of array has enormous potential in drug discovery.

The detection of CD20 surface antigen in lymphoma patients by immunohistochemistry or flow cytometry aids the follow-up of patients treated with Mabthera, a monoclonal antibody infusion with rituximab as active ingredient.

SELDI-TOF

While protein expression and quantitative protein measurements can still be carried out with electrophoresis-based techniques, mass spectrometry has increased the sensitivity and specificity of results and allows a high-throughput analysis of protein samples.

SELDI-TOF stands for surface-enhanced laser desorption/ionization with time of flight mass spectrometry. The principle of the technique is the exploitation of differential binding of different proteins to different surfaces. The 'chips' capture different types of protein (acidic, basic, antigens, etc.), depending on the nature of their surface properties; this provides a degree of pre-purification of proteins from the sample, which helps in the final resolution of the proteins by mass spectrometry. The chips are then bombarded using a laser, so that the bound proteins and peptides become ionized and unbound. The released proteins are then characterized

Table 6.1
Tyrosine kinase inhibitors used in the treatment of cancer

Name	Indication	Mechanism of action
Gefitinib (Iressa®)	Lung and pancreas	Inhibits a mutated EGFR
Erlotinib (Tarceva®)	Lung and pancreas	Inhibits a mutated EGFR
Imatinib (Gleevec®)	GIST and chronic myeloid leukaemia	Inhibits EGFR with a specific mutation found in some leukaemias and gastrointestinal tumours
Sorafenib (Nexavar®)	Renal cell	Targets multiple tyrosine kinase receptors
Sunitinib (Sutent®)	Renal cell	A multi-targeted tyrosine kinase inhibitor which targets VEGFR, PDGFR, KIT, RET and FLT3. The agent has both anti-tumour and anti-angiogenic activity

(GIST = gastrointestinal stromal tumour)

using time of flight analysis in a mass spectrometer. The dedicated software quantifies the mass and relative abundance of each protein in a sample. Using this technology, the analysis of 300–800 proteins from 20 microlitres of plasma counts as a 'routine procedure'.

SELDI-TOF is a versatile proteomic tool but provides information only on the molecular weight, abundance and biophysical characteristics of the proteins. Further techniques, e.g. sequencing, are required for the identification of particular protein species identified using this technique.

Proteomic markers of disease

Most diseases are multifactorial, with different genetic and environmental components, each of which could potentially alter the function or expression of different proteins. Therefore it is perhaps not surprising that most disease conditions seem to be associated with changes in many proteins (protein maps) rather than with alteration of a single protein marker. Large protein mapping studies indicate that it is often not realistic to envisage the clinical usefulness of a single protein marker for diagnostic purposes, or to monitor disease progression and response to therapy.

An increasing number of studies indicate that the analysis of complex protein maps from cerebrospinal fluid (CSF) could greatly help the diagnosis and follow-up of patients with nervous system diseases. Similar studies from plasma have led to the discovery of several cancer-related biomarkers and markers of rheumatoid arthritis from synovial fluid.

Advances in therapeutic approaches

Besides the development of new diagnostic biomarkers, proteomics research has also led to advances in therapy. These advances include the use as therapeutic agents of:

- monoclonal antibodies
- specific tyrosine kinase inhibitors
- vaccines.

Monoclonal antibodies in therapy

The discovery of the up-regulation of specific proteins in certain cancers resulted in the development of humanized monoclonal antibodies targeting these molecules (see Ch. 10). Some of these antibodies (such as Herceptin®; see Box 6.2) bind to receptor proteins and block pathways essential for cell proliferation, metastasis and tissue invasion. Additionally, once bound to the cancer cell, these antibodies help to mobilize the patient's own immune mechanisms against the tumour. Antibodies have been conjugated with radioactive isotopes or toxins to kill directly the cells they recognize.

Tyrosine kinase inhibitors as therapeutic agents

The proliferation, invasiveness and metastatic ability of many tumour cells are growth factor-dependent. Indeed, mutation of growth factor receptors or over-expression of growth factors can contribute greatly to the growth of tumour cells. Tumour-specific expression of mutated growth factor receptors has enabled the development of therapies which inhibit the function of these receptors (see also Ch. 9). Examples of some of these tyrosine kinase inhibitors are shown in Table 6.1.

Vaccines as drugs

Vaccines are traditionally regarded as a way of preventing disease (see Ch. 7). Some of the new vaccines, however, are designed to be curative, and are being developed for use in such conditions as cancer and Alzheimer's disease (Box 6.4).

A vaccine against Alzheimer's disease?

The idea behind the design of a vaccine against Alzheimer's disease was relatively simple. It seems likely that β-amyloid accumulation in the brain is the cause of Alzheimer-type neurodegeneration and subsequent cognitive decline. It seemed possible, therefore, that 'vaccination' with β-amyloid could produce an immune response against this protein which would help to treat the disease. Unfortunately, active immunization against β-amyloid led to catastrophic consequences in patients and the clinical trials had to be aborted; the patients developed a dramatic immune response which resulted in encephalitis. This serves as a strong reminder that the targets for biological therapies have to be very carefully selected and, even then, may not always be easy to develop in clinically useful interventions (see also Ch. 10).

Metabolomics

The newest of the '-omic' sciences is metabolomics. Just as genomics, transcriptomics and proteomics are already providing promising medical advances, metabolomics promises a new level of insight into the functioning of complex biological systems.

What is metabolomics?

Metabolomics is broadly defined as the quantitative study of global metabolite profiles in biofluids, cells, tissues or organisms, and the response of these metabolites to numerous stimuli such as toxicants, disease, genetic modification, ageing or medication. Of particular interest are those low-molecular-weight metabolites (up to 1000 daltons) that serve as substrates and products in the metabolic processes by which energy is extracted from nutrient material and used to maintain the chemical and physiological processes that sustain life. We are probably all familiar with the hugely complex metabolic pathway charts that adorn the walls of many biochemistry student's study.

Indeed, it can be argued that it is the metabolite profile that represents the true cellular conditions and functioning at the time of sampling, and that DNA, transcripts and proteins are the upstream entities predictive of this. In other words, to quote Bill Lasley of the University of California, 'genomics and proteomics tell you what might happen, metabolomics tells you what actually did happen.'

How many metabolites are there?

The Human Genome Project has revealed that man has around 30 000 genes that can make around 100 000 different proteins. However, the number of metabolites known in man is far smaller, maybe in the order of 3–4000, although, for the reasons explained below, the exact number is unknown. This collection of metabolites is referred to as the metabolome, and may include numerous classes of compound such as carbohydrates, amino acids, lipids, purine and pyrimidine bases, antioxidants, enzyme cofactors, hormones, nutrients, neurotransmitters and vitamins. In addition, clinical samples may also contain drugs and their metabolites, and dietary components, as well as metabolites derived from gut bacteria.

But don't we already measure metabolite levels?

Levels of specific metabolites form the basis of many clinical diagnostic tests — for example, measuring blood glucose in diabetic patients. However, in these instances we target specific metabolites known to be of relevance.

In contrast, metabolomics approaches metabolism in a unified and completely unbiased multi-pathway fashion. For example, in relation to medicine, examination of the dynamic changes in the metabolite profiles between normal and diseased systems may give insight into disease processes. These profiles, and any subsequently identified biomarkers, may then be linked back to their genetic origins. In this way, metabolomic studies, rather than being unfocused, may more quickly generate hypotheses that can then be tested using classical research tools.

So how can we study the metabolome?

The wide structural diversity of the metabolome means that, unlike genes or proteins, there is no single analytical platform available at present that can detect and measure the full complement of metabolites in a clinical sample such as plasma or a cell or tissue extract. Indeed, it is for this reason that the exact number of metabolites is unknown. Although it is perfectly possible to profile metabolite patterns in samples of tissue such as biopsy material, initial metabolomics investigations in medicine have tended to focus on biofluids such as plasma, serum or urine that are available with minimal invasion. With most analytical platforms, some preliminary sample preparation, such as protein precipitation, desalting or solid phase extraction, is required. The next consideration is whether the clinical sample can be analysed directly, or whether it is necessary first to separate the metabolites by chromatographic or other means. In most cases, the complexity of the metabolome requires that a separation stage is carried out before analysis.

Separation techniques

If prior separation is required, three techniques predominate:

- *Gas chromatography (GC).* This is arguably the most mature separation technique and offers very high chromatographic resolution. However, GC can only analyse volatile molecules and this excludes many important classes of biomolecule. Chemical derivatization of non-volatile metabolites can increase the range of substances detectable, but this adds a new layer of complexity to the analysis of metabolomic data.
- *High-performance liquid chromatography (HPLC).* 'This can measure a much wider range of metabolites, both with and without chemical derivatization, but has poorer chromatographic resolution than GC.' However, as we shall see when discussing the analytical platforms below, overlapping chromatographic metabolite peaks may still be discriminated on the basis of other physical properties.
- *Capillary electrophoresis (CE).* This final separation technique has been far less widely used to date but is likely to grow in popularity in coming years. The most common configuration is capillary zone electrophoresis (CZE) but this is only suitable for ionic species. Charged and neutral molecules can also be separated by micellar electrokinetic chromatography (MEKC), in which a surfactant is added to the running buffer. The major advantages of CE-based separation techniques are very high separation efficiency, application to a wide range of metabolite classes, and the ability to use very small, even sub-microlitre, sample volumes.

Analytical techniques in metabolomics

Two analytical techniques (nuclear magnetic resonance (NMR) and mass spectrometry (MS)) have predominated in metabolomic studies, and indeed will continue to do so, although there is an increasing awareness that the addition of complementary techniques is needed to expand the number of metabolites covered. Detailed explanation of the principles of these analytical platforms is beyond the scope of this chapter, but basic explanations are provided and can be built upon by reference to analytical chemistry textbooks.

NMR spectroscopy

NMR spectroscopy exploits the magnetic properties of an atom's nucleus, such as ^1H or ^{13}C, and can provide important information on the identity and structure of

 Box 6.5

NMR metabolomics in the study of coronary heart disease

Pattern recognition techniques have been applied to ^1H-NMR spectra obtained from human serum samples and correlated with the patients' coronary heart disease status. This technique was able to predict not only the presence of coronary heart disease, but also its severity. The differences between the diseased patients and those with angiographically normal coronary arteries arose from changes in lipoprotein composition. These are present in serum in relatively high concentration, making direct NMR analysis of serum samples the appropriate investigative tool. Diagnosis of coronary heart disease would normally be made on the basis of angiographic examination, which is both invasive and costly, so here metabolomics offers a much cheaper and much less invasive diagnostic alternative.

Source: Brindle JT, et al. 2002

biomolecules. Clinical samples, such as plasma or urine, require little sample preparation prior to analysis, and there is no requirement for chromatographic separation. In addition, high-throughput sample delivery systems make the technique applicable to longitudinal studies. However, although many metabolites can be measured simultaneously, and whilst NMR is close to being a universal detection system, it is a relatively insensitive technique and is thus limited to the detection and analysis of only highly abundant metabolites accounting for less than 10% of the metabolome.

An illustration of the value of NMR metabolomics in clinical science is described in Box 6.5.

Mass spectrometry

With MS, molecules are ionized and can subsequently be dissociated into fragments characteristic of the parent molecule. Analysis of the ions (and fragments) in the resulting mass spectrum, on the basis of their mass-to-charge (m/z) ratios, can produce spectral fingerprints that can be matched to library data to assist metabolite identification. There are several variations of mass analyser, with the most sophisticated, Fourier Transform Ion Cyclotron Resonance (FT-ICR), producing such high mass accuracy that empirical formulae can theoretically be determined unequivocally in samples directly infused into the mass spectrometer without prior chromatographic separation; this makes it ideal for metabolomic analysis of biological samples. However, such equipment is extremely costly. Much more widely available are mass spectrometers that can be directly coupled to separation systems, as described above. Of these, GC-MS is the most developed, as the separated metabolites are already in the gaseous phase. With HPLC-MS, or indeed CE-MS, there is the additional challenge of interfacing a liquid flow to the mass spectrometer. Such interfaces must have a high ionization efficiency, should not confer any further chemical modification to the separated analytes, should produce no background signal from evaporated mobile phase components, and should not diminish MS function — for example, by ion suppression. All of these pose significant analytical challenges.

In contrast to the relative insensitivity of NMR, MS-based techniques are highly sensitive and versatile, but the range of detectable substances in a single run may be limited by the choice of instrumental parameters such as ionization mode, acquisition mode and the type of mass analyser employed.

An example of the value of MS metabolomics within a clinical scenario is described in Box 6.6.

Electrochemistry

Electrochemical oxidation or reduction has been used as the basis of a selective and highly sensitive detection system for redox-active biomolecules when coupled to HPLC separations. Although several configurations of electrochemical flow-cells are available, coulometric cells utilize high surface area porous graphite carbon working electrodes, and are capable of near to 100% electrolysis, giving high sensitivity and a stable and reproducible response. Coulometric electrochemical array detection (CEAD) is a more recent development of this technology, in which multiple coulometric cells (up to 16) are used in series. Coupled to an appropriate HPLC separation system, CEAD allows the resolution of a wide range of redox-active compounds, both on the basis of their chromatographic properties and on their intrinsic electrochemical behaviour across the range of the array, and is thus ideally suited to metabolite profiling. In many clinical conditions in which ischaemia occurs or in several neurodegenerative disorders, an imbalance between cellular oxidative and antioxidant mechanisms has been shown to be a key factor. The resulting oxidative stress leads not only to damage to macromolecules, such as proteins, lipids and DNA, but also to the production of abnormal redox-active metabolite patterns, so CEAD targets a particularly relevant group of metabolites when used in clinical studies. However, as with other analytical platforms, there are also disadvantages to this analytical approach. Because of the chromatographic separation stage, it is not readily applicable to high-throughput metabolomic studies, and only provides very limited structural information on key metabolites identified, in contrast to both NMR and MS.

The potential value of measuring redox-active metabolites in a neurodegenerative disease is illustrated in Box 6.7.

How do we analyse and interpret metabolomics data?

Whichever of the analytical platforms described above is used to obtain the data, the resulting dataset is extremely dense, with each individual sample providing hundreds, if not thousands, of datapoints. In addition, it is not necessarily the concentrations of individual metabolites that are important, but rather the relationships and fluxes between metabolites that need to be characterized and considered. To draw such information out of such complex datasets, advanced multivariate statistical analysis and pattern recognition techniques are employed, and this is commonly referred to as

Box 6.6

Metabolomics and mass spectrometry in the study of pre-eclampsia

Pre-eclampsia is a disorder of pregnancy, characterized by maternal hypertension and proteinuria, and is a significant cause of maternal and perinatal morbidity and mortality. However, it is clear the condition originates very early during pregnancy and long before clinical symptoms are evident. There is therefore a need for early diagnosis so that appropriate treatment can be instigated. Using a combination of gas chromatography as the separation technique and mass spectrometry as the analytical platform, these investigators were able to discriminate pre-eclampsia from normal pregnant controls on the basis of just three metabolite peaks in the GC-MS ion chromatogram from plasma samples. The study showed that one peak was raised in the disease while two further peaks were lowered relative to controls, thus illustrating the importance of the high sensitivity of the GC-MS analytical platform.

Source: Kenny LC, et al. 2005

Box 6.7

CEAD metabolomics in the study of motor neuron disease

Motor neuron disease (MND) is a rare but rapidly progressive disease that can affect both upper and lower motor neurons in adults. This study employed HPLC coupled to CEAD to profile redox-active metabolites in plasma samples from MND patients, and was able not only to demonstrate differences between patient and control groups, but also to identify a group of metabolites that correlated strongly with disease associated with the lower motor neurons only. Once again, some of the metabolites that distinguished between the patient groups were present at very low concentration, highlighting the importance of sensitive detection techniques.

Source: Rozen S, et al. 2005

chemometrics. Whilst it is beyond the scope of this chapter to consider such techniques in detail, they can be subdivided into unsupervised and the more powerful supervised methods.

Unsupervised chemometric analysis

This assumes no previous knowledge as to the category of the samples (for example, disease versus controls); hence the term unsupervised. The most commonly employed technique is principal components analysis (PCA): that is, a method of simplifying a dataset by reducing its dimensions. In PCA, the first principal component is that which contributes most of the variance to the overall dataset, with the second highest contributor to the variance being plotted on an orthogonal coordinate to it. Commonly, this representation of the data variation is displayed as a figure in two or three dimensions, with clustering of related sample categories within this graphical representation being indicative of commonalities within the metabolic profile.

Supervised chemometric analysis

These techniques allow modelling of multiparametric data on the basis of what is known about the category of the sample (for example, knowing whether the sample is from a 'disease' or 'control' group). Typically, part of a large dataset is used as a 'training' set, with mathematical models being derived to maximize separation between the known distinct sample categories. These models can then be applied to the remainder of the dataset to assess their ability to discriminate between the sample categories. Examples of commonly employed supervised techniques include partial least squares (PLS) analysis and partial least squares discriminant analysis (PLS-DA).

How do we apply metabolomics to clinical studies?

Suppose, for example, we want to use metabolomics to identify potential biomarkers that may discriminate between our 'disease' and 'control' groups. We can break down the investigation into four separate phases.

- In the first, appropriate biological sample types and analytical platforms are chosen, and the resulting datasets are then subjected to multivariate statistical analysis, as described above, to identify those metabolites that appear to discriminate between the 'disease' and 'control' groups.
- The second stage is to seek to identify these potential biomarkers, most commonly using MS-based techniques.
- Having achieved this, the utility of the new biomarker to discriminate between patient groups should then be tested on different patient populations using multi-centre studies.

- Finally, once the value of this diagnostic biomarker has been confirmed, conventional hypothesis-driven research techniques can then be applied to answer questions such as its genetic origin, its compartmentation within a cellular system, and why it is present in abnormal amounts in the disease situation. This may then give insight into the pathophysiology of the disease process itself.

Conclusion

Proteomics and metabolomics study very different types of molecules, using very different techniques. However, their underlying philosophies are similar; they both represent a 'model-free' approach to finding changes in cell function in disease, with the hope that these changes will prove useful as disease biomarkers and in the elucidation of disease aetiology and the development of new treatment strategies.

FURTHER READING

Brindle JT, Antti H, Holmes E et al. 2002 Rapid and noninvasive diagnosis of the presence and severity of coronary heart disease using ^{1}H-NMR-based metabonomics. Nat Med 8:1439–1444.

de Seny D, Fillet M, Meuwis M-A et al. 2005 Discovery of new rheumatoid arthritis biomarkers using the surface-enhanced laser desorption/ionization time-of-flight mass spectrometry ProteinChip approach. Arthritis Rheum 52:3801–3812.

Glazyrin A, Shen X, Blanc V, Eliason JF 2007 Direct detection of herceptin/trastuzumab binding on breast tissue sections. J Histochem Cytochem 55:25–33.

Greenbaum D, Luscombe NM, Jansen R et al. 2001 Interrelating different types of genomic data, from proteome to secretome: 'oming in on function. Genome Res 11:1463–1468.

Huang RP, Chen L-P, Yang W, Huang R 2004 ELISA-based protein arrays: multiplexed sandwich immunoassays. Current Proteomics 1:199–210.

Kenny LC, Dunn WB, Ellis DI et al. 2005 Novel biomarkers for pre-eclampsia detected using metabolomics and machine learning. Metabolomics 1:227–234.

Khwaja FW, Nolen JDL, Mendrinos SE 2006 Proteomic analysis of cerebrospinal fluid discriminates malignant and nonmalignant disease of the central nervous system and identifies specific protein markers. Proteomics 6:6277–6287.

Maier M, Seabrook TJ, Lemere CA 2005 Developing novel immunogens for an effective, safe Alzheimer's disease vaccine. Neurodegener Dis 2:267–272.

Rozen S, Cudkowicz ME, Bogdanov M et al. 2005 Metabolomic analysis and signatures in motor neuron disease. Metabolomics 1:101–108.

7

Vaccines
D. Bartis

Vaccination is one of the great success stories of modern medicine. Widespread mass vaccination projects have led to the virtual eradication of once-feared diseases, such as smallpox or poliomyelitis, from the world.

Vaccination was first applied by Edward Jenner in the 18th century. He noticed that milkmaids who had acquired cowpox became immune to the much more serious disease of smallpox. Using this observation, he postulated that immunity must be the result of direct contact with the discharge from papules of infected cows. To test his theory, he inoculated a young boy with the discharge of cowpox papules then intentionally exposed him to smallpox. Fortunately, the boy did not fall ill, and Jenner's theory was proved correct.

The predecessors of many current vaccines were developed during the late 19th and early 20th centuries by pioneer immunologists such as Louis Pasteur, who developed the first vaccines against anthrax, rabies and cholera; Albert Sabin, who developed the oral polio vaccine; and Albert Calmette and Camille Guérin who developed the bacillus Calmette–Guérin (BCG) vaccine against tuberculosis. Developed in the 1920s, BCG is still the only licensed vaccine against tuberculosis.

Nowadays, however, the comprehensive use of modern biotechnology has enabled the design of new vaccines which provide efficient protection against a number of pathogens (e.g. hepatitis B virus and *Neisseria meningitidis*) that was not possible with the use of conventional methods.

This chapter will briefly consider the immunological principles which underlie vaccination, and how these have been exploited by some conventional vaccines. It will then consider how biotechnology is impacting on the design of new and improved vaccines.

Immunological principles

To achieve more than just a hit-and-miss chance of success during vaccination, an understanding of the cellular and molecular principles of pathogenic infections and the resulting immune responses is a prerequisite for effective vaccine design. These principles are considered briefly here; a more detailed consideration can be found in Abbas and Lichtman (2005).

The first line of defence during infections with many common microorganisms is formed by the macrophages, neutrophils and natural killer (NK) cells of the innate immune system. However, the innate immune response can rarely eliminate a massive invasion and it

is primarily there to 'buy some time' (4–7 days) until the adaptive immune response can stage a more effective and concentrated attack on the invading pathogen. As the innate immune response has no 'memory' and treats each pathogenic invasion as new, it is an inappropriate target for vaccination and induction of immunological protection. The adaptive immune system, however, produces a pathogen-specific immune reaction which leads to the elimination of pathogen, and this reaction is 'remembered' by an immunological memory. Activation of the adaptive immune system is thus the primary target in vaccination.

Vaccination traditionally aims for protection against bacterial (e.g. tuberculosis) and viral (e.g. measles) infections, although attempts have also been made to develop vaccines against parasite infections (e.g. malaria) and even tumours (see below). The sites of pathogen invasion are usually the 'linings' of the body: the skin and the mucous membranes. Infection of the lymph or blood can also occur, and these are especially dangerous conditions, as the risk of the infection spreading is much greater. The invading pathogens can cause either intracellular or extracellular infections that lead to the activation of both innate and adaptive immune responses (see above). The various immune responses triggered by invading pathogens are listed in Table 7.1.

Activation of the immune system is dependent on molecular patterns on the surface of invading pathogens which activate the innate immune system. For an adaptive immune response, unique molecular sequences, specific for the infecting pathogen, have to be presented to cells of the immune system, together with major histocompatibility complex (MHC) class II molecules by professional antigen-presenting cells (APCs). APCs are mainly dendritic cells and macrophages that phagocytose the extracellular pathogen and process their proteins into smaller fragments to be presented. If the pathogen is intracellular — most often viral — then the foreign proteins are presented to the surrounding immune system by the host cell with MHC I molecules which can also be recognized by the adaptive immune system. In the case of molecular changes during tumour development, altered self-proteins are also presented together with MHC I molecules and can activate an immune response, MHC I molecules being the ones advertising selfness on the surface of all nucleated cells and platelets.

These specific molecular sequences that are recognized by the immune system are the antigens. Antigens were originally defined as molecules or specific parts of molecules that stimulate an immune response (*anti*body *gener*ation). The modern definition includes all substances that can be recognized by the adaptive immune system. The

Table 7.1
Characteristics of different types of immune response

	Extracellular pathogens	Intracellular pathogens
Pathogen types	Fungi; protozoa; parasites; bacteria	Viruses; bacteria; protozoa
Antigen presentation	MHC class II	MHC class I
Immunoresponse	Mainly humoral	Mainly cellular
Th cytokine pattern	Th2	Th1
Effector cells dominating the response	B cells; plasma cells	Cytotoxic T cells; macrophages
Effector molecules	Antibody; complement	Cytolytic and cytotoxic proteins secreted by effector cells

important features of antigens are the epitopes: antigenic parts of the larger antigen molecule. A single antigen can contain several epitopes that are not only antigenic due to their primary (amino acid sequences), but also their secondary or tertiary structures. Some epitopes/antigens are more effective than others at triggering an immune response and these characteristics of antigens are important, as they aid the selection of the most antigenic sequences to be used as vaccines, for example.

In the adaptive immune reaction, APCs and antigen-specific T and B cells all participate. The different location of pathogens (namely extracellular or intracellular) can determine the combination of immune cells involved in the reaction. While extracellular pathogens trigger mainly humoral-type immune response, intracellular pathogens are eliminated mostly by cell-mediated immune response (CMI), although any effective immune response relies on both cellular and humoral immune mechanisms. The main principles of these immune mechanisms are summarized in Figure 7.1.

Studies of immune responses have also led to the realization that certain types of antigen are capable of activating B cells without the contribution of T-helper-derived cytokines. These antigens are called T-independent (TI) antigens and are characterized by multiple tandem repeat carbohydrate epitopes. Typical TI antigens are the different polysaccharides of the bacterial cell wall. In contrast, T-dependent (TD), typically protein, antigens require the co-stimulatory signals provided by helper T cells to induce effective B-cell response. Based on the pattern of cytokines secreted by the T-helper cells, two basic types of immune response can be distinguished: Th1 and Th2.

- Th1-type response activates mainly the cellular immune response.
- Th2-type response shifts the balance towards humoral immune response (see Table 7.1).

The aim of vaccination is to induce a T-dependent immune response, as:

- the titre of the generated antibodies is higher
- the effector mechanisms are more effective
- the immunological memory lasts longer
- efficient CMI can be induced (Box 7.1).

Deciphering the mechanisms of antigen recognition and presentation has become very important for vaccine design, as it has led to the realization that inoculation may not require the presence of the whole virus or bacterium. Rather, individual molecules can be used which can be modified to achieve the desired effect.

Additionally, discovering various ways of pathogen elimination has also aided vaccine design. In principle, pathogen elimination can be divided into two main groups:

- the antibody-independent mechanisms
- the antibody-mediated mechanisms.

Antibody-mediated effector mechanisms are summarized in Table 7.2. As we have described above, there is no strict divide between types of immune response. However, as antibody-dependent immune responses are more effective in pathogen elimination, it is desirable to use vaccines that trigger a high level of antibody production. Antibody production is the typical representation of the humoral immune response, in which activated and differentiated B cells produce antibodies.

In the primary immune response, when the host encounters the pathogen for the first time, low-affinity IgM antibodies are secreted by short-lived plasma cells. However, as the immune response advances, B-cell clones differentiate further in the newly formed follicles of the peripheral lymphoid organs. During this follicular reaction, B cells undergo affinity maturation and isotype change, governed by T-helper cell-derived cytokines. This will result in the production of non-IgM (IgG, IgA, IgE) antibodies of higher affinity. Most of these B cells differentiate into plasma cells, secreting vast amounts of antibodies, and some of them will persist as memory B cells of considerably long lifespan.

The most effective of all antibodies capable of facilitating pathogen elimination is the IgG type; therefore one of the aims of vaccination is to trigger IgG production.

Following the successful elimination of the pathogens, antigen-specific, long-living memory cells (both T and B cells) persist in the body. These memory cells are selected because they bear antigen receptors with the highest affinity towards the antigen.

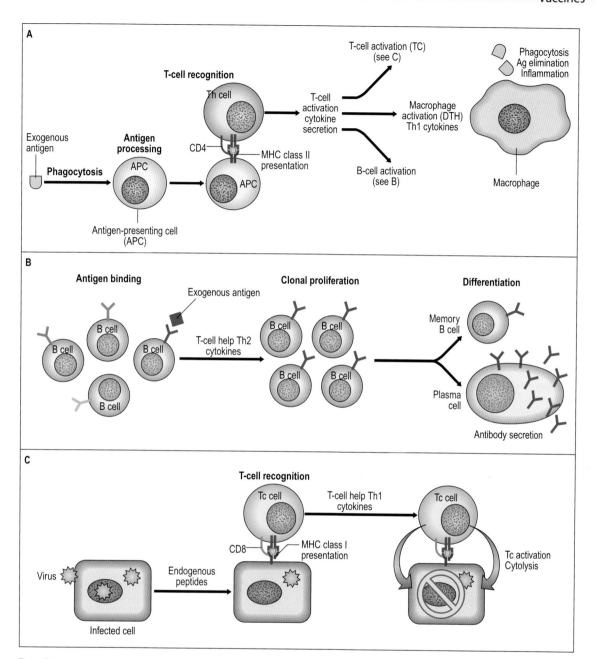

Figure 7.1
Schematic representation of antigen-induced immunoresponse. (A) The exogenous antigens (bacteria or soluble antigens) are engulfed by phagocytosis by antigen-presenting cells (APCs; dendritic cells and macrophages). Degradation of the antigen occurs and the fragments of antigen are presented via MHC class II for Th cells. Th cells bearing antigen-specific receptor and CD4 recognize the presented antigen and become activated. T-cell activation results in the secretion of various cytokines which are required for the activation of macrophages (Th1 help, panel A), B cells (Th2 help, panel B) and cytotoxic T cells (Th1 help, panel C). (B) Antibody production. B-cell clones bearing antigen-specific B-cell receptor proliferate and differentiate with the help of Th2 cytokines. Most activated B cells differentiate into plasma cells, secreting a vast amount of antigen-specific antibodies; a few activated B cells differentiate into long-living memory B cells. (C) Virus-infected or tumorous cells present endogenous antigens via MHC class I. Antigen-specific CD8[+] cytotoxic T cells recognize the foreign antigen and become activated. Activation results in the lysis of the target cell and also in clonal proliferation of antigen-specific Tc cells.

As a result of immunological memory, the next time the pathogen is encountered, a secondary or memory-type immune response will be elicited. This is characterized by rapid clonal proliferation of the pre-formed memory cells, quick production of high-affinity pathogen-specific antibodies and an effective cellular immune response. This will ideally prevent the establishment of infection or — if infection still occurs — the course of the disease is markedly milder.

The special ability to develop a pathogen (antigen)-specific 'immunological memory' is a prerequisite for long-lasting protection from a specific pathogen and is the primary aim of vaccination.

Box 7.1

TI and TD responses to pneumococcal vaccines

A good example of how changing a TI antigen to a TD antigen can improve a vaccine is shown by the new pneumococcal conjugate vaccine (PCV). The original pneumococcus polysaccharide vaccine (PPV) contained purified bacterial polysaccharides, a typical TI antigen. Unfortunately, PPV proved to be ineffective in infants, who are prone to pneumococcal infections. Moreover, even in adults, the protection provided by PPV lasted only for a very limited period. The new vaccine, PCV, however, contains bacterial polysaccharides conjugated to a protein carrier (namely diphtheria toxoid). As the new PCV induces efficient TD immune response instead of the original TI response against pneumococcal antigens, the protection is more effective and lasts considerably longer than that afforded by PPV.

Active and passive immunization

There are two main mechanisms by which the response of the immune system to an infection can be improved: namely, passive and active immunization. In passive immunization preformed antibodies are administered, while during active immunization the immunogenic substance(s) is administered that requires the active participation of the host's immune system, leading to long-lasting memory. The terms 'active immunization' and 'vaccination' mean essentially the same thing.

- *Passive immunization* tends to be used when the patient needs immediate protection or is immunocompromised. For example, patients with symptoms of tetanus (lockjaw) are treated with antibodies against tetanus toxin. In the past, these antibodies were obtained from horse or cow serum, but this had the potential for serious allergic responses to the non-human proteins. Today purified human immunoglobulins are used for passive immunization.
- *Active vaccination* is administered for preventive purposes. While passive immunization provides protection for only a few weeks (the half-life of human IgG in the serum is approximately 23 days), a good vaccine may provide protection for a lifetime. Some of the differences between active and passive immunization are summarized in Table 7.3.

Conventional vaccines

Live-attenuated vaccines

The initial approach to vaccination involved the administration of live pathogens that had been weakened (attenuated) in order to reduce their pathogenicity.

Table 7.2
Antibody-mediated effector mechanisms

Effector mechanism	Complement activation	Antibody-dependent cellular cytotoxicity (ADCC)	Neutralization	Opsonization
Antibody isotype	$IgM > IgG_3 > IgG_1$	IgG_1; IgG_3; IgE	IgG; IgA	IgG_1; IgG_3
Short description	Complement proteins activated by antibodies (classical pathway) are able to kill microorganisms by cytolysis	Antibodies direct and activate cytotoxic cells (NK cells, macrophages, neutrophils, mast cells, eosinophils); pathogens are killed by cytolysis	Antibodies bind to distinguished protective epitopes of the microorganism, thus inhibiting the pathogen from attaching to and/or infecting host cells	Antibodies (and complement proteins) cover the surface of the pathogen, thus facilitating phagocytosis
Partner molecules	Complement proteins	Fc receptors; secreted cytolytic proteins	N/A	Complement proteins; Fc receptors; complement receptors

Table 7.3
Differences between active and passive immunization

	Active vaccination	Passive vaccination
Immunization with	Antigen	Preformed antibodies
Required time until protection occurs	Weeks–months	Minutes–hours
Duration of protection	Ideally, for a lifetime	Few weeks
Role of host immune system	Develops own protective immunity	Only effector mechanisms are activated by administered antibodies
Cells participating	Ideally, all cells of the immune system	No cells or effector cells only are activated
Induction of immunological memory	Yes	No

Jenner, of course, used a different virus (vaccinia) which happened to induce cross-immunity to the smallpox virus (variola). In fact, attempts to reduce the risk of smallpox infection by deliberate exposure to the disease have a very long history. In the Far East, dried smallpox scabs were blown into the noses of individuals in order to induce a (hopefully) mild form of the disease which would confer immunity against subsequent exposure; in Europe and the US it was more common to inoculate discharge from a scab under the skin. If you survived this process of 'variolation' you would indeed become immune to smallpox, but unfortunately the risks of the procedure were very high; many subjects died from the initial infection and there was a further risk that this source of infection could initiate a smallpox epidemic. Unsurprisingly, following Jenner's discovery, variolation was quickly superseded by the much safer process of vaccination.

Live-attenuated vaccines are still in use and are among the most potent vaccines developed with conventional methods. Examples include the BCG vaccine and all the components of the combined MMR vaccine against mumps, measles and rubella. The pathogens in these vaccines were attenuated by growing them in non-human hosts or cell cultures so that the microorganisms become adapted to these hosts. Strains for use in the vaccine are then carefully selected for reduced virulence and a low risk of reversion to the pathogenic form. Another method for attenuating pathogens is chemical mutagenesis. *Salmonella typhi*, for example, was attenuated by nitrosoguanidine treatment and used for oral vaccination. These mutant bacteria lack some enzymes which are needed for virulence.

A list of live-attenuated vaccines in current use is shown in Table 7.4; one of the live-attenuated vaccines, the oral polio vaccine, is described in more detail in Box 7.2.

Live-attenuated vaccines have a number of advantages. They may infect the host via the natural route and show a controlled proliferation very similar to the virulent pathogen. Moreover, these vaccines clearly contain all the antigenic components of the pathogen and the 'natural' combination of these antigens is sustained.

As a result, the immune response is stronger than that typically produced by inactivated vaccines (see below), the immunological memory lasts longer, and both humoral and cellular components of the immune system are activated. A single dose of this type of vaccine may provide a sufficient level of immunity against the disease.

However, there are also clear risks with these vaccines, the most significant of which is the risk of virulent reversion, whereby the attenuated pathogen mutates in such a way that it regains its virulence and the vaccinee succumbs to the disease. Fortunately, this risk is very low with the live-attenuated vaccines in current use. Nevertheless, immunocompromised individuals should not receive these vaccines, as their weakened immune systems may not be capable of controlling the replication of even these attenuated microorganisms.

Inactivated vaccines

The risk of virulent reversion can be avoided by administering killed pathogens as a vaccine. The 'first-generation' inactivated vaccines were developed during the late 19th and early 20th centuries. A common feature of these vaccines was that they contained the entire inactivated organism. Inactivation was usually achieved chemically (using formaldehyde or glutaraldehyde, for example; Fig. 7.2) or by heat. Such vaccines were developed against diphtheria (croup), pertussis (whooping cough), cholera, typhoid fever and poliomyelitis.

Although vaccinations with inactivated organisms abolish the risk of virulent reversion, the first-generation inactivated vaccines proved to be poor immunogens and therefore less effective than live-attenuated vaccines. Moreover, constituents of some of the inactivated organisms are associated with severe adverse reactions; such constituents include the bacterial endotoxins which produce high fever and even endotoxic shock. The constituents of viruses seem much less likely to cause adverse reactions than those of bacteria, however, and there are some first-generation inactivated viral vaccines still in use, including the inactivated polio vaccine (IPV; Box 7.3).

'Second-generation' inactivated vaccines or 'subunit vaccines' consist of purified preparations of inactivated

Table 7.4
Currently available conventional live-attenuated vaccines

Vaccine	Disease	Symptoms/forms of the disease	Vaccination risks/side-effects	Epidemiological trends	Remarks
BCG	Tuberculosis (TB)	Pulmonary symptoms, meningitis	Lymphadenitis, osteitis, meningitis, systemic BCGitis	TB is a re-emerging disease, increasing occurrence of multidrug-resistant (MDR) strains	Discontinued in USA and in most Western European countries
Mumps (MMR vaccine)	Mumps	Parotitis, orchitis, meningitis	Fever, mild rash, temporary joint pain, thrombocytopenia, encephalitis	Rare in developed countries	Recommended for all children
Measles (MMR vaccine)	Measles (Morbilli)	Rash, Koplik-spots, pneumonia, encephalitis	Same as above	Rare in developed countries	Recommended for all children
Rubella (MMR vaccine)	Rubella (German measles)	Rash, swollen glands, congenital rubella syndrome	Same as above	Rare in developed countries	Recommended for all children
Varicella (MMRV vaccine)	Varicella (chickenpox), Zoster (shingles)	Rash, pneumonitis, encephalitis, zoster	Same as above, if given together with MMR vaccine	Decreasing incidence	Recommended for all children
OPV (oral polio vaccine)	Poliomyelitis (infantile paralysis)	Flu-like symptoms, leg pain, flaccid paralysis, respiratory paralysis	Fever, nausea/vomiting, diarrhoea, CNS symptoms, VAPP	Extremely rare in developed countries	Discontinued in USA and UK; recommended to be given after immunization with IPV
Yellow fever vaccine	Yellow fever	High fever, bradycardia, jaundice, kidney failure, haemorrhages	Fever, headache, muscle pain, vaccine-associated neurologic disease, or viscerotopic disease	Temporary outbreaks in endemic areas	Advised for travellers
Typhoid vaccine	Typhoid fever	High fever, abdominal pain, rash, constipation/diarrhoea, CNS symptoms	Fever, gastrointestinal symptoms	Common in developing countries	Advised for travellers
Vaccinia vaccine	Smallpox	High fever, pustules all over the body, including palms and soles	Fever, pustule at injection site, lymphadenitis, skin lesions, encephalitis	Eradicated worldwide; risk of outbreak as a result of malevolent action	Excellent vector for recombinant proteins for vaccination
Adenovirus types 4 and 7	Acute adenoviral respiratory infection	Rhinitis, conjunctivitis, pharyngitis, atypical pneumonia	Flu-like symptoms	Adenoviruses 4 and 7 responsible for 60% of all acute respiratory diseases among US military recruits	Currently available only for US military services

Box 7.2

Oral polio vaccine — a live-attenuated virus

Poliovirus is the cause of poliomyelitis (polio) or infantile paralysis. Polio is an acute viral infectious disease, spread from person to person via the faecal–oral route. Despite polio's fearsome reputation, approximately 90% of polio infections are asymptomatic and about 9% develop mild, flu-like symptoms. Less than 1% of the infected have CNS symptoms: headache, neck stiffness, and paralysis, which usually affects the lower extremities.

The oral polio vaccine (OPV) was developed by Albert Sabin in the late 1950s. The vaccine consists of wild-type human polio virus attenuated by serial passages on simian kidney epithelial cells at lower than normal temperatures. This treatment leads to mutations in the virus that reduce its ability to infect nervous tissue. The vaccine is administered orally, with a few drops of the vaccine being swallowed. This has the advantage of developing a local mucosal immunity and the formation of neutralizing IgA antibodies against polio, which is considered to be the most effective protection, since the wild-type infection also occurs via the oral pathway. The virus can replicate in the person vaccinated, so his or her close contacts are also exposed to the virus; this is clearly a risk but can also be seen as an advantage, as these contacts are also likely to become immune. Children are advised to have two doses of OPV between 4 and 6 months of age and a booster OPV dose later, around 12–15 months. The vaccine is effective and provides a life-long immunity against poliomyelitis.

The main risk with this vaccine is the development of vaccine-associated polio paralysis (VAPP), in which the person vaccinated succumbs to full-blown, paralysing polio. The incidence of VAPP is small, at around one case per 1 million vaccinations. However, as the incidence of polio infection in the developed world has decreased dramatically, it had been thought that the risk of the vaccine might outweigh the risk from the disease and regular OPV vaccination has been discontinued in the USA since 2000. In many countries, it is recommended that OPV vaccination should take place after IPV (inactivated polio vaccine; see Box 7.3 below) vaccination to reduce the risk of VAPP.

Claims have been made that AIDS may have arisen due to mass vaccination in Central Africa in the 1950s with an experimental OPV contaminated with simian immunodeficiency virus from the simian kidney cells used in its production. This hypothesis is not generally supported within the scientific community.

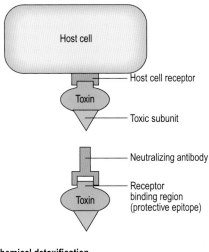

Chemical detoxification

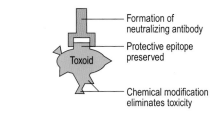

Genetic detoxification

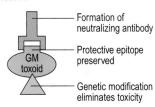

Figure 7.2
Pathogen detoxification. Bacterial exotoxins usually have a region responsible for toxicity and another region responsible for host-cell binding. The toxin has to bind to a cell-surface receptor to exert its toxic effects. The formation of a neutralizing antibody prevents the toxin from binding the cell surface receptor, thus abolishing its toxic nature. Chemical modification eliminates the toxic effects through formaldehyde groups bound to the toxin (represented by green triangles here) but the protective epitope is preserved; thus the formation of the protective antibody can be induced. Genetic inactivation is performed through modifications introduced in the DNA sequence encoding the region responsible for toxicity. The protective epitope is left unaltered so the potential of inducing neutralizing antibodies is retained.

The preparation of the so-called 'third-generation' inactivated vaccines involves precise purification steps to leave the resultant vaccine devoid of toxic remnants. Examples are the new acellular pertussis vaccines (Box 7.4) and the *Haemophilus influenzae* b (Hib) vaccine, which consists of bacterial polysaccharide components conjugated to carrier proteins, such as tetanus toxoid. Table 7.5 shows some of the other inactivated vaccines currently in use.

In general, inactivated vaccines tend to be safer than live-attenuated vaccines, especially as they do not cause

pathogens, with the aim of retaining useful antigens whilst eliminating harmful constituents of the organism, such as the bacterial endotoxins. Many of these vaccines consist of chemically inactivated bacterial exotoxins, or toxoids, such as those involved in diphtheria or tetanus.

Box 7.3

Inactivated polio vaccine

The first polio vaccine was an inactivated vaccine (IPV) developed by Jonas Salk in 1955. IPV is administered by injection. It contains three pathogenic polio strains inactivated by formaldehyde treatment. Originally it was cultured on simian kidney cells but in the 1980s a new IPV was developed. In this new vaccine, the virus is cultured on human cells. The new vaccine is very effective, producing seroconversion in 99–100% of the vaccinated individuals after three doses, with protective levels of neutralizing antibodies against all three virus strains. However, while these antibodies provide systemic immunity, the level of mucosal immunity provided by neutralizing IgA antibodies remains low.

Despite the availability of the inactivated vaccine, live-attenuated OPV (see Box 7.2) was the vaccine of choice for most countries from 1963 until the 1990s, as OPV is much more effective than IPV. However, naturally occurring polio infections have become extremely rare in the developed world and the vaccination policy of some Western countries has shifted in favour of the use of IPV, which provides less effective protection than OPV but with no risk of causing polio.

In some countries, sequential IPV-OPV vaccination is recommended, the rationale being that IPV will protect against VAPP (see Box 7.2), whilst OPV will provide enhanced immunity against polio infection.

Box 7.4

Pertussis vaccines

Pertussis or whooping cough is a bacterial disease caused by *Bordetella pertussis*. This is a highly contagious bacterium, spreading by droplet infection. After the initial flu-like symptoms, paroxysms of numerous rapid coughs emerge. At the end of the paroxysms a long inhaling period occurs, which is characterized by a high-pitched whoop (hence the name 'whooping cough'). Pertussis can be very serious, especially in younger infants who are prone to developing serious complications. These include pneumonia, secondary bacterial infections and CNS complications (seizures and encephalopathy) related to reduced oxygen supply.

The earliest pertussis vaccine was inactivated *Bordetella pertussis*, which was often combined with the diphtheria and tetanus toxoids in the combined DTP vaccine. However, the use of DTP was occasionally associated with seizures or encephalopathy, which seemed to be due to the pertussis component of the vaccine.

Today, the recommended pertussis vaccines are the 'third-generation' acellular pertussis vaccines. These are highly purified preparations that only contain pertussis toxoid, filamentous haemagglutinin (both of which are secreted by the bacterium) and one or more other defined components of *Bordetella pertussis* which aid in the generation of the protective immune response. Acellular pertussis vaccines seem to cause about ten times fewer adverse effects than their predecessors but they are somewhat less effective than the complete inactivated bacterium at inducing immunity.

infection. Side-effects of vaccination are usually mild and in most cases confined to local injection reactions or mild fever. However, inactivated vaccines often do not induce a sufficient level of cellular immune response. Inactivated vaccines always require at least two booster immunizations, and even then, protection declines within a few years.

Careful risk–benefit analysis is needed to decide whether to use a live-attenuated or an inactivated vaccine against a particular pathogen.

The use of biotechnology in vaccine design and production

Despite the undoubted success of the conventional approaches to vaccine production, they are not without their limitations. The live-attenuated vaccines tend to be effective but rather dangerous, whilst the inactivated vaccines are safer but also less effective, and the period of protection provided may be limited.

There are still a large number of important diseases, such as malaria, for which it has so far proved impossible to develop an effective vaccine. Moreover, the rapid evolution of many pathogens, such as the influenza viruses, can quickly render existing vaccines ineffective. With the contribution of biotechnology, it is hoped that modern vaccine technologies will be able to overcome many of these limitations.

Another potential benefit of biotechnology would be to decrease the cost of vaccine production, distribution and administration, making the advantages of vaccination much more widely available in the developing world.

Modern vaccine technologies

Biotechnology can be applied to vaccines in a number of ways and is allowing the development of a number of novel strategies for vaccination. These include genetically improved live-attenuated vaccines (see Fig. 7.2), recombinant vector vaccines, dendritic cell vaccines,

Table 7.5
Currently available conventional inactivated vaccines

Vaccine	Disease	Symptoms/forms of the disease	Vaccination risks/ side-effects	Epidemiological trends	Remarks
Diphtheria vaccine	Diphtheria or croup	Fever, sore throat, pseudomembrane in the throat, neuritis, arrhythmia, heart failure, diaphragm paralysis	DTaP: Mild local injection reaction, fever, vomiting, prolonged crying	Rare in developed countries	Recommended for all children
Tetanus vaccine	Tetanus or lockjaw	Muscle spasms, bone and joint damages due to spasms, spasm of laryngeal and respiratory muscles	DTaP: Mild local injection reaction, fever, vomiting, prolonged crying	Rare in developed countries	Recommended for all children
Pertussis vaccine	Pertussis or whooping cough	Coughing paroxysms, pneumonia, encephalopathy, seizures	DTaP: Mild local injection reaction, fever, vomiting, prolonged crying	Rare in developed countries	Recommended for all children
Inactivated polio vaccine (IPV)	Poliomyelitis or infantile paralysis	Flu-like symptoms, leg pain, flaccid paralysis, respiratory paralysis	Mild local injection reactions	Extremely rare in developed countries	Increased use instead of OPV in some countries
Haemophilus influenzae b vaccine (Hib)	Meningitis and other invasive Hib infections	Respiratory infections, ear infections, meningitis, epiglottitis, osteitis, purulent arthritis	Mild fever, local injection reactions	Greatly decreased since regular immunization was introduced	Recommended for all children; efficiently prevents Hib infections
Hepatitis A vaccine	Hepatitis A (acute hepatitis)	Malaise, gastrointestinal symptoms, dark urine, jaundice	Local injection reactions	Endemic areas in Asia, Central and South America	Advised for certain high-risk groups; routine vaccination in USA
Rabies vaccine	Rabies or lyssa or canine madness	Anxiety, confusion, agitation, abnormal behaviour, delirium and hallucinations, hydrophobia	Local injection reactions, headache, nausea, muscle pain	Wild animal reservoirs persist	Advised for certain high-risk groups; post-exposure treatment
Influenza vaccine	Influenza or flu	Fever, sore throat, muscle pain, secondary bacterial pneumonia, myocarditis	Local injection reactions, mild fever	Common disease; seasonal outbreaks	Annual vaccination recommended
Pneumococcus vaccine	Pneumococcal disease	Airway infections, midear infection, pneumonia, meningitis, sepsis	Local injection reactions, mild fever	Common disease; children, elderly and chronically ill are at risk	PPV23: purified bacterial polysaccharides PCV7: polysaccharides conjugated to carrier protein
Meningococcus vaccine	Meningococcal disease	Airway infections, midear infection, pneumonia, meningitis, sepsis	Local injection reactions, mild fever	Local outbreaks; young children, students in dormitories or military recruits are at risk	MPSV: purified capsular polysaccharides MCV: bacterial polysaccharides conjugated to carrier protein

recombinant antigen vaccines and nucleic acid vaccines. These strategies are considered in more detail below and are summarized in Table 7.6.

Genetically improved live-attenuated vaccines

Our growing insights into molecular pathogenesis are enabling the design of genetically attenuated microorganisms. Virulence can be reduced by the introduction of multiple, function-losing mutations into the DNA regions encoding pathogenic factors. Live-attenuated vaccines against the influenza viruses and rotaviruses are currently being developed using these approaches.

A genetically engineered live-attenuated oral cholera vaccine is already on the market. This vaccine contains a *Vibrio cholerae* strain which secretes a genetically modified cholera toxoid. The mutant toxoid retains its immunogenicity and is thus capable of inducing the formation of protective antibodies. However, the toxicity

Table 7.6
Comparison of different types of modern vaccine

Vaccine technology	General features	Advantages	Drawbacks	Examples
Genetically improved live microorganisms	Genetic inactivation of virulence factors while retaining immunogenicity	Sustained antigen presence; long-lasting cellular and humoral immunity induced	Risk of virulent reversion; nucleic acid incorporation into host's genome; not applicable in immunocompromised patients	Live-attenuated rotavirus vaccine, live-attenuated influenza vaccine
Genetically detoxified proteins	Genetic inactivation of toxicity while retaining immunogenic protective epitopes	Protein retains original conformation and therefore immunogenicity; highly safe vaccines	Subunit vaccines do not induce effective cellular immunoresponse; exact knowledge of nature and mechanism of toxicity is essential	Genetically detoxified diphtheria, tetanus, pertussis and cholera toxoids are now available
Live vectors expressing foreign antigens	Expression of pathogen antigens in harmless bacteria or viruses	Sustained antigen presence; possibility of expression of multiple antigens	Careful selection of foreign antigen needed; induced immunoresponse by vector may be different from that of original pathogen	Mycobacterial or HIV antigens expressed by poxviruses
Recombinant proteins	Recombinant proteins produced in bacterial, yeast and mammalian cells	High yield, consistent quality, safe production	Subunit vaccines do not induce effective cellular immunoresponse	HBsAg, HPV vaccines, recombinant gp120 (HIV envelope antigen)
Recombinant peptide vaccines	Protective epitope fused into a carrier protein; recombinant proteins expressed in bacterial, yeast and mammalian cells	High yield, consistent quality, safe production	Exact information on protective epitope is needed; subunit vaccines do not induce effective cellular immune response	Plasmodium antigen sequence fused with HBsAg
Synthetic peptide vaccines	Synthetic peptide corresponding to protective epitope	High production yield; safe and cheap production; easy purification; no contamination with toxic bacterial products	Exact information on protective epitope is needed; subunit vaccines do not induce effective cellular immune response	Experimental malaria vaccine, canine parvovirus vaccine
Nucleic acid vaccines	Plasmid DNA is injected into host	Safety of subunit vaccines combined with advantages of live recombinant vaccines; muscle cells of host express encoded protein	Nucleic acid incorporation into host's genome; long-term safety unknown; regulatory and ethical concerns; application restricted to protein and peptide antigens	Equine West Nile virus vaccine, experimental HIV vaccines

of the mutant toxoid is abolished by the introduction of site-directed mutations in the toxin subunit.

A genetically modified BCG vaccine termed rBCG30 is currently undergoing clinical trials. This BCG strain is genetically altered to over-express the highly immunogenic Ag85B protein. This antigen has been shown to induce a protective immunoresponse against TB in animal models.

Another genetically modified BCG-based vaccine under development is rBCGΔUreC:hly. This organism has been transfected with HLY or listeriolysin, a protein derived from *Listeria monocytogenes* which facilitates antigen-processing and cross-presentation and thus increases the activation of the immune system. The *ureaseC* gene has also been deleted from this strain in order to maintain the function of HLY (See Fig 7.4). The rBCGΔUreC:hly strain seems to induce a remarkable degree of protection not only against a laboratory strain of *M. tuberculosis*, but also against a clinical isolate of the Beijing/W *Mycobacterium tuberculosis* family; standard BCG vaccination is completely ineffective against this latter genotype.

The genetically modified live-attenuated vaccines may well be an improvement on conventional vaccines, but they still present a risk of virulent reversion. Therefore the live-attenuated approach has not been considered a suitable strategy for the production of an HIV vaccine, for example.

Recombinant vector vaccines

A variation on the theme of genetically modified live-attenuated viruses is the use of recombinant vectors as vaccines. In this approach a non-pathogen or attenuated microorganism is transfected with the gene for an antigen from another, more virulent organism so that they act as 'carriers' for the pathogen-derived antigen (Fig. 7.3). The viruses used most commonly as vectors are vaccinia, avipox and the adenoviruses; the most common bacterial vectors are BCG and *Salmonella* species.

An example of a recombinant vector vaccine is an experimental tuberculosis vaccine, which consists of a recombinant, replication-defective vaccinia virus, expressing the Ag85A antigen. This vaccine induces protective immunity in animal models and phase I clinical data have demonstrated its immunogenicity in both naïve and BCG-primed individuals.

A similar approach has been used to develop two candidate HIV vaccines. One vaccine is a recombinant, live canarypox vector, expressing the genetically modified HIV antigen gp120. The other vaccine candidate is a replication-defective, recombinant type 5 adenovirus vector (Ad5) expressing the *gag, pol* and *nef* genes of HIV.

The recombinant vector vaccines share many of the advantages of the live-attenuated vaccines and large amounts of antigens can be expressed. It should also be possible to express multiple pathogen-derived antigens in a single vector, so that a single vaccine can produce protective immunization against several different pathogens.

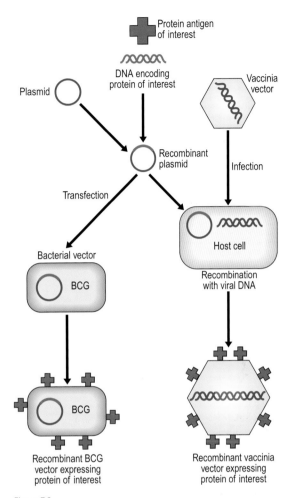

Figure 7.3
Recombinant vector vaccines. The DNA sequence encoding the protein of interest is inserted into an expression plasmid. The plasmid is used for transfection of either bacterial or eukaryotic host cells. When bacteria are used as vectors, the harmless bacteria (e.g. BCG) serve as a carrier for the foreign antigen. Then the recombinant bacteria expressing the foreign antigen can be used for vaccination. A frequently used viral vector is the vaccinia virus. A plasmid encoding the foreign protein and the vaccinia virus is co-transfected into host cells, and recombination of the foreign DNA sequence and the wild-type vaccinia vector occurs in the host cells. The new recombinant vaccinia viruses expressing the foreign protein will be secreted by the infected host cells. These harmless viruses are suitable for vaccination.

Dendritic cell vaccines

Production of antibodies as well as cellular immunoresponse relies heavily on the presentation of antigen by dedicated 'antigen-presenting cells', so it seems possible that the ultimate vector for a vaccine antigen would be one of these APCs. Dendritic cells are the main APCs in the immune system and are thus able to induce strong and sustained T- and B-cell responses against various antigens.

This is being exploited in an experimental vaccine against hepatitis C virus (HCV). Dendritic cells were derived from murine bone marrow and transfected *in vitro* with a replication-defective adenovirus vector expressing HCV core antigen. The modified dendritic cells were then injected back into mice. As a result, the mice exhibited a substantial degree of anti-HCV core cellular immunity. Moreover, the vaccinated mice became resistant to infection with recombinant HCV core-expressing vaccinia virus. These murine vaccination studies suggest that dendritic cell-based vaccination may be a promising new approach for vaccine design.

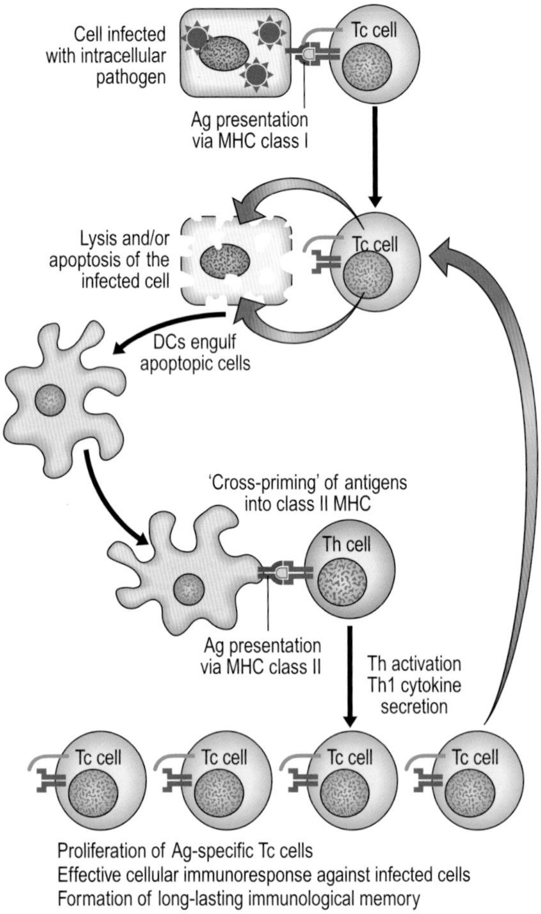

A dendritic cell vaccine is also being developed for the treatment of kidney cancer.

Recombinant antigen vaccines

Modern subunit vaccines are produced as recombinant proteins. This technique has the advantage of higher production yield, increased safety, constant and reproducible quality. The encoding DNA sequence is inserted into an expression vector, most often in *Escherichia coli*, yeast or a mammalian cell line. The cells are cultured *in vitro* in large industrial bioreactors and the product is purified from the supernatant or directly from the cells (see Fig. 7.5 and Ch. 11).

The hepatitis B vaccine is one of the most successful of these vaccines. It consists of recombinant HBV surface

Cell infected with intracellular pathogen

Tc cell

Ag presentation via MHC class I

Lysis and/or apoptosis of the infected cell

Tc cell

DCs engulf apoptopic cells

'Cross-priming' of antigens into class II MHC

Th cell

Ag presentation via MHC class II

Th activation Th1 cytokine secretion

Tc cell Tc cell Tc cell Tc cell

Proliferation of Ag-specific Tc cells
Effective cellular immunoresponse against infected cells
Formation of long-lasting immunological memory

Figure 7.4

Cross-priming enhances the immunoresponse. Cross-priming means that the presentation of a certain antigen of intracellular origin shifts from the original MHC class I pathway to the MHC class II pathway, thus initiating the formation of armed effector Th cells. This is a desirable process, since T-helper-derived cytokines induce the effective proliferation of ag-specific Tc cells, which mediate a more effective immunoresponse. Moreover, the formation of ag-specific memory Tc cells is also enhanced. The process is initiated when a cell infected by a virus of other intracellular pathogen undergoes apoptosis. Beside Tc or NK cells, this can also be induced by cytotoxic cytokines, such as tumour necrosis factor (TNF) or interferons. Apoptotic cells containing the intracellular pathogens are engulfed by APCs, primarily dendritic cells (DCs) or macrophages which treat them as extracellular antigens; thus antigen presentation occurs via the MHC class II pathway. As a result, antigens derived from intracellular pathogens will be presented via MHC class II for Th cells, thus greatly enhancing both cellular and humoral immunoresponse towards the pathogen.

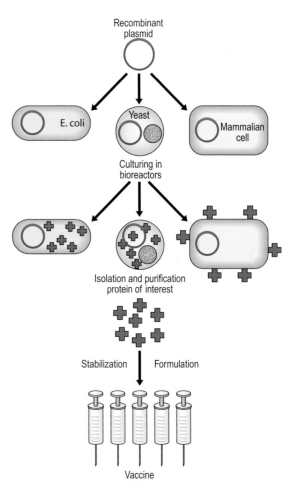

Recombinant plasmid

E. coli   Yeast   Mammalian cell

Culturing in bioreactors

Isolation and purification protein of interest

Stabilization   Formulation

Vaccine

Figure 7.5

Production of a recombinant vaccine. The DNA sequence encoding the recombinant protein is inserted into an expression plasmid. The plasmid is transfected into *E. coli*, yeast or mammalian cells. The recombinant cells are cultured in industrial bioreactors, allowing the large-scale synthesis of the protein of interest. The protein is then isolated either from the cells or from the cell culture supernatant. After appropriate purification and formulation the protein is used for vaccine production.

antigen (HBsAg) expressed in yeast cells. HBsAg particles self-assemble into virus-like particles (VLPs). These VLPs are very immunogenic, but as they do not contain the genetic material of the virus, they are not infectious. This vaccine is highly safe and relatively cheap, and induces a protective immunoresponse in high percentage of the immunized individuals.

A similar approach is used in the new vaccine against human papillomavirus (HPV), which is responsible for genital warts and cervical cancer. The vaccine consists of VLPs formed from the major capsid proteins of HPV serotypes 6, 11, 16 and 18. These four serotypes are responsible for 70% of cervical cancers and 90% of genital warts. The viral capsid proteins are expressed in yeast cells and self-assemble into VLPs. The vaccine also contains immunogenic proteins absorbed to amorphous aluminium hydroxyphosphate sulphate which acts as an adjuvant to increase immunogenicity.

An attractive idea for vaccine production is to express pathogen-derived antigens in edible plants. Experiments have been conducted with bananas expressing HBsAg, but this research remains at an early stage (see also Ch. 11).

Synthetic peptide vaccines

Instead of vaccines expressing a whole pathogen protein, it should also be possible to make effective vaccines that contain just the key epitope to be targeted by protective antibodies.

Synthetic peptides, produced in the laboratory rather than in living cells, have the advantage of cheap, safe production in unlimited quantities. Purification of the final product is also much easier than when produced in a pathogen or other cell. However, peptides are usually poor immunogens and the conformation of linear peptides does not always correspond to the 3D structure of native antigens. Cyclization of linear peptides may help to stabilize the conformation. Immunogenicity can be enhanced using a poly-L-lysine core and branching peptides to produce multiple antigenic peptides or by the conjugation of low molecular weight peptides to an appropriate carrier protein.

The epitope sequence may be inserted into the DNA encoding a carrier protein. This approach has been used in an experimental recombinant malaria vaccine, in which a malaria parasite-derived antigenic sequence is inserted into the encoding sequence of the HBsAg carrier protein. However, while this approach improves the immunogenicity of the epitope peptide sequence, it of course loses the advantages of a synthetic peptide.

In some cases the exact amino acid sequence of the protective epitope is not known, or it is a 'conformation epitope' formed by multiple non-continuous polypeptide regions. In this case, an initial peptide library-screening step is used, to detect which of a whole variety of peptides interact with the protective antibody. The peptides reacting with the protective antibodies can then be sequenced and put into large-scale synthesis for vaccine production.

Reverse vaccinology

Traditionally, the first step in developing a vaccine would require culture of the pathogen of interest. 'Reverse vaccinology' exploits the availability of the genome sequence of many pathogens to avoid this step. The sequence can be examined and likely antigen candidates identified using bioinformatics techniques. These antigens can then be screened as potential vaccines.

This approach has been used in the development of novel vaccines against type B meningococci. More than 600 potential immunogenic proteins were identified by genetic analysis of *N. meningitidis* B genome. Of these, 350 as tagged fusion proteins in *E. coli*. The fusion proteins were purified and used to immunize mice. Within a short period, 25 of these novel antigens were shown to induce bactericidal antibodies in the mice. Recently, a number of genome-derived neisserial antigens, which seem well conserved among the various *Neisseria* strains, have been tested as vaccine candidates. Since these antigens share high homology in various *Neisseria* strains, the vaccine might offer universal protection against meningococci. Clinical trials of these vaccines are expected to begin shortly.

Nucleic acid vaccination

Nucleic acid vaccination does away entirely with the need to produce proteins. Purified plasmids of DNA, encoding the antigen of interest, are injected into muscle. Some of the plasmids get taken up into cells, which then hopefully express the antigen on the cell surface and stimulate an immune response.

The first DNA vaccine was licensed in 2005, for the protection of horses from West Nile virus. A human vaccine against West Nile virus has also entered clinical trials. This vaccine consists of a single plasmid which encodes both the West Nile virus precursor membrane protein and envelope protein.

A number of studies have been investigating the application of DNA vaccination against HCV. The best results were obtained with plasmids encoding the HCV core protein. Researchers demonstrated that intramuscular immunization of mice with these plasmids elicited both cellular and humoral immune responses against the HCV core protein. Priming with DNA encoding HCV core protein and boosting with the recombinant protein itself proved to be even more effective. More recent experiments were conducted on mouse models with plasmids encoding non-structural (NS) HCV proteins; these were also able to elicit both cellular and humoral immune responses. A new method of DNA vaccination, using DNA-coated microparticles, has also been tested on mice and monkeys and found to be superior to naked DNA.

Compared with protein, DNA is much simpler and easier to produce and purify, and is much more stable in storage. These properties offer considerable advantages for vaccine production and distribution, particularly in the developing world. Moreover, DNA vaccines promise to combine the advantages of continuous antigen production, usually associated with live-attenuated vaccines, with the safety profile of the highly purified subunit vaccines, whilst also eliciting a substantial degree of cellular immunity. However, DNA vaccines only produce a low level of antigen expression, such that the immune response may be insufficient to provide protection. Currently intensive research efforts are being made to:

- find an appropriate immunostimulatory adjuvant
- improve the DNA delivery technique in order to enhance antigen expression.

There are some serious safety and ethical concerns regarding the use of DNA vaccines. These include:

- the risk of formation of antinucleic acid antibodies
- the possible incorporation of foreign DNA into the host's genome
- possible adverse effects of the long-term expression of a foreign antigen (see also Ch. 10).

Malaria vaccine candidates

Experimental malaria vaccines are good examples to demonstrate the great diversity of modern vaccine technologies. Worldwide, malaria is still among the leading causes of death, and an effective vaccine against malaria has been sought for a great many years. A number of obstacles tower before malaria vaccine developers. These involve:

- the poor knowledge about the nature of the protective immune response against *Plasmodium* spp.
- the lack of reliable and predictive animal models
- the great developmental and antigenic variability of the parasite.

Despite the great efforts made in this field, the release of a new vaccine does not seem imminent. Part of the problem is that the malarial parasite spends most of its time in the human body within either liver cells or red blood cells, where it is inaccessible to antibodies. Successful immunization is likely to require a potent cellular immune response.

The most advanced and well-documented vaccine candidates are aimed at the liver stage of the parasite (circumsporozoite). The antigen used for immunization is a repeating peptide sequence derived from a circumsporozoite protein (CSP) which is a known B-cell epitope. The CSP is found on the surface of both the circumsporozoite and the infected hepatocytes.

Perhaps the most advanced vaccine, RTS,S/AS02A, uses a VLP consisting of a recombinant protein containing the tandem repeat sequences of CSP fused with HBsAg. The recombinant protein is expressed in yeast and the purified VLPs are formulated with an adjuvant called AS02A for use as a vaccine. This vaccine is currently at the phase I/II field trial stage. However, while initial trial results showed that this vaccine produces an immune response in 30–70% of individuals, the protection from malaria wanes rapidly. Heterologous prime-boost immunization studies were also conducted with RTS,S/AS02A and an attenuated vaccinia vector also expressing the CSP antigen. Sadly, this approach failed to induce any increased protection against malaria.

Another strategy using the CSP protective epitope involved the synthesis of multiple antigenic peptides (MAPs) using the tandem amino acid repeats. This synthetic peptide vaccine also failed to induce efficient protection, possibly because only individuals with particular HLA haplotypes may have a sufficient immune response. Other synthetic peptide vaccine trials have been conducted using the CSP epitope linked to the 'universal T-cell epitope' sequences in order to 'bypass' MHC restriction.

Recently, field trials have been conducted using live vectors expressing the plasmodium antigen, TRAP (thrombospondin-related adhesion protein). A vaccination regime following a prime-boost strategy was used, with TRAP expressed in fowlpox virus (FPV-TRAP) used as the primer, and TRAP expressed in attenuated vaccinia (MVA-TRAP) used as the boost. Strong T-cell responses were elicited using FPV-TRAP priming and MVA-TRAP boosting immunizations, but the partial cross-reactivity between poxvirus antigens might reduce the effectiveness of the immunizations.

A DNA vaccine is also being developed which consists of a plasmid-encoding TRAP and a string of several malarial epitopes which are believed to be important in generating a T-cell response. The same malarial epitopes plus TRAP have also been expressed in MVA as a recombinant vector vaccine.

A number of other candidate vaccines targeted at the erythrocytic phase of the disease are also undergoing clinical trials. Details of these are summarized in Table 7.7.

Tumour vaccines

A number of companies are attempting to develop effective cancer vaccines, targeted against specific tumour antigens. Unlike vaccines against bacterial or viral infections, which are aimed at preventing disease, cancer vaccines are designed to be curative, helping the immune system to eliminate pre-existing cancer cells. Most studies have so far concentrated on melanoma and renal cancer, as these two cancers are most often associated with an effective immune response.

An experimental vaccine against melanoma is a protein–peptide complex consisting of a 96-kDa heat shock protein (Hsp), gp96 and an array of gp96-associated cellular peptides. The precise sequence of these proteins and peptides varies within individual tumours and the vaccine has to be 'personalized' using a sample of the patient's melanoma cells to ensure that the epitopes used are precisely those of the individual cancer.

Sadly, most of the early trials of tumour vaccines have not been a great success, but work in this area is ongoing.

Ethical aspects of vaccination

Vaccination programmes are most effective when a very high proportion of the population are immunized. Mass vaccination against a variety of infectious diseases

Table 7.7
Malaria vaccines currently under clinical development

Antigen(s) used for immunization	Type of vaccine	Type of expected protection	Current stage	Remarks
CSP-HBsAg fusion protein (RTS,S/ AS02A vaccine)	Recombinant peptide vaccine	Pre-erythrocytic (liver stage)	Phase I/II field trials	No long-term protection
FPV-TRAP/ MVA-TRAP	Recombinant live vector	Pre-erythrocytic (liver stage)	Phase I/II field trials	Results under evaluation
CSP linked to special core	Synthetic peptide vaccine	Pre-erythrocytic (liver stage)	Pre-clinical	Strong T-cell response elicited
MSP-1 and 2 with RESA	Recombinant peptide vaccine	Erythrocytic	Phase I/IIa	Efficient against one genotype
MSP-1	Recombinant peptide vaccine	Erythrocytic	Phase I field trials	Results under evaluation
MSP-1/AMA-1 fusion protein	Recombinant peptide vaccine	Erythrocytic	Passed phase I trials	Results under evaluation
MSP-3	Synthetic peptide vaccine	Erythrocytic	Phase I	Results under evaluation
GLURP	Synthetic peptide vaccine	Erythrocytic	Phase I	Results under evaluation
SERA	Synthetic peptide vaccine	Erythrocytic	Phase I	Results under evaluation

(CSP = circumsporozoite protein; HBsAg = Hepatitis B virus surface antigen; FPV = fowlpox virus; MVA = modified vaccinia Ankara; TRAP = thrombospondin-related adhesion protein; MSP = merozoite surface protein; RESA = ring-stage infected–erythrocyte surface antigen; AMA = apical membrane antigen; GLURP = glutamate-rich protein; SERA = serine repeat antigen)

was introduced in developed countries during the 20th century with enormous success. Thanks to these efforts, diseases such as measles, whooping cough and poliomyelitis are virtually unknown.

However, vaccination is not without risk, and some have questioned whether general obligatory vaccination contravenes basic human rights. It is probably because of the success of vaccination, however, that we enjoy the luxury of asking such a question; as the incidence of disease has fallen, some may now feel that the side-effects of some vaccines pose a greater risk than infection with the wild-type virus. This is a difficult issue, but it seems likely that if take-up of vaccination is decreased, the incidence of disease will increase.

The situation is not helped by controversies surrounding the safety of vaccination. In the 1990s it was suggested that there was a causal link between vaccination with the MMR combined vaccine and the development of autism. Wakefield and colleagues published a hypothesis that the MMR vaccine causes intestinal inflammation and consequent loss of intestinal barrier function. The damaged gut barrier might then result in the leakage of encephalopathic proteins into the blood and subsequent autism. They later claimed that the virus genome could be detected significantly more frequently in children with autism than in healthy controls. The controversy was widely reported and use of the MMR vaccine declined as a result.

The claims relating to a role for the MMR vaccine in the development of autism seem unsubstantiated. One Danish study included more than half a million children, representing more than 2 million person-years of study. Approximately 82% of children had received the MMR vaccine. The risk of autism in the group of vaccinated children was the same as that in unvaccinated children. Furthermore, there was no association between the age at the time of vaccination, the time since vaccination or the date of vaccination and the development of autism. Nevertheless, public confidence in the MMR vaccine has not fully recovered and vaccination rates remain low in many places.

It is essential to emphasize that the benefits of general vaccination greatly outweigh the risk of unwanted side-effects caused by vaccines. As soon as the ratio of vaccinated individuals falls below a certain limit, the susceptibility of the population increases and the disease will re-emerge. In the former Soviet Union, vaccination was compulsory and tightly regulated. However, vaccination programmes were neglected following the break-up of the USSR and a large-scale diphtheria epidemic occurred during the 1990s — the first such epidemic in an industrialized country for over 30 years.

There are other factors that put emphasis on the importance of mass vaccination and the efforts of developing new vaccines. A number of factors suggest that the death toll from infectious disease will rise in the near future. These factors include:

- increasing migration from the developing nations to the West
- the irresponsible and extensive use of antibiotics, which has led to the rising incidence of antibiotic resistance
- the increasing number of immunocompromised patients due to the HIV pandemic and immunosuppressive therapies.

There clearly remains an important place for vaccination in 21st-century medicine.

FURTHER READING

Abbas AK, Lichtman AH 2005 Cellular and molecular immunology, 5th edn. WB Saunders. Philadelphia, PA.

Banchereau J, Palucka KA 2005 Dendritic cells as therapeutic vaccines against cancer. Nat Rev 5(4):296–308.

Baumann S, Eddine AN, Kaufmann SHE 2006 Progress in tuberculosis vaccine development. Curr Opin Immunol 18(4):438–448.

Girard MP, Preziosi M-P, Aguado M-T, Kieny MP 2006 A review of vaccine research and development: meningococcal disease. Vaccine 24(22):4692–4700.

Greenland JR, Letvin NL 2007 Chemical adjuvants for plasmid DNA vaccines. Vaccine 25(19):3731–3741.

Kaiser J 2006 A one-size-fits-all flu vaccine? Science 312(5772):380–382.

Kanoi BN, Egwang TG 2007 New concepts in vaccine development in malaria. Curr Opin Infect Dis 20:311–316.

Martin C 2005 The dream of a vaccine against tuberculosis: new vaccines improving or replacing BCG? Eur Respir J 26(1):162–167.

Rappouli R 2000 Reverse vaccinology. Curr Opin Microbiol 3:445–450.

Schlom J, Arlen PM, Gulley JL 2007 Cancer vaccines: moving beyond current paradigms. Clin Cancer Res 13(13):3776–3782.

8

Transgenics

A. Bacon and J. Frampton

The study of medical genetics over the last 25 years, and more recently the completion of the Human Genome Project, have together raised the possibility of identifying inherited and acquired DNA sequence differences that are associated with many human diseases. Loss or mutation of an essential protein can directly cause disease, as seen with the absence of the β-globin gene expression in zero thalassaemia or aberrant function of mutated CTFR protein in cystic fibrosis, and it is now at least relatively straightforward to identify the genetic change underlying such diseases (see Ch. 2).

In contrast, disease susceptibility manifested as an increased life-long risk (e.g. cardiovascular disease) may result from a genetic 'profile' involving more subtle differences in several — perhaps many — genes and it will be a considerable challenge to elucidate the crucially different sequences.

Although genetic mapping and comparative sequencing projects can identify associations between DNA sequence and a disease or human trait (see Ch. 2), it remains necessary to test this link in a relevant model. Moreover, once DNA sequence differences in a gene or genes have been identified as the cause of disease, how can we move forward towards the development of therapies? The incredible advances over the last 20 years in our ability to manipulate the genome of inbred strains of laboratory mice have given us the opportunity to address these issues. Our aim in this chapter is to show how models generated using mouse genetics can form the cornerstone of investigative and translational biomedical research during the coming decade. More detailed discussion on the topics covered can be found in a number of excellent reviews and books on the subject (see, for example, Bedell et al., 1997; Hardouin and Nagy, 2000).

Prerequisites for the creation of a mouse model

A number of conditions must be met in order for a mouse model to be used to investigate a human inherited or acquired genetic disease:

- Homologous genes must be identified between human and mouse. Largely speaking, this condition is met for most genes, since determination of the mouse genome sequence and its comparison to the human genome reveal that more than 98% of genes are shared.

- Measurable biological parameters must be able to be compared between human and mouse. This requirement has been made possible by recent advances in phenotypic analysis of mice, including, for example, the ability to make measurements of heart and lung function and blood pressure in freely moving animals, and the use of imaging techniques such as magnetic resonance imaging (MRI), computed tomography (CT), ultrasound and dual-energy X-ray absorptiometry (DEXA) bone density scanning.
- Genetic changes in a specific gene in the mouse must result in a phenotype that correlates with the disease in humans.

The scope of mouse models and types of genetic modification

Increases in the efficiency with which a genetically engineered mouse can be generated and ever-advancing complexities in the nature of the modifications that are possible mean that mouse models can be created to test a wide variety of human conditions.

- Single gene defects
  Inherited
  Acquired
- Multigene defects
- Chromosome defects.

Although the mouse provides an excellent model for numerous human diseases, ranging from relatively simple inherited single-gene defects and acquired mutations (e.g. cancer) to more complex multigene or even whole chromosome defects, one note of caution is necessary, as it is not always possible to mimic human disease in the mouse. A mouse model cannot be used if:

- Homologous genes do not exist between mouse and man.
- The gene defect does not have the same effect in mouse and man. For example, mutation or loss of the retinoblastoma gene causes retinoblastoma in humans but not in mice.
- Physiological differences between mice and humans mean that disease progression is not the same. For example, the development of atherosclerotic plaques in ApoE-deficient mice does not lead to thrombosis.

Basically, two strategies can be adopted in the creation of a mouse model of human disease. These are:

- *Disease-driven, directed genetics*, in which a human mutation is identified and then a specific mouse model is made to mimic it. The models employ three broad types of genetic modification: transgenesis, gene targeting and chromosome engineering.
- *Mutagenesis-driven, non-directed genetics*, which relies on the selection of disease phenotypes following random mutagenesis, induced by chemicals of gene trapping.

Transgenesis and gene targeting generally involve the introduction of changes into one or a small number of genes. Some confusion can arise, as the term 'transgenesis' also tends to be used much less specifically to refer to any type of genetic modification that we will discuss. Here, we will use transgenesis to mean the integration of copies of DNA sequences encoding a protein of interest (the 'transgene') randomly into the genome, so as to distinguish it from gene targeting, in which a precise modification is introduced into a gene in its normal genomic location.

Non-directed genetics has considerable potential for the identification of genes that lead to a particular disease phenotype and it is being adopted in a number of large-scale projects. We will discuss approaches that involve chemical mutagenesis as well as a specialized version of transgenesis, i.e. gene trapping, in which the transgene acts as the mutagen.

Mouse models are becoming increasingly important in drug development and testing, and in the final section of this chapter we will examine how this is likely to revolutionize the pharmaceutical industry.

Disease-driven, directed genetics

Transgenesis

Transgenesis entails the integration of the exogenous transgene essentially at random within the genome. This integration must be heritable and therefore present in every cell, including the gametes. To achieve this, the transgene must become integrated at the one-cell stage of development. The number of copies may vary widely and the site of integration can determine the specificity and level of transgene expression.

The best-defined and most frequently applied method of transgenesis involves pronuclear injection of fertilized mouse oocytes with the linearized DNA transgene (Fig. 8.1). Large numbers of oocytes are produced from immature female mice by administering hormones which lead to 'superovulation'. The now-fertilized oocytes are harvested from the fallopian tubes approximately 0.5 days post-coitum (dpc). The oocytes are immobilized by a holding pipette in a position that allows clear imaging of either or both of the pronucleii. A micropipette containing the linearized transgene DNA is then inserted into one or both pronucleii and a small volume of DNA is ejected. The oocyte is then transferred into

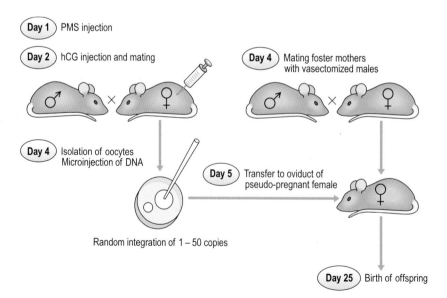

Figure 8.1
Pronuclear injection of transgene DNA. Superovulation is induced by successive injection of pregnant mare serum (PMS) and human chorionic gonadotrophin (hCG). The superovulated female is then mated and one-cell stage embryos are collected. These are injected with the transgenic DNA into the large pronucleus and are then reimplanted into the uterus of a pseudo-pregnant female; thereafter, they develop as a normal embryo.

Transgenic expression of luciferase

Transgenes capable of expressing firefly luciferase are proving to be excellent models to study the dynamics of clinically relevant biological processes ranging from tumour growth to the testing of drug therapies.

Luciferase protein, expressed from the cDNA under the control of a tissue-specific or inducible promoter, will catalyse the release of photons in a reaction requiring ATP, oxygen and the cofactor luciferin.

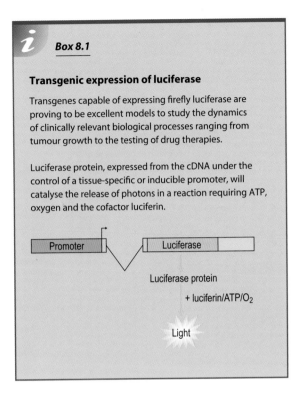

Conventional transgenes

The essential features of the transgene are:

- a promoter
- an intron element to mimic normal gene structure
- the coding sequences of the molecule under investigation
- a polyadenylation signal (Fig. 8.2).

The choice of promoter used to drive expression of the sequence encoded in the transgene is of crucial importance. Promoters that give rise to widespread expression of the exogenous gene are of limited use because of the likelihood of problems associated with inappropriate expression. Usually, the transgene is designed so that it should be expressed in specific cell types. Limiting expression of transgenes to a specific cell lineage can be achieved by harnessing the control elements of genes that are exclusively, or at least predominantly, expressed in that cell type.

More subtle use of a transgene: regulated expression

An alternative way of limiting transgene expression is to make use of a promoter that can be expressed in all cell types but is under the control of a regulator, which is expressed from a second transgene created separately, but brought together with the first transgene by breeding. The activity of the regulator is controlled by the *in vivo* administration of a small molecule that can be taken up by all cells.

There are a number of systems of this type, but by far the most widely exploited makes use of the tetracycline-dependent reversal of the binding of the bacterial tet repressor (TetR) to its DNA recognition motif, the tet operator (*tetO*). There are several possible permutations of this system using different engineered variants of TetR. Fusion of TetR to the transactivation domain of the HSV-1 viral regulatory protein VP16 creates a transactivator (tTA) that binds *tetO* in the absence of tetracycline. Wider applicability *in vivo* has been achieved by mutation of tTA so that it binds to *tetO* only in the presence of tetracycline. Therefore, by linking the gene of interest to an essentially inactive promoter element containing multimers of *tetO*, a transgene is created that should only be expressed when cells encounter tetracycline (Fig. 8.3 and Box 8.2).

However, there are two drawbacks to this approach.

- Firstly, induced expression will be in all cell types, perhaps leading to some of the same problems that might be encountered with a constitutive transgene.
- Secondly, it is difficult to limit the basal expression of the transgene in the absence of tetracycline.

the oviduct of a pseudo-pregnant female — obtained by mating females in oestrus with either vasectomized or genetically sterile males. After birth, a small sample of tissue is taken from each pup and tested for incorporation of the transgene using Southern blotting or PCR (see Appendix 2). The rate of transgene integration is highly variable and dependent on factors such as transgene size and sequence and DNA purity. In the hands of a skilled operator, approximately 5–20% of pups born alive should contain the transgene. Initial transgene-positive animals ('founders') are bred to ensure that the transgene can be transmitted to the next generation and phenotypic testing can then commence.

Since a transgene integrates into the genome at random, this can lead to spurious or inadequate expression patterns. Effects of the integration site, perhaps due to the vicinity of a powerful gene enhancer or repressor element, necessitate the generation of multiple founders in order to ensure acceptable transgene expression. Comparison of multiple founders also avoids confusion on those occasions when transgene insertion occurs around or within the body of another gene, leading to a change in that gene's expression and a phenotype that is not related to the effect of the protein encoded by the transgene. Transgenes are most frequently integrated as multiple copies in concatamers, which can be an advantage if over-expression is required, but can also be undesirable if the level of expression vastly exceeds that of the normal gene product. Examples of the use of transgenes can be found in Boxes 8.1 and 8.2.

Box 8.2

Over-expression of nitric oxide synthase-2

The concentration of nitric oxide (NO) in exhaled air of untreated asthmatic patients is increased compared with individuals without asthma. NO may be toxic to airway tissues and may increase inflammation and airway hyperresponsiveness in asthmatic subjects, although it is also possible that it may have beneficial effects by inducing bronchodilation.

Nitric oxide synthase 2 (NOS-2) induced in airway epithelial cells by inflammatory cytokines is thought to be the major source of increased NO in asthmatic patients.

To explore the roles of NO in airway biology, Hjoberg et al. (2004) developed a mouse strain that can be induced to over-express NOS-2 in airways. The CC10-rtTA-NOS-2 mouse contains a reverse tetracycline transactivator (rtTA) under the control of the Clara cell 10-kDa protein (CC10) promoter and the mouse NOS-2 cDNA under control of a tetracycline operator/minimal CMV promoter (tetO/pCMV min).

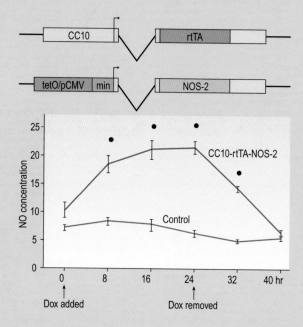

Addition of doxycline to the drinking water leads to an increase in NOS-2 activity and an accumulation of NO in the lungs. This is reversible upon removal of the doxycline.

CC10-rtTA-NOS-2 mice treated with doxycline exhibited decreased airway resistance and were hyporesponsive to methacholine. This suggests that NO has no proinflammatory effects and may even have beneficial effects on pulmonary function.

Hjoberg J, Shore S, Kobzik L, Okinaga S, Hallock A, Vallone J, Subramaniam V, De Sanctis GT, Elias JA, Drazen JM, Silverman ES. Expression of nitric oxide synthase-2 in the lungs decreases airway resistance and responsiveness. J Appl Physiol. 2004 Jul;97(1):249–59.

More subtle use of a transgene: RNA knockdown

Silencing of gene expression by RNA interference (RNAi) has become a powerful experimental tool for analysing the function of mammalian genes, both *in vitro* and *in vivo* (see Appendix 2). Double-stranded RNA is used to bind to and promote the degradation of target RNAs, resulting in knockdown of the expression of specific genes. RNAi can be induced by the introduction of synthetic double-stranded small interfering RNAs (siRNAs) 21–23 bp in length, or by plasmid and viral vector

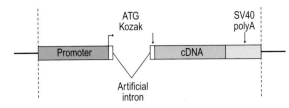

Figure 8.2
Transgene structure. A conventional transgene consists of a promoter and the coding sequences (cDNA) of the gene of interest separated by a small intron. A consensus Kozak ATG and a polyadenylation signal sequence ensure correct translational initiation and transcriptional termination, respectively.

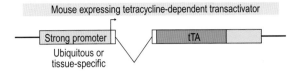

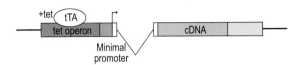

Figure 8.3
Tetracycline-regulated transgenes. Tetracycline (tet)-regulated systems require a combination of two distinct transgenes that have essentially the structure described in the top diagram. One transgene expresses a tet-dependent transactivator (tTA) protein from either a ubiquitous or a tissue-specific promoter. The tTA protein consists of a fusion between the tet-binding domain of the bacterial tetR repressor and the transactivation domain of the HSV-1 VP16 protein. A second transgene encodes the gene of interest driven from a minimal promoter containing binding sites for tTA that are derived from the tet operon (*tetO*). In the example illustrated, tTA binds to *tetO* when tetracycline is present, leading to activation of expression of the sequences encoding the gene of interest. Variants of tTA can be used that behave in the opposite manner; that is, they bind constitutively to *tetO* unless tetracycline is present.

systems that express double-stranded short hairpin RNAs (shRNAs); these are subsequently processed to siRNAs by the cellular machinery (Fig. 8.4). Both siRNA and shRNA libraries have been developed to allow the systematic analysis of genes using high-throughput RNAi screens.

Potentially, knockdown animals can be generated more rapidly and more cheaply using transgenesis than with gene targeting approaches (see below). The use of lentivirus-based vectors that express shRNAs seems to be particularly promising. However, the prerequisites for ubiquitous and reproducible shRNA expression are as yet not well defined, and future developments will certainly aim towards achieving tissue-specific and inducible shRNA knockdown of genes.

Gene targeting

Gene targeting in the mouse enables the removal or replacement of specific gene sequences and thereby avoids some of the problems of transgenesis, such as the multiple and random nature of transgene integrations; however, the two approaches should definitely be regarded as complementary. Key to the whole technology is the embryonic stem (ES) cell. These cells, which can be derived from the early 3.5 dpc pre-implantation embryo ('blastocyst'), can be grown indefinitely in culture while retaining the ability to give rise to a mouse if injected back into a blastocyst (the 'host'). Once reimplanted into the uterus of a pseudo-pregnant foster mother, the injected ('donor') ES cells compete with cells in the host blastocyst to form the developing embryo and ultimately lead to a chimeric mouse. If the germ cells (sperm or eggs) of the chimera also contain cells derived from the donor ES cells, some progeny resulting from mating will have one set of chromosomes derived completely from the donor, thereby establishing a 'line' (Fig. 8.5).

In order to distinguish the contribution of ES cells in a resulting chimera easily, use is made of differences in coat colour genes encoded by the ES cells and the host blastocysts. The majority of ES cells employed are derived from the 129Sv strain that has a dominant agouti (brown) coat colour. When such ES cells are injected into C57/BL6 blastocysts, which contain genes encoding a black coat colour, the resultant chimera will have a coat

that is both agouti and black. The higher the extent of agouti colouring, the greater the degree of incorporation of the donor ES cells. To establish whether or not the ES cells have contributed to the germ cells of the chimera, it is crossed with a C57/BL6 animal, and because the agouti coat colour of the 129Sv strain is dominant, transmission of the ES cell-derived genetic material is apparent in the generation of agouti pups. If agouti pups are seen, these have to be genotyped to detect any genetic modification introduced into the ES cells, since this will usually have been at only one of the two alleles of the relevant gene and will therefore be inherited by half of the progeny.

The other feature of ES cells that is crucial to their use in mouse genetics is that an introduced segment of mouse genome can recombine precisely with the corresponding sequences in the ES cell genome ('homologous recombination'; see also Ch. 10). If the introduced segment contains an alteration, such as a deletion, insertion or small sequence change, this will become a part of the ES cell genome and therefore ultimately can be included in the genome of a mouse.

'Simple' genetic alterations

The simplest, and so far most widely applied, use of homologous recombination in ES cells has been the generation of mice that no longer express a particular gene. This is commonly termed a 'knockout' or null allele of a gene. Usually, all or part of the protein coding sequences is deleted or an insertion is made into an exon encoding an essential domain. In practice, this is achieved by generating a targeting vector that consists of DNA 'isogenic' with the ES cells to be modified and designed to carry

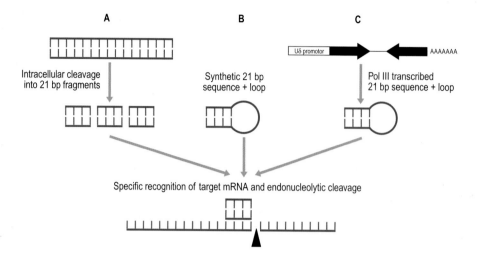

Figure 8.4
RNA interference (RNAi). Three routes for the generation of 21 bp double-stranded RNAi molecules are illustrated. (A) Large double-stranded RNAs are introduced by injection or transfection and are cleaved into fragments by a non-specific endonuclease (the 'Dicer' complex). (B) Synthetic oligonucleotides can be introduced by injection or transfection. These are most efficient if the two strands are connected by a small loop. (C) The 21-base sequence and its complement, separated by a small 'intron', are transcribed from plasmid DNA utilizing a Pol III promoter (e.g. from the *U6 RNA* gene). A short run of Ts at the end of the construct ensures correct termination. The 21 bp double-stranded molecule produced by any of these means is then incorporated into an RNA–protein complex ('RISC') that recognizes the target RNA and catalyses its cleavage.

the required modifications as well as flanking arms of unmodified DNA that are necessary for homologous recombination. The vector bears:

- a constitutively active antibiotic resistance gene (usually *neo*^R conferring resistance to G418) for selection of targeted cells
- a negative selection cassette (usually the HSV-1 *tk* gene conferring sensitivity to ganciclovir) for elimination of those integration events that have occurred through non-homologous recombination (Fig. 8.6).

The targeting vector is introduced into ES cells by subjecting a cell suspension in a solution of the DNA to a short electric pulse; positive and negative selections are then applied. The efficiency of homologous recombination is greatly enhanced if:

- the DNA of the targeting vector and the ES cell line are from the same strain ('isogenic')
- the genomic segments flanking the sequence modification(s) are as long as is compatible with the cloning and screening strategies.

ES cells that successfully exchange the targeting sequences by homologous recombination for one of its two corresponding genomic sequences are able to grow in the presence of the selective antibiotic and can expand as a clone. Potential clones are expanded and analysed by Southern blotting and PCR to determine whether homologous recombination has occurred. A correctly targeted ES clone is then injected into blastocysts to produce a chimeric founder. If the ES clone has retained pluripotent potential and contributes significantly to

the chimera, the modified gene should be transferable to the next generation and a line will have been created. The consequences of loss of function of the gene are then assessed by breeding mice so that both of their gene copies are the knockout allele (homozygous null, or 'nullizygous').

Gene knockouts cannot yet be regarded as a standard laboratory technique and a timescale of about a year to obtain a knockout mouse is probably realistic. The making of simple gene knockouts by individual laboratories may soon be a thing of the past, as a number of companies develop high-throughput technologies for ES cell targeting aiming to provide 'off-the-shelf' knockouts of every single gene. Examples of the use of single-gene knockouts are presented in Boxes 8.3 and 8.4.

The effect of homozygosity for the knockout allele of a gene depends on the encoded protein's role. If related proteins can perform a similar function, then the absence of one of the corresponding genes may have little or no effect. This often means that several members of a gene 'family' have to be deleted individually and then brought together in one mouse by lengthy crossbreeding, before a phenotype is apparent. Even if a gene is not part of a family, its deletion may have very subtle effects that can only be teased out by careful observation or by subjecting the animal to specific conditions. Alternatively, the essential function of some gene products means that homozygous knockout animals may die at some point in their development. Such a lethal effect is clearly informative, but may reflect the function of the protein in only a subset of the tissues in which it plays a role. Moreover, the death of a knockout animal at some stage during its development precludes analysis of the protein's role in the adult.

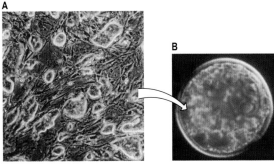

Genetically altered 'Donor'   Day 3.5 blastocyst 'Host'

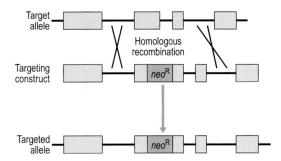

Figure 8.6
A simple gene knockout. A cloned gene segment is modified to prevent expression of functional protein. In the example illustrated, this is achieved by insertion of the neomycin resistance cassette (neo^R) into an exon (grey box). After introduction into ES cells, the targeting construct recombines with homologous sequences in one allele of the gene.

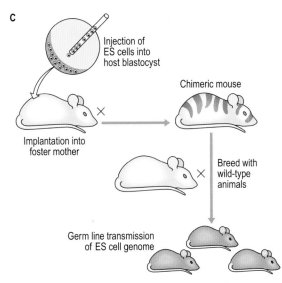

Figure 8.5
Embryonic stem cells are able to give rise to a mouse. (A) The appearance of cultured ES cells growing on a layer of supportive fibroblasts. (B) A day 3.5 embryo, or blastocyst. (C) ES cells are injected into the cavity at the centre of the blastocyst and become incorporated into the cell mass located along one edge of the embryo. Normal development continues after reimplantation into a foster mother. A contribution from donor ES cells in the resulting chimera can be seen because the donor and host carry distinct coat colour genes.

Tricks of the trade: getting beyond a lethal phenotype

A number of elegant genetic methods are available to meet the challenge of investigating genes that have a lethal phenotype when knocked out. We will concentrate on the most widely used technology: namely, conditional gene deletion. The basic principle is simple; a gene is engineered by homologous recombination in ES cells so that the whole gene, or an exon encoding a crucial protein domain, is flanked by recognition sites for a recombinase enzyme that can delete the intervening sequences. Gene knockout is restricted by expressing the recombinase in specific tissues or at a particular time. Several recombinase systems have been characterized from bacteria or yeast, but by far the most widely used at

the moment employs the λ bacteriophage phage-derived Cre recombinase and its 32 base recognition element loxP (Fig. 8.7). The Cre-loxP approach has been applied to a wide range of genes. Although the principle of the method is simple, its application is not. Generation of the targeting construct is much more complicated than for a simple knockout. Since the aim of such targeting is to generate an allele that behaves in the same way as the wild type until Cre recombinase brings about its deletion, provision is included for removal of the selection cassette using a second recombinase, Flp (Fig. 8.8). An important aspect of the technology is to express Cre recombinase where and when you want, at sufficient levels to bring about efficient recombination. This involves crossing mice containing the loxP modification to strains that express Cre in a particular cell type. Alternatively, the recombinase can have the potential to be expressed in all tissues, but only when an inducer is provided. An example of the latter makes use of a transgene containing an interferon-inducible promoter to drive Cre expression. Further examples of conditional Cre-mediated gene deletion can be found in Boxes 8.1 and 8.4.

Gene targeting can achieve more than gene deletion

Although deletion is a very useful way of investigating the importance of a gene, the majority of diseases with a genetic basis involve small sequence changes. The same ES cell-based approaches can be used to create mouse lines to model such mutations (so-called 'knock-ins'; Fig. 8.9).

Knock-in of transgenes

As we have already discussed, the random integration of multiple copies of transgenic DNA into the genome often leads to expression that is not ideal, either in terms of cell type restriction or the level of transcription. A possible solution is to insert the transgenic cassette directly into a gene locus that is expressed specifically or

Box 8.3

Knock-in mutation of a mitochondrial DNA polymerase

Mitochondria accumulate mutations during ageing. These mutations can lead to accumulation of reactive oxygen species (ROS) and proton leakage. ROS may in turn induce more mutations thereby setting up a vicious circle of events.

In order to address the question of whether the mitochodrial mutations are a cause or a consequence of ageing, Trifunovic et al. (2004) engineered a mouse strain containing a knock-in mutation (D257A) in the mitochondrial DNA (mtDNA) polymerase γ. The D257A mutation abolishes the proof reading activity of DNA polymerase γ that normally corrects defects introduced during mtDNA replication. As a consequence, the D257A mice accumulate multiple mtDNA mutations (3–5 fold above average).

The phenotype of the mutant mice includes a decreased life span and signs of premature ageing such as weight loss, reduced subcutaneous fat, hair loss, curvature of the spine, osteoporosis, anaemia, reduced fertility and heart enlargement.

Trifunovic A, Wredenberg A, Falkenberg M, Spelbrink JN, Rovio AT, Bruder CE, Bohlooly-Y M, Gidlof S, Oldfors A, Wibom R, Tornell J, Jacobs HT, Larsson NG. Premature ageing in mice expressing defective mitochondrial DNA polymerase. Nature. 2004 May 27;429(6990):417–23.

predominantly in the cell type of interest. This is a labour-intensive strategy and should perhaps only be undertaken if transgenesis using a specific promoter fails. Another possible disadvantage is that the sequences being 'knocked in' can so disrupt the target gene that a null allele is generated. In this case, modified animals could only be used as heterozygotes.

BAC transgenes and recombineering

Problems associated with inappropriate expression due to the presence of insufficient gene regulatory elements in a conventional transgene, or problems with the manipulation of large segments of DNA *in vitro* to produce transgenes or vectors for gene targeting (including the presence of suitable restriction enzyme sites and difficulties in fragment isolation and cloning) have been substantially overcome through the combined development of specialized bacterial vectors and systems for recombination directly within bacteria. Bacterial artificial chromosomes (BACs) make use of the replication and chromosome partitioning systems from the F-plasmid of *E. coli*, and enable the cloning of fragments of 200–300 kbp, which are maintained at low copy number and can be purified for use in either pronuclear injection or introduction into ES cells. The great step forward, in an approach that has been termed 'recombineering', has been the application of phage-encoded recombination to enable manipulation of BAC DNA within bacteria, without the need for *in vitro* molecular biology. The precise details of strategies for recombineering are beyond the scope of this chapter and we refer readers to recent articles on the topic (see, for example, Copeland et al., 2001). In essence, recombineering entails recombination within bacteria between the BAC DNA and an introduced fragment that has short regions of homology (40–50 bp) with the target genomic sequence at either end. The fragment,

which may contain additional sequences for the purpose of selection, is generated by PCR, using primers that contain the short regions of genomic homology as well as regions complementary with whatever other DNA segments are to be introduced. The precise design of the homology 'arms' of the fragment allows introduction of point mutations, or the generation of a deletion of genomic sequences following recombination. If a selection cassette has been incorporated into the fragment recombined with the BAC, this can ultimately be removed, if recombination target sites have been included that can be recognized by one of the systems used for conditional gene modification, such as Cre-loxP.

Although recombineering in BACs has many advantages, one major potential problem to be aware of is that, when using a BAC for gene targeting in ES cells, the size of the genomic sequence makes it very difficult to ascertain whether homologous recombination has been absolutely faithful on both sides of the introduced alteration.

Chromosome engineering

Aberrations in human chromosome copy number and structure are common and extremely deleterious, both as development-associated defects and as acquired events in tumours. Their effects on phenotype can be the result of aberrant dosage of sequences in the affected regions (e.g. trisomy of chromosome 21 in Down syndrome) or because the resulting juxtaposition of sequences leads to abnormal gene expression (e.g. activation of Bcl2 expression in lymphoid cells following translocation to an immunoglobulin gene locus) or to the creation of a novel fusion containing portions of two distinct proteins (e.g. the Bcr-Abl fusion oncoprotein associated with many cases of chronic myeloid leukaemia; see also Ch. 9). The combination of gene targeting in

Box 8.4

Mouse models of deafness

The inner ear sensory epithelia are responsible for the transduction of sound. The cells that sense sound waves are called hair cells and are characterized by cytoskeletal projects on their apical surface called stereocilia. These respond to movement, causing channel opening and ion influx that results in depolarization and propagation of a signal to the brain.

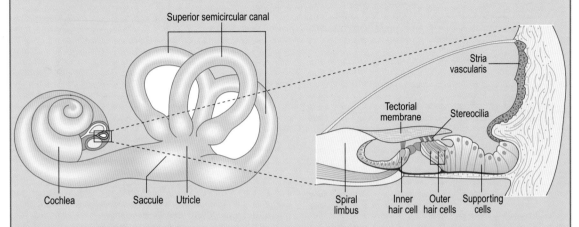

The complexity of the inner ear makes hearing loss the most common form of sensory loss. A multitude of genes have been described, encoding many different types of protein, that have been implicated in hereditary hearing loss. There are a large number of mouse mutants that serve as models for human hearing defects. Some of these have arisen spontaneously, such as the waltzer strain, which has a mutation in the cadherin 23 gene causing stereocilia disorganization (Di Palma et al., 2001). Other mouse strains have been generated to model defects that have been identified in humans. These include both simple gene knockouts and more elaborate conditional gene modifications. For example, constitutive ablation of the gene encoding Collagen type XIα2 causes deafness by influencing the extracellular matrix of the tectorial membrane (McGuirt et al., 1999). More elaborate models are typified by the conditional knockout of the connexin 26 gene, using Cre recombinase expression driven specifically in the developing ear from the otogelin promoter, which causes defects in stereocilia gap junctions (Cohen-Salmon et al., 2002).

Cohen-Salmon M, Ott T, Michel V, Hardelin JP, Perfettini I, Eybalin M, Wu T, Marcus DC, Wangemann P, Willecke K, Petit C. Targeted ablation of connexin26 in the inner ear epithelial gap junction network causes hearing impairment and cell death. Curr Biol. 2002 Jul 9;12(13):1106–11.

Di Palma F, Holme RH, Bryda EC, Belyantseva IA, Pellegrino R, Kachar B, Steel KP, Noben-Trauth K. Mutations in Cdh23, encoding a new type of cadherin, cause stereocilia disorganization in waltzer, the mouse model for Usher syndrome type 1D. Nat Genet. 2001 Jan;27(1):103–7.

McGuirt WT, Prasad SD, Griffith AJ, Kunst HP, Green GE, Shpargel KB, Runge C, Huybrechts C, Mueller RF, Lynch E, King MC, Brunner HG, Cremers CW, Takanosu M, Li SW, Arita M, Mayne R, Prockop DJ, Van Camp G, Smith RJ. Mutations in COL11A2 cause non-syndromic hearing loss (DFNA13). Nat Genet. 1999 Dec;23(4):413–9.

ES cells, recombinase technology and other techniques makes it possible to generate new chromosomes carrying specific and defined deletions, duplications, inversions and translocations, which can serve as models for human chromosomal aberrations.

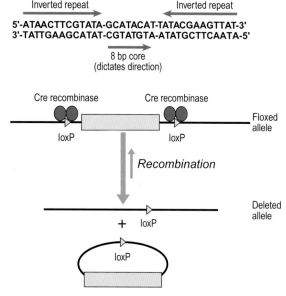

Figure 8.7
Using recombinases to delete engineered gene segments. The loxP recognition site (orange arrow) for Cre recombinase is a 32-bp sequence consisting of a 12-nucleotide inverted repeat separated by 8 residues. LoxP sites are engineered on either side of the sequence to be deleted. A dimer of Cre (represented by red circles) binds to each loxP site and catalyses recombination. The deleted allele retains one copy of the loxP site.

Chromosomal rearrangements

Cre-loxP technology can be used:

- to create very large deletions or inversions on a single chromosome
- to bring about specific recombination between two different chromosomes.

The latter requires two separate loxP sites in the regions that are to be linked. This can be achieved either:

- by two successive independent targeting events in ES cells, *or*
- through crossing of mice, each with one of the loxP modifications.

The relative positioning and orientation of the loxP sites will dictate the exact form of rearrangement elicited by Cre recombinase, while the distance between the loxP sites affects the efficiency of recombination. The precise details of the different rearrangements possible are beyond the scope of this chapter and we refer readers to a recent review for further information on this topic (Brault et al., 2006).

Transchromosomal lines

Microcell-mediated chromosomal transfer (MMCT) enables manipulation of large chromosome fragments or even whole chromosomes. It is being successfully applied to generate transchromosomal mouse lines in which the additional chromosomal material is human-derived. Microcells containing a single or small number of human chromosomes can be fused with ES cells, which can then be used to produce chimeras and

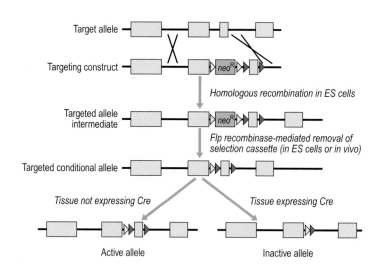

Figure 8.8
Generation of a conditional allele. LoxP sites (blue arrows) are engineered on either side of sequences encoding a crucial domain. The selection cassette is flanked by Flp recombinase sites (white arrows), allowing for its removal. The conditional allele functions like the wild-type allele until exposed to Cre recombinase.

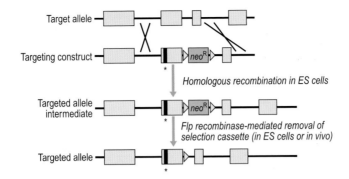

Figure 8.9
Knock-in mutation. Small mutational changes (asterisk) can be introduced by targeting, and usually it is desirable to remove the selection cassette as described in Figure 8.7.

stable germline transmitting lines, as described above. Recently, and most impressively, this approach has been adopted to create a model of Down syndrome in which the normal complement of mouse chromosomes is supplemented by a copy of human chromosome 21.

Mutagenesis-driven, non-directed genetics

This approach requires selection of phenotypes following either spontaneous or induced random mutation. Spontaneous mutations in genes have occasionally been recognized during the maintenance of mouse strains because of characteristic changes in phenotype, and a few of these have proven to be useful as models of genetic diseases in man. More importantly, considerable effort is presently being expended to induce random mutations throughout the genome with the aim of revealing all genes that yield a defined phenotype as a result of alterations to either the level or the functional activity of their encoded protein. These large-scale screens are generally undertaken with a limited set of physiological processes in mind; for example, one screen is looking for developmental defects caused by single gene defects, while another is trying to identify novel genes involved in cardiac development and function.

Random mutagenesis strategies can be broadly divided on the basis of the mutagen used, and here we will consider the two principal approaches, namely:

- chemical mutagenesis
- gene trapping using transgene insertion as the mutagen.

Chemical mutagenesis

Random chemical mutagenesis is generally achieved using the powerful alkylating mutagen, N-ethyl-N-nitrosourea (ENU). Males are injected with ENU at

concentrations that lead to approximately 1 in 175 sperm carrying a mutation in any given gene. ENU-treated males are mated with females, and the progeny are then put into a breeding programme, the exact nature of which is determined by whether the phenotypic screening is geared towards dominant or recessive mutations (see Ch. 2). Depending on the position of the mutation within a gene, this may affect:

- protein levels through changes in gene expression or splicing, *or*
- protein function through changes in specific amino acid residues.

Many mutations within the protein coding sequence will, of course, be silent because of redundancies within the genetic code. Those mutations that elicit a change in amino acid sequence can have an effect ranging from partial loss of function through to extreme loss of function. More unusually, an amino acid alteration might even result in a gain of function.

- Simplistically, it might be expected that a dominant mutation might arise from a gain-of-function mutation.
- Conversely, and much more likely, a recessive mutation might occur if protein function is partially or completely compromised.

Gene trapping

Gene trapping, which is essentially a modified version of transgene insertion (see above), offers a method of creating random mutations in ES cells, with a direct route to cloning and defining the expression pattern and function of a gene. Gene trapping involves the use of a reporter gene that is activated following insertion into an endogenous transcription unit. A number of vectors have been developed, which differ in their requirements for reporter gene activation. Hence, 'promoter trap' vectors simply consist of a promoterless reporter gene that is activated following insertions in exons of other genes. In contrast, 'gene trap' vectors contain a splice acceptor sequence upstream of a reporter and are activated

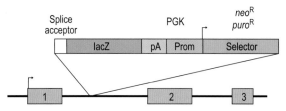

Figure 8.10
Gene trap vector. A standard gene trap transgene consists of a reporter (usually the lacZ gene encoding β-galactosidase), flanked by splice acceptor and polyadenylation sequences. A downstream-strong, ubiquitous promoter (e.g. PGK) is used to drive expression of a selectable gene (usually for antibiotic resistance). When randomly integrated into an intron, the gene trap cassette is transcribed under the control of the endogenous regulatory elements of the gene and, through transcriptional termination, prevents expression of gene sequences downstream of the site of insertion.

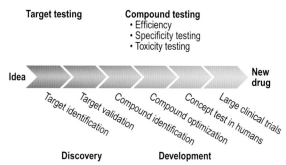

Figure 8.11
Drug discovery pipeline.

following insertions into introns of genes (Fig. 8.10). Both promoter and gene trap insertions create a fusion transcript from which a portion of the endogenous gene may be readily cloned. After introduction of the trap vector into ES cells, individual clones may be screened — for example, for expression of the reporter — either in undifferentiated ES cells or following differentiation *in vitro* towards a specific cell lineage. Usually based on the pattern of reporter expression *in vitro*, ES cell clones are then tested *in vivo*:

- firstly, for expression of the reporter in chimeric embryos following introduction into blastocysts
- subsequently, for both reporter expression and function of the trapped gene in embryos and adults, if germline transmission can be achieved.

Several large-scale projects are making available libraries of gene-trapped ES cell clones, and these may be accessed through a number of websites including that provided by the Sanger Institute Gene Trap Resource (SIGTR; www.sanger.ac.uk/PostGenomics/genetrap).

Drug target validation and drug testing using mouse models

The pharmaceutical industry is increasingly turning towards mouse models as a means to increase the efficiency of drug research and development. A typical

drug discovery 'pipeline' (Fig. 8.11) involves several stages at which mouse models have already proven effective or show great promise for future application. Mouse models have found use in drug target identification, and this will become an increasingly important area as high-throughput strategies for screening for individual gene function, such as RNAi knockdown, become easier and cheaper. An illustration of the power of mouse models in screening drug effects *in vivo* can be found in the example described in Box 8.1, in which anti-inflammatory mediators are assessed by their effect in alleviating induction of the iNOS promoter.

Genetically altered mice are also ideal models for target validation; in other words, if a drug candidate is thought to operate through a particular gene product, this can be tested by comparing the effect of the compound in wild-type mice and in animals that only differ by being mutated at the relevant gene locus.

A mouse model of a human disease may also be used to study *in vivo* efficacy of candidate compounds, and this will certainly become a more widely used approach as it becomes easier to 'humanize' individual genes or even whole sets of genes. Since roughly 40% of clinical drug failures are for pharmacokinetic reasons, there is great interest in using mouse models as a more efficient way of predicting drug absorption, distribution, metabolism and elimination (ADME) early in the drug development process. Hence, even though key enzymes and factors involved in ADME exhibit species-specific differences, mice can be humanized with respect to small subgroups of proteins responsible for the major routes of transport and metabolism of a large proportion of drugs (see also Ch. 9).

FURTHER READING

Bedell MA, Jenkins NA, Copeland NG 1997 Mouse models of human disease. Part I: techniques and resources for genetic analysis in mice. Genes Dev 11(1):1–10.

Bedell MA, Largaespada DA, Jenkins NA, Copeland NG 1997 Mouse models of human disease. Part II: recent progress and future directions. Genes Dev 11(1):11–43.

Brault V, Pereira P, Duchon A, Herault Y 2006 Modeling chromosomes in mouse to explore the function of genes, genomic disorders, and chromosomal organization. PLoS Genet 2(7):e86.

Brennan J, Skarnes WC 1999 Gene trapping in mouse embryonic stem cells. Methods Mol Biol 97:123–138.

Bujard H 1999 Controlling genes with tetracyclines. J Gene Med 1(5):372–374.

Cohen-Salmon M, Ott T, Michel V et al. 2002 Targeted ablation of connexin26 in the inner ear epithelial gap junction network causes hearing impairment and cell death. Curr Biol 12(13):1106–1111.

Copeland NG, Jenkins NA, Court DL 2001 Recombineering: a powerful new tool for mouse functional genomics. Nat Rev Genet 2(10):769–779.

Di Palma F, Holme RH, Bryda EC et al. 2001 Mutations in Cdh23, encoding a new type of cadherin, cause stereocilia disorganization in waltzer, the mouse model for Usher syndrome type 1D. Nat Genet 27(1):103–107.

Hardouin SN, Nagy A 2000 Mouse models for human disease. Clin Genet 57(4):237–244.

Hjoberg J, Shore S, Kobzik L et al. 2004 Expression of nitric oxide synthase-2 in the lungs decreases airway resistance and responsiveness. J Appl Physiol 97(1):249–259.

Justice MJ, Noveroske JK, Weber JS et al. 1999 Mouse ENU mutagenesis. Hum Mol Genet 8(10):1955–1963.

Kwan KM 2002 Conditional alleles in mice: practical considerations for tissue-specific knockouts. Genesis 32(2):49–62.

McGuirt WT, Prasad SD, Griffith AJ et al. 1999 Mutations in COL11A2 cause non-syndromic hearing loss (DFNA13). Nat Genet 23(4):413–419.

Sandy P, Ventura A, Jacks T 2005 Mammalian RNAi: a practical guide. Biotechniques 39(2):215–224.

Testa G, Zhang Y, Vintersten K et al. 2003 Engineering the mouse genome with bacterial artificial chromosomes to create multipurpose alleles. Nat Biotechnol 21(4):443–447.

Trifunovic A, Wredenberg A, Falkenberg M et al. 2004 Premature ageing in mice expressing defective mitochondrial DNA polymerase. Nature 429(6990):417–423.

Valenzuela DM, Murphy AJ, Frendewey D et al. 2003 High-throughput engineering of the mouse genome coupled with high-resolution expression analysis. Nat Biotechnol 21(6):652–659.

Vooijs M, Jonkers J, Lyons S, Berns A 2002 Noninvasive imaging of spontaneous retinoblastoma pathway-dependent tumors in mice. Cancer Res 62(6):1862–1867.

Zhang N, Weber A, Li B et al. 2003 An inducible nitric oxide synthase-luciferase reporter system for *in vivo* testing of anti-inflammatory compounds in transgenic mice. J Immunol 170(12):6307–6319.

9

Pharmacogenetics
M. Keen

Pharmacogenetics is the study of how our genes influence the way in which we respond to drugs.

Individuals differ markedly in their responsiveness to drugs; the 'standard' dose may be fine in many individuals, but in others may be ineffective or produce unacceptable side-effects. Many factors underlie this variation, including age, weight, disease, other drugs and the environment (Fig. 9.1). However, a substantial component of the difference between individuals is due to genetic influences, and it is these genetic influences that are the preserve of pharmacogenetics. In an ideal future, you will be able to undergo a simple test to determine your pharmacogenetic profile, and on the basis of this test, doctors will be able to prescribe the ideal medications for you, at the ideal dose.

The history of pharmacogenetics

The realization that genes can affect responsiveness to drugs is not new. In fact, the science of pharmacogenetics dates back to the 1950s, when three important and independent discoveries regarding the inheritance of unusual drug responsiveness were made. These were:

- glucose-6-phosphate dehydrogenase (G6PD) deficiency
- impaired metabolism of suxamethonium
- variation in the rate of metabolism of isoniazid.

The term 'pharmacogenetics' was first used to describe the field in 1959 by the German geneticist, Friedrich Vogel.

The early discoveries of inherited differences in responsiveness to drugs started with the identification of a phenotype, usually based on unexpected drug toxicity. Further studies determined the underlying biochemical cause of the abnormality, and finally the gene responsible. Now, in the post-genome era, it is possible to identify genetic polymorphisms and then seek to establish whether they affect responsiveness to drugs.

The simplest and most common form of polymorphism is the single nucleotide polymorphism (SNP; see Ch. 1), in which a single nucleotide varies between alleles. The current estimate for the number of SNPs in the human genome is over 10 million, and the tables in this chapter demonstrate the fact that SNPs underlie many of the observed polymorphisms in drug responsiveness. The joint public-private SNP Consortium initiative represents a coordinated effort to identify, analyse and catalogue SNPs throughout the human genome.

With the explosion of information regarding the human genome, allelic variants and single nucleotide polymorphisms, pharmacogenetics is becoming increasingly important and has gained the new name of 'pharmacogenomics'. However, as yet, the impact of the field on clinical practice remains limited.

Glucose-6-phosphate dehydrogenase deficiency

This condition was also first characterized in the 1950s, following investigation into why some black servicemen in the US army developed an unusual haemolytic reaction to the antimalarial drug, primaquine. G6PD catalyses the step by which glucose-6-phosphate enters the pentose phosphate shunt, providing a source of NADPH. Despite the fact that G6PD is present in all/many cells, it seems to be almost exclusively the red blood cells that are affected in G6PD deficiency. This appears to be for two reasons:

- The pentose phosphate pathway is the only source of NADPH in the red blood cell.
- Many of the variant forms of G6PD appear to be inactivated more rapidly than the normal enzyme; this will have a particular impact in the enucleate red blood cells, which are unable to synthesize new protein.

The gene for G6PD is located on the X chromosome and G6PD is a sex-linked characteristic, occurring much more frequently in males. Females homozygous for an abnormal gene will exhibit the condition, and in heterozygous females random inactivation of one or other of the two X chromosomes can result in mosaicism with some aspects of the condition.

There are an enormous number of different polymorphisms that underlie G6PD deficiency; a few of these are described in more detail in Table 9.1. However, there are still many phenotypes, such as the 'Gambia' and 'Wakayama' variants, for which the underlying molecular cause has yet to be established. The degree to which enzyme activity is affected influences the severity of the condition and the World Health Organization classifies G6PD deficiency into four kinds:

- *type 1* — associated with chronic haemolytic anaemia, even in the absence of precipitating drugs or infection
- *type 2* — associated with less than 10% of normal enzyme activity and haemolytic reactions to various drugs and/or infections
- *type 3* — associated with 10–60% of normal enzyme activity and less severe haemolytic reactions to drugs and/or infection

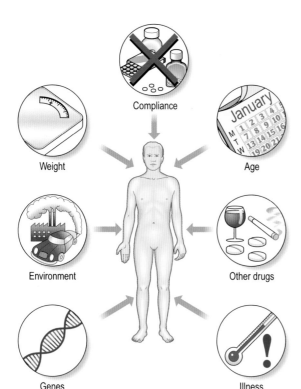

Figure 9.1
Some of the factors that may influence the way in which an individual responds to a drug.

- *type 4* — associated with more than 60% of normal enzyme activity and no apparent clinical problem.

Complete absence of G6PD activity appears to be lethal.

The number and prevalence of these different alleles, coupled with the relative frequency of G6PD deficiency in, for example, African, Asian and Mediterranean populations, hint at the selection advantage that G6PD deficiency can confer under certain conditions. It is, in fact, well established that G6PD helps protect against malaria (see Ch. 1). Biochemical tests for G6PD deficiency are available and are used fairly widely among populations where deficiency is likely to occur.

Impaired metabolism of suxamethonium

A prolonged effect of suxamethonium was one of the first inherited variations in drug responsiveness to be identified. Suxamethonium is a depolarizing neuromuscular blocking drug used as a paralysing agent during general anaesthesia. Its chief advantage is that it is very short-acting, being rapidly metabolized by the butyryl cholinesterase enzyme present in the plasma. This means that patients recover from its paralysing effects very rapidly after surgery. However, in a minority of individuals (about 1 in 35 000) suxamethonium is not rapidly eliminated, and these patients require prolonged support after its administration; artificial ventilation is essential, as the respiratory muscles are paralysed.

There are several phenotypes which exhibit deficient plasma cholinesterase activity and thus unusual sensitivity to suxamethonium, and several alleles of the butyryl cholinesterase gene (*BCHE*) have been identified. Of these, several exhibit reduced cholinesterase activity and unusual substrate specificity, and there are also 'silent genes' in which cholinesterase activity is completely absent. In at least some individuals with

Table 9.1
Some mutations of the G6PD gene which result in reduced enzyme activity

Nucleotide substitution	Amino acid substitution	Phenotype
Deletion of 105–107	Deletion of ile-35	'Sunderland' type 1, chronic haemolytic anaemia
G-1228 to T	gly-410 to cys	'Riverside' type 1, chronic haemolytic anaemia
A-493 to G	asn-165 to asp	'Chinese-3' type 2, < 10% normal enzyme activity
G-1376 to C	arg-459 to pro	'Cosenza' type 2, < 10% normal enzyme activity
G-172 to A	asp-58 to asn	'Metaponto' type 3, 10–60% normal enzyme activity
G-949 to A	glu-317 to lys	'Kalyam' type 3, 10–60% normal enzyme activity
G-337 to A	asp-113 to asn	'Sao Borga' type 4, > 60% normal enzyme activity
A-376 to G	asn-126 to asp	'A' type 4, > 60% normal enzyme activity

Table 9.2
Some of the SNPs of the *BCHE* gene which result in reduced or absent plasma cholinesterase activity

Nucleotide substitution	Amino acid substitution	Phenotype
GGT to GGAG	Reading frame shift at gly-117 leading to premature stop codon	Inactive enzyme
A-290 to G	asp-70 to gly	Dibucaine resistance and decreased catalytic activity
C to T	thr-245 to met	Fluoride resistance and decreased catalytic activity
G to T	gly-390 to val	Fluoride resistance and decreased catalytic activity
A-1490 to T	glu-497 to val	Quantitative J variant; 60% decrease in enzyme expression
G-1615 to A	ala-593 to thr	Quantitative K variant; 30% decrease in enzyme expression

the silent gene, there is a mutation in the codon for gly-117, in which the normal GGT sequence becomes GGAG; this results in a +1 shift in the reading frame, so that a TGA stop codon is encountered at position 129 and a greatly truncated mRNA is generated; thus inactive protein is produced.

Some of the polymorphisms resulting in butyryl cholinesterase deficiency are summarized in Table 9.2.

N-acetyl transferase polymorphism: slow and fast acetylators

In the late 1950s, it was discovered that there was common genetic variability in the ability of individuals to metabolize isoniazid, an anti-tubercular drug. This resulted in marked differences in the plasma concentration and half-life of isoniazid, and also of other drugs metabolized by the same enzyme, including hydralazine (a vasodilator) and procainamide (an anti-arrhythmic). The effect on metabolism is so marked that there appear to be three distinct populations: the 'normal' population and those who are abnormally slow or fast acetylators. This triphasic distribution can be seen in Figure 9.2.

- In slow acetylators, high plasma concentrations of isoniazid and the other drugs are achieved, and these individuals are at a much greater risk of an adverse reaction to these drugs; there may also be an increase in susceptibility to some diseases, such as bladder cancer, in slow acetylators.
- In rapid acetylators, only low plasma concentrations are achieved and the therapeutic effectiveness of these drugs is reduced. A number of allelic variants of the

N-acetyl transferase genes (*NAT2*) have been identified and some of these are summarized in Table 9.3.

How do genes influence responsiveness to drugs?

There are two main ways in which genes can alter the response to a drug:

- *Variations in the drug target*, such as a variant form of a receptor. This may be a variant of the drug's intended target, or a target responsible for some of the unintended (side)-effects of the drug.
- *Variations in pharmacokinetics* — the processes of absorption, distribution, metabolism and excretion by which the drug gets into the body, is distributed around it and is finally eliminated from it. As you can see in Figure 9.3, a change in the rate at which the drug is absorbed into the body or eliminated from it can have profound effects on the maximum concentration that any given dose of a drug will achieve in the plasma. This, in turn, will influence the response that the drug produces; too low a plasma concentration may mean that the drug is ineffective, while too high a plasma concentration may mean that the drug produces unacceptable toxic effects.

However, there are some instances in which it is not easy to classify a polymorphism in drug responsiveness into one of these two groups; G6PD deficiency is a good example (see below).

Examples of both of these types of variation are described in this chapter (see below). At the moment, however, we have by far the most information regarding the genetics of drug-metabolizing enzymes.

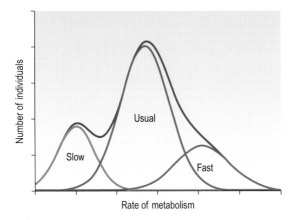

Figure 9.2
A triphasic distribution such as that seen for isoniazid metabolism.
To generate this type of graph, many people would have the rate at which they metabolize isoniazid measured. The data have been plotted with rate of metabolism on the *x*-axis and the number of people who metabolize the drug at that particular rate on the *y*-axis. For any characteristic like this, there will be a degree of variation. However, the majority of the population would be expected to fall into a single normal distribution, as shown by the curve marked 'usual'. Deviation from a normal distribution may suggest that the data consist of more than one population. In this case, the data can be best described as the sum of three individual but overlapping populations: the 'usual', 'slow' and 'fast' acetylators, shown here. This type of discontinuous variation occurs because mutations of the *NAT2* gene produce such a marked effect on the ability to metabolize isoniazid.

Table 9.3
Some of the SNPs of the *NAT2* gene that result in the slow acetylator phenotype

Nucleotide substitution	Amino acid substitution	Phenotype
G-590 to A	arg-197 to gln	Slow
T-341 to C	ile-114 to thr	Very slow
A-803 to G	lys- 268 to arg	Slow
G-857 to A	gly to glu	Slow

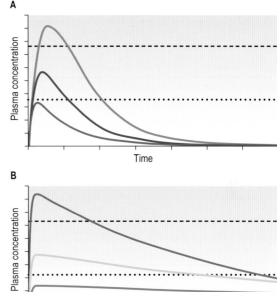

- - - - Toxic concentration
· · · · · Effective concentration

Figure 9.3
The effect of changes in the rate of absorption or elimination of a drug on plasma concentration. These graphs show the predicted plasma concentrations for an orally administered drug, for which both absorption and elimination are first-order rate processes. (A) The effect of altering the rate of elimination. The middle curve represents the normal rate of elimination; the upper and lower curves represent the effect of halving or doubling this rate, respectively. Decreasing the rate of elimination causes the plasma concentration to be higher, and may result in toxicity. Increasing the rate of elimination causes the plasma concentration to be lower, and may result in a lack of therapeutic effect. (B) The effect of altering the rate of absorption. The middle curve represents the normal rate of absorption; the upper and lower curves represent the effect of doubling or halving this rate, respectively. Decreasing the rate of absorption causes the plasma concentration to be lower, and may result in a lack of therapeutic effect. Increasing the rate of absorption causes the plasma concentration to be higher, and may result in toxicity.

Genetic polymorphisms of drug-metabolizing enzymes

The first polymorphisms of drug-metabolizing enzymes to be identified were those of butyryl cholinesterase and N-acetyl transferase (both discussed in more detail below). Since then, a great number of polymorphisms in a large number of enzymes have been characterized.

In the mid-1980s, several patients treated with standard doses of the anticancer drug, 5-fluorouracil, developed fatal CNS toxicity, which was found to be associated with excessive plasma concentrations of the drug. These unfortunate patients were later shown to have had an inherited deficiency of dihydropyrimidine dehydrogenase, the rate-limiting step in the metabolism of 5-fluorouracil. Many cases of dihydropyrimidine dehydrogenase deficiency have since been shown to

be caused by an SNP: a G to A transition in the 14th intron. This transition is an 'exon-skipping mutation' which results in the complete absence of exon 14 from the finished protein and an almost complete lack of enzyme activity. Life-threatening toxicity of 5-fluorouracil occurs with regard to nerves, bone marrow and the gastrointestinal tract of patients who are homozygous or heterozygous for this SNP.

Polymorphisms in the metabolism of anticancer drugs attract particular attention because of the potential toxicity of these aggressive drugs. Thiopurine S-methyl transferase (TPMT) metabolizes mercaptopurine and azathioprine (a 'pro-drug' which converts to the active mercaptopurine in the body); these are used as anticancer drugs and immunosuppressants. Caucasians can be separated into three groups on the basis of TPMT activity in their red blood cells, and this is inherited in an autosomal co-dominant fashion. A low rate of enzyme activity leads to a markedly enhanced risk of bone marrow suppression, whereas high rates are associated with decreased effectiveness of the drug. Two common SNPs in the *TPMT* gene have been identified, both of which lead to markedly reduced amounts of the enzyme, presumably because the variant protein is unstable and is more rapidly degraded. Tests are available to detect these inactivating SNPs in the *TPMT* gene, but although the tests are now mentioned in the prescribing literature, their use is not mandatory. However, this sort of test is potentially particularly useful in the case of drugs, such as many of the anticancer drugs, for which there is a small difference between the concentrations of the drug needed to be effective and the concentrations that will be toxic. For these drugs, anything that could help in achieving the correct dose for an individual may be of great importance.

Why is there so much interest in polymorphisms of drug-metabolizing enzymes? Most of these enzymes are responsible for metabolizing more than one drug. Thus these polymorphisms are likely to affect more people, more frequently, than a polymorphism of a target for only one type of drug. The widespread impact of these polymorphisms also makes them of greater economic interest to pharmaceutical companies, and nowhere is this more true than in the case of polymorphisms of the cytochrome P450 enzymes.

The cytochrome P450 system

The cytochrome P450 system is a superfamily of microsomal enzymes, capable of metabolizing a very wide range of compounds, including a great many drugs (Box 9.1). A number of the P450 enzymes exhibit polymorphisms which affect the rate of elimination of a number of drugs, and this are considered in more detail in Boxes 9.1 and 9.2.

Individual variation in the ability of the cytochrome P450 enzymes to eliminate drugs has already had an impact on drug development; pharmaceutical companies tend to avoid potential new drugs that are substrates for the P450 system, as a degree of variability in their metabolism by the population is virtually inevitable.

One of the cytochrome P450 enzymes, CYP2D6, is responsible for metabolizing many drugs, including codeine, dextromethorphan, metoprolol, nortriptyline, debrisoquine and spartein. Around 5–10% of Caucasians have a relative deficiency in their ability to metabolize these drugs, and this is inherited as an autosomal recessive trait. Other polymorphisms of this enzyme can increase the rate of drug metabolism. Polymorphisms of CYP2D6 are considered in more detail in Box 9.2.

A gene-based microarray test for CYP2D6 alleles that allows identification of poor, intermediate, extensive and ultra-rapid metabolizers is available from Roche Diagnostics. Given the number of psychiatric drugs that are substrates for CYP2D6, the UK Department of Health has suggested that it would be cost-effective to introduce routine testing for psychiatric in-patients, in order to tailor the dose of drug better to an individual and to reduce the incidence of both severe side-effects and ineffectiveness of the drug.

Box 9.1

The cytochrome P450 system

The liver has evolved a complex system of enzymes involved in the metabolism and elimination of a variety of drugs and other exogenous and endogenous substances. One of the best-studied of these enzyme systems is the hepatic cytochrome P450 system, responsible for the oxidation or hydroxylation of a wide range of substances. The cytochrome P450 enzymes are a large superfamily of haem-containing enzymes which were originally designated '450' due to their characteristic absorption peak at 450 nm. Humans possess around 60 separate genes for cytochrome P450 enzymes, which can be grouped into a number of subfamilies. The functions of these enzymes are varied, and a number are involved in steroid biosynthesis in gonads, adrenal glands and other tissues. It is the subset involved in the hepatic metabolism of the overwhelming majority of drugs with which pharmacogenetics is particularly concerned.

The fact that these enzymes are responsible for the metabolism of so many different drugs means that they underlie many important drug interactions; for example, components within grapefruit juice can inhibit the activity of the enzyme(s) responsible for the metabolism of erythromycin and terfenadine, and fatal toxicity of standard doses of terfenadine has occurred in patients who were also taking erythromycin and/or grapefruit juice. The P450 enzymes can also be 'induced' by a variety of drugs and other chemicals, so that greater levels of the enzyme are expressed and the rate of drug metabolism is increased. For example, exposure to rifampicin can speed up the elimination of phenytoin, reducing its efficacy in the prevention of epileptic seizures. Moreover, individuals who consume large amounts of brassicas and chargrilled meat — both of which induce the P450 system — have higher levels of some of the P450 enzymes.

The naming convention for the cytochrome P450s is explained in Figure 9.4. The ones that have a well-established role in drug metabolism include CYP1A2, CYP2A6, CYP2B6, CYPC8, CYPC9, CYP2C19, CYP2D6, CYP2E1, CYP3A5 and CYP4A11; a number of these (CYP2B6, CYPC9, CYP2C19 and CYP2D6) exhibit considerable polymorphism which can impact the rate of drug metabolism and thus the therapeutic effects of the drug and the risk of drug interactions. Furthermore, about 75% of Caucasians and 50% of blacks do not express functional CYP3A5; fortunately, many of the substrates for this enzyme can also be metabolized by other P450 enzymes. Table 9.4 shows some of the drugs metabolized by the various P450 enzymes, along with some of the substances that can inhibit or induce these enzymes.

Genetic polymorphisms of drug targets

Up until now, the emerging field of pharmacogenetics has had very little impact on clinical practice, but there are a handful of products on the market for which there

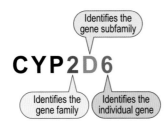

Figure 9.4
The naming convention for enzymes in the cytochrome P450 system.

is good evidence that pharmacogenetic testing is of use. Despite the widespread impact of polymorphisms of drug-metabolizing enzymes on human responsiveness to drugs, the main area in which tests for a specific gene or phenotype are currently used is to test for a particular drug target, especially in cancer. It is now clear that even cancers that appear the same can arise from a variety of different mutations, and as such can and/or should be treated differently. Moreover, elucidation of the nature of the somatic mutations underlying various tumours provides an obvious target for drug development. Drugs for which it may be useful to use genetic tests to determine whether an individual is a suitable candidate for therapy include the following anticancer drugs:

- specific tyrosine kinase inhibitors, such as imatinib and trastuzumab
- retinoic acid in acute promyelocytic leukaemia.

Table 9.4
Examples of selected substrates, inhibitors and inducers of some of the cytochrome P450 enzymes, with an indication as to whether there are known genetic polymorphisms of these enzymes

Enzyme	Substrates	Inhibitors	Inducers	Polymorphisms?
CYP1A2	Amitriptyline Haloperidol Paracetamol Warfarin	Cimetidine Ciprofloxacin	Broccoli Omeprazole Tobacco	
CYP2B6	Bupropion Cyclophosphamide Methadone	Ticlopidine	Phenobarbital Rifampicin	Yes: 3–4% Caucasians slow metabolizers
CYP2C8	Paclitaxel Cerivastatin Repaglinide	Trimethoprim Glitazones	Rifampicin	
CYP2C19	Omeprazole Diazepam Phenytoin Indometacin	Chloramphenicol Cimetidine	Carbamazepine Rifampicin	Yes: 3–5% Caucasians and 15–20% Asians slow metabolizers
CYP2C9	Diclofenac Ibuprofen Losartan Tolbutamide	Fluconazole Isoniazid	Rifampicin Secobarbital	Yes: 1–3% Caucasians slow metabolizers
CYP2D6	Alprenolol Amitriptyline Chlorphenamine Chlorpromazine Haloperidol	Chlorpromazine Chlorphenamine Cimetidine	Dexamethasone Rifampicin	Yes: 5–10% Caucasians slow metabolizers
CYP2E1	Ethanol Halothane Paracetamol Theophylline	Disulfiram	Ethanol Isoniazid	
CYP3A4,5,7	Caffeine Chlorphenamine Clarithromycin Nifedipine	Grapefruit juice Ketoconazole Verapamil	Phenobarbital Rifampicin St John's wort	Yes: 75% Caucasians and 50% blacks do not express functional CYP3A5

CYP2D6

CYP2D6 is the P450 enzyme that is involved in the metabolism of a number of drugs, including various β-adrenoreceptor-blocking drugs, antidepressants such as amitriptyline, paroxetine and fluoxetine, antipsychotic drugs such as haloperidol, thioridazine and risperidone, and a variety of other drugs such as codeine. In fact, CYP2D6 is involved in the metabolism of around 25% of all prescribed drugs. Among Caucasians, 5–10% of individuals have polymorphisms in the *CYP2D6* gene, and these polymorphisms are associated with alterations in the rate of metabolism of the drug substrates, with corresponding alterations in the clinical effectiveness of the drugs. There appear to be almost 80 distinct alleles of the *CYP2D6* gene. In one of the polymorphic forms, known as CYP2D6*5 or CYP2D6(D), there is homozygous deletion of the entire CYPD6 locus and a complete absence of the CYP2D6 protein in the liver. Unsurprisingly, this is associated with poor metabolism of a number of drugs. This deletion is the second most common inactivation allele in the UK population. It is noteworthy that the human genetic sequence produced by the Human Genome Project does not contain the sequence for CYP2D6, as the copy of chromosome 22 sequenced happened to have the deletion allele. A few of the other CYP2D6 polymorphisms are summarized in Table 9.5.

Whilst under-activity of CYP2D6 can be a problem, leading to excessive (and potentially lethal) side-effects of a variety of drugs, over-activity of the enzyme can also be a problem. CYP2D6 metabolizes the analgesic drug codeine to the more active morphine. In a notable case, a patient given a small dose of codeine to control cough developed a life-threatening opiate 'overdose' due in part at least to ultra-rapid metabolism of codeine to morphine (see Table 9.5). In contrast, poor metabolizers convert codeine to morphine poorly or not at all, and achieve very little analgesia from this particular drug.

Imatinib

Imatinib (Glivec® or Gleevec®) is a drug that can be used in the treatment of chronic myeloid leukaemia. In contrast to the vast majority of anticancer drugs, which target all rapidly dividing cells, imatinib specifically targets one aspect of the cancer cells; it is a selective inhibitor of a tyrosine kinase enzyme which is deregulated in the cancer cells and thus acts as a powerful stimulus for growth. Imatinib is a particularly good inhibitor of the fusion protein, Bcr-Abl, which is formed in the majority of cases of chronic myeloid leukaemia. These cases are characterized by the presence of the so-called 'Philadelphia chromosome', which results from a reciprocal translocation between chromosomes 9 and 22. This translocation leads to the insertion of the *Bcr* gene into the first exon of the normal c-Abl tyrosine kinase. The resulting Bcr-Abl kinase is permanently active and appears to have a key role in the development of disease. Thus inhibition of this enzyme is an excellent target for drugs and imatinib has proved extremely effective, producing complete remission in over 80% of patients with the Philadelphia chromosome who were in the chronic phase of chronic myeloid leukaemia. Unfortunately, the development of resistance to imatinib is becoming a problem in clinical use, but this drug still represents a real advance in the treatment of this disease.

Trastuzumab

Another tyrosine kinase with an established role in cancer is HER2. This is found to be expressed at high levels in about 25–30% of breast cancers. A normal cell possesses two copies of the *HER2* gene, over-expression resulting from the presence of multiple copies of the gene. *HER2* is inhibited by trastuzumab (Herceptin®), a monoclonal antibody which has been shown to be of benefit in the treatment of *HER2*-positive cancers. Trastuzumab is very much less effective in cancers that do not express high levels of *HER2*, and so the drug can only be used in combination with a diagnostic test to establish the *HER2* status of the tumour. The main way in which the *HER2* status of a tumour is established is currently immunohistochemistry to detect the expression of the HER2 protein (see Ch. 6), but this technique yields notoriously variable results both between different laboratories and from within a single laboratory. Other tests have been developed which detect the presence of the *HER2* gene or mRNA using fluorescence in situ hybridization (FISH), reverse transcriptase polymerase chain reaction (RT-PCR) and microarrays, and these are gradually replacing immunohistochemistry in the diagnostic laboratory. The FISH assay in particular is now accepted as a standard method of establishing *HER2* over-expression.

Retinoic acid

Retinoic acid is licensed for the induction of remission in acute promyelocytic leukaemia. In some forms of this disease, there is a balanced translocation between chromosomes 15 and 17, which results in the fusion of the *PML* gene with the retinoic acid receptor α (*RARα*) gene. Activation of the resulting fusion protein, PML/RARα, with retinoic acid leads to decreased growth and increased differentiation of the cancer cells.

Polymorphisms of other drug targets

An ever-increasing number of polymorphisms of well-established drug targets are being discovered. These include polymorphisms of receptors, such as the β₁ and β₂ adrenoreceptors, molecules responsible for adverse drug reactions, such as HERG (see below), and a number of targets in microorganisms.

β₁ and β₂ adrenoreceptors

A large number of β receptor polymorphisms have been discovered and some of these have been shown to affect receptor activity and/or desensitization in *in vitro*

Table 9.5
Some of the allelic variants of CYP2D6

Name	Mutation	Effect	Protein	Phenotype
CYP2D6*4	G-1934 to A	Aberrant splicing of mRNA	Inactive	Poor metabolizer
CYP2D6*5	Deletion		None	Poor metabolizer
CYP2D6*6	Deletion of T-1795	Premature stop codon	Inactive	Poor metabolizer
CYP2D6*10	C-188 to T	pro-34 to ser	Reduced catalytic activity and reduced thermal stability	Poor metabolizer
CYP2D6*2	C-2938 to T G-4268 to C	Associated with multiple copies of the gene	Over-expression	Ultra-rapid metabolizer

experiments. Given the fact that a number of clinically important drugs target these receptors (the β-blockers such as propranolol and atenolol used in hypertension and angina, and the β_2 agonists such as salbutamol used in asthma), there have been many suggestions that these polymorphisms may have a role in unusual responses to drugs acting at these receptors, or in susceptibility to diseases such as asthma. However, there is as yet very little convincing evidence to support these hypotheses.

HERG

Another drug target that is currently the focus of great interest on the part of the pharmaceutical industry is the cardiac potassium channel encoded by the human ether-a-go-go related gene, HERG. A number of drugs are capable of blocking this channel and producing potentially fatal cardiac arrhythmias. These include anti-arrhythmics such as quinidine and procainamide, but also a wide range of other drugs, including antipsychotics such as chlorpromazine and haloperidol, antihistamines such as terfenadine and loratadine, the antibacterial drug clarithromycin, the prokinetic cisapride (recently removed from the US market), and cocaine. It is now reasonably routine for pharmaceutical companies to screen new drugs for an interaction with HERG at an early stage in development.

Polymorphisms of HERG are well established. Rare mutations in HERG result in familial long-QT syndrome, which is associated with arrhythmias and sudden death. However, there are also a number of other HERG polymorphisms. The most common is K897T, a substitution of threonine for lysine at position 897, which is present in 25–30% of humans. These polymorphisms are associated with subtle changes in channel behaviour, which may well predispose individuals to the adverse channel-blocking effects of a variety of drugs.

Targets for antimicrobial drugs

It is not just knowledge of the human genome that has the potential to improve drug therapy. The genome of numerous pathogens, including *Haemophilus influenzae*, *Mycobacterium leprae*, *Mycobacterium tuberculosis*, *Escherichia coli O157*, *Plasmodium falciparum*, *Trypanosoma brucei*, *Trypanosoma cruzi* and *Bacillus anthrax*, have all been, or are in the process of being, sequenced as part of various pathogen genome projects. This is yielding an enormous amount of information which is highly relevant to the pharmacological therapy of diseases caused by these organisms. For example, it has been shown that a mutation in the chloroquine transporter gene, *pfcrt*, can render the malarial parasite, *Plasmodium falciparum*, resistant to chloroquine. Field studies in Mali suggest that there is a stable relationship between chloroquine resistance and the presence of this mutation. Thus in future it may be possible to use a relatively simple DNA test to determine the drug sensitivity of a range of disease-causing organisms (see Ch. 3).

Knowledge of pathogen genes has also revealed new drug targets. Sequencing of the *Plasmodium falciparum* genome revealed that this organism appeared to use the DOXP pathway: an enzyme system known to be present in plants and bacteria, but not in humans. A drug that targets the DOXP pathway had already been developed, as a potential treatment for urinary tract infections. Unfortunately, although this drug, fosmidomycin, was well tolerated, it was ineffective in the infection model used. The discovery of the DOXP pathway in *Plasmodium falciparum* prompted the trial of fosmidomycin in malaria, and the early results of clinical trials are encouraging.

Why are polymorphisms tolerated?

The question arises as to why there should be so much individual variation in the sequence of key genes. Mutations will persist in the population if the mutation has no impact on function, at least into young adulthood, by which time the genes will, in all likelihood, have been passed on to the next generation. This is presumably what has happened in most cases of pharmacogenetic polymorphisms; the variant has no discernable impact on 'fitness' unless the individual survives into old age (in which case increased susceptibility to various diseases may become apparent) or is subject to treatment with one of the multitude of weird and wonderful drugs that have been developed by modern medicine.

In some cases, the polymorphism may actually confer some selective advantage. The best-characterized example of this is the resistance to malaria conferred by G6PD deficiency. Other polymorphisms also appear to have undergone positive selection. Long-range haplotype studies to define linkage disequilibrium in the region of chromosome 8 that encodes the genes for N-acetyl transferase (NAT2) have suggested that a particular haplotype (NAT2*5B) has been under recent positive selection in Western and Central Europeans. This haplotype contains the T-341 to C mutation which encodes for the 'slowest acetylator' NAT2 enzyme (see Table 9.3); the positive selection suggests that slow acetylation has conferred some survival advantage during the past 6500 years. Oddly, this haplotype is the one most strongly associated with adverse drug reactions and also susceptibility to bladder cancer.

How soon are we likely to see routine pharmacogenetic testing?

It has been known for many years that potentially lethal differences in responsiveness to drugs can be inherited. In the post-genome era, we are now identifying more and more polymorphisms which impact on the effectiveness and toxicity of drugs. The World Health Organization is actively promoting the use of DNA tests to assess the drug resistance of common parasites in the developing world, with a view to improving the efficacy and cost-effectiveness of drug treatment. In the UK, the government has devoted £4 million to a pharmacogenetic programme aimed at identifying patients at risk from adverse reactions to drugs currently in widespread use. There is clearly a huge potential benefit from targeting therapies more appropriately on the basis of pharmacogenetic testing, but at the moment testing remains rare. Why is this?

Tests are currently expensive and many are logistically complicated. However, their cost is reducing all the time as technology improves and economies of scale become possible. There could well be a time when an individual would only need to undergo a battery of genetic tests once. This information could then be stored in that person's medical record for future reference; after all, one's genes are not going to change. Testing the entire genome for all possible

polymorphisms would obviously be a huge job, but the observation that our chromosomes contain a number of reasonably invariant haplotype blocks (see Ch. 2) could mean that the entire genotype could be predicted by testing for a smaller number of well-chosen 'tag' SNPs to characterize the various blocks. One (possibly over-optimistic) estimate suggests that a single microarray testing for 100 000 SNPs might be sufficient to predict each individual's responsiveness to drugs. However, this estimate is likely to need to be revised as we understand more about the polymorphisms' underlying drug responsiveness.

Of course, this kind of genetic testing raises issues of confidentiality and consent. What if a particular polymorphism is known to be associated with an increased risk of cancer? Should a patient's insurance company be informed of the results of these tests?

Alongside the problem of cataloguing and testing for every possible polymorphism, there is the substantial problem of understanding the effect of all these possible polymorphisms on the efficacy of drugs and their likely side-effects, toxicity and interactions. While the amount of information that we possess regarding this is increasing all the time, it is still very far from complete and will require an enormous amount of work before the possibility of determining an individual's drug phenotype becomes a reality. It is clearly an enormous logistic task to correlate all reported adverse drug reactions with the genotype of the individuals affected. Moreover, as adverse reactions are, by their very nature, fairly rare, achieving statistically meaningful results will be extremely difficult. However, more focused tests are already a reality and it is very likely that more and more of them will be used, and more widely, to inform the prescription of drugs in the near future.

Public pressure seems likely to increase the demand for pharmacogenetic testing. There are already companies offering testing for CYP polymorphisms, for example, to members of the public who are becoming increasingly knowledgeable about the impact of genetics on their health.

Even with reliable, simple and cost-effective tests, it is essential to have medical personnel sufficiently knowledgeable to put the results of these tests into practice. It is widely accepted that medical education has lagged far behind the technical advances in the field of molecular genetics; hence the importance of this book!

Given the complexity and expense of testing individuals for polymorphisms, are there any 'short cuts' that could be used? For example, should drugs be prescribed for particular ethnic groups, who are more likely to possess a particular polymorphism? Some drugs may well be used in this way already by individual prescribers, and recently BiDil™ has been licensed by the US Food and Drug Administration (FDA) as an adjunct in the treatment of heart failure, but only in patients who identify themselves as black (Box 9.3). However, racial prescribing, as well as being ethically sensitive, is unlikely to be a widely applicable solution, as there appears to be much greater genetic variability within an ethnic group than between different groups.

Box 9.3

BiDil

BiDil is a fixed-dose combination of two vasodilator drugs, hydralazine and isosorbide dinitrate, developed as a treatment for heart failure. In initial clinical trials it was not shown to produce any significant improvement and was abandoned. However, close inspection of the data suggested that, while no effect was apparent in patients who identified themselves as white, improvement was seen in patients who identified themselves as black. Based on this observation, a further trial was conducted, using only black patients; the results were so convincing that the trial was terminated early so that the control group could also receive the drugs. The US FDA has now licensed BiDil as a treatment for heart failure only in those patients who identify themselves as black — the first instance of a drug licensed according to race.

Despite the initial success of this 'race-based prescribing' approach, it is recognized that race is at best a crude indicator of particular genetic polymorphisms. All participants in the BiDil trial donated DNA samples and these are being analysed in an attempt to identify a more specific biomarker that predicts efficacy of this drug combination.

The widespread use of pharmacogenetic testing will inevitably increase the costs involved in drug therapy. Whether or not the improvements in health and efficiency of prescribing (fewer adverse drug reactions, less prescribing of ineffective drugs) are capable of offsetting these increased costs remains to be seen. Clearly, cost–benefit analysis of these new approaches will be extremely important. The situation is further complicated by the fact that the incidence of polymorphisms is generally fairly low, but everyone might need to be tested in order to detect the few individuals affected. Moreover, genetics is not the only reason for individual variation in responsiveness to drugs; age, disease, other drugs and compliance all have a significant impact. These factors are considered in more detail in relation to responsiveness to warfarin (below).

What is the likely impact of pharmacogenetics on drug development?

Pharmacogenetics could clearly be of benefit to individuals and to a society which aims to make the best use of limited healthcare resources. However, its benefits to the pharmaceutical industry are not always so obvious.

Pharmaceutical companies are already using pharmacogenetic tests to identify polymorphisms of drug-metabolizing enzymes in the subjects used in clinical trials. The US FDA has published a guidance document regarding the submission of these data for the purposes of drug licensing. In general, drugs that are likely to prove problematic in individuals with common polymorphisms, such as those in CYP2D6 or HERG, are avoided. Thus pharmacogenetics appears to have already been embraced by the industry to some extent.

Drugs targeted to particular populations on the basis of their genetic makeup inevitably means a smaller market for each drug. The current trial and error approach to prescribing means sales of unnecessary drugs and therefore profit for the drug manufacturers. However, if targeting could be done at the clinical trial stage, it could result in smaller, cheaper trials, with fewer drugs 'failing' due to adverse side-effects. Indeed it has already been the case that 'failed' drugs, such as BiDil and fosmidomycin, have been 'rescued' on the basis of pharmacogenetic information.

An increased role for pharmacogenetic testing will mean an increased role for the growing diagnostics industry, which will be intimately linked with the development, testing and everyday use of drugs. Regulation and licensing of the tests will be as important as the regulation and licensing of the drugs themselves, especially if use of a pharmacogenetic test is incorporated into the licence for a drug. At present only a handful of polymorphisms (e.g. cytochrome P450 polymorphisms) are considered by regulatory agencies such as the FDA to be valid biomarkers, able to predict drug response with confidence.

Variability in response to warfarin

The impact of genetics on drug response is, of course, likely to be complex and, what is more, genetics is not the only factor that influences responsiveness to drugs (see Fig. 9.1). This can be illustrated by considering the factors that influence the variation observed in an individual's responsiveness to warfarin.

Warfarin is an orally active anticoagulant, used to reduce the risk of inappropriate blood clotting in, for example, patients immobilized after surgery, at risk of stroke or with artificial heart valves. About 750 000 people in the UK currently receive warfarin each year and this number is increasing annually. It has been estimated that up to a quarter of patients treated with warfarin for over 12 months will experience a serious side-effect, usually haemorrhage.

Each individual differs in his or her response to warfarin. It is routine for patients to be started on a low dose of the drug, which is then gradually increased until the appropriate inhibition of blood clotting is achieved. In the first week of therapy, patients should have their blood clotting monitored every other day at least, but even if a patient has been stabilized on warfarin for many years, he or she will still need to have blood clotting monitored every 4–8 weeks to check that the dose of warfarin is still appropriate. So what are the causes of the variation in responsiveness to warfarin both between and within individuals?

Genetic effects on warfarin metabolism

Warfarin is metabolized by CYP2C9, and polymorphisms associated with reduced activity of this enzyme are known to cause an increased risk of haemorrhage and an increased susceptibility to interactions with certain drugs, such as the anti-epileptic, phenytoin. The usual average dose of warfarin is around 5 mg per day; people with low levels of CYP2C9 activity normally require doses as low as 1–5 mg per *week*.

Genetic effects on the target for warfarin

The gene for warfarin's target, vitamin K epoxide reductase complex 1, has recently been identified; it is *VKORC1*. There are different alleles of this gene, which allow patients to be grouped in low-, intermediate- and high-dosage groups on the basis of the maintenance doses of warfarin required to achieve an appropriate anticoagulant effect. Thus not only are at least two genes involved in determining response to warfarin, but also a host of environmental and other factors.

Environmental factors and drug interactions

Warfarin is subject to interaction with a wide range of drugs and dietary factors that will alter its effectiveness. It is essential that patients maintained on warfarin are educated about these various factors and seek professional advice whenever appropriate.

- *Vitamin K levels.* Warfarin works by inhibiting the reduction of vitamin K epoxide, and thus inhibiting the synthesis of various clotting factors. Increased availability of vitamin K will offset the effect of warfarin, whereas decreased vitamin K levels enhance warfarin's anticoagulant effect. Vitamin K is obtained from two sources: the diet (in leafy green vegetables such as spinach and broccoli) and synthesis by gut bacteria. Changes in the amount of vitamin K in the diet will necessitate a change in the maintenance dose of warfarin, as will the use of antibacterial drugs, which kill some of the gut bacteria and reduce the availability of vitamin K.
- *Liver metabolism.* As well as genetic effects on CYP2C9 activity, the presence of other drugs and chemicals will alter the rate at which this enzyme metabolizes warfarin. For example, phenytoin, tolbutamide and diclofenac inhibit the metabolism of warfarin, enhancing its effects and requiring a reduction in dose. On the other hand, rifampicin and phenobarbital induce levels of CYP2C9 activity in liver, reducing the effectiveness of warfarin and requiring an increase in maintenance dose.
- *Plasma protein-binding.* In common with many other drugs, warfarin is extensively bound to plasma proteins in the blood stream, which reduces the amount of drug available to produce its effects. However, if another drug, such as aspirin, is taken which binds to the same sites on the plasma proteins, warfarin will be displaced from its binding sites, increasing the free concentration and therefore the effect.

Effect of age

Elderly people are more sensitive to the effects of warfarin. They require lower maintenance doses than younger people to achieve the same level of anticoagulant effect.

Effects of disease

It is well recognized that the response to warfarin is affected by intercurrent illness. Fever increases the effect of warfarin and thus increases the risk of excessive bleeding, as does hyperthyroidism; hypothyroidism decreases the effectiveness of warfarin and increases the risk of thrombosis.

Compliance

One of the main factors that influences whether or not a drug is effective is whether or not the patient takes it appropriately. Missing one or several doses will obviously decrease efficacy, whereas taking too much, either by accident or design, will increase the likelihood of toxicity. We are a very long way indeed from understanding the genetic basis of this complex factor.

Thus, while pharmacogenetic testing may seem likely to improve therapy with drugs such as warfarin, these tests may well not obviate the need for routine testing, as so many other factors are also involved in determining the drug's effectiveness. If it is necessary to monitor patients carefully in any case, is there any added benefit of administering a (possibly expensive) genetic test?

Conclusion

Undoubtedly pharmacogenetics is having an increasing impact on the use and development of drugs. However, testing is costly, and genetic variation is only one of the many sources of individual variation in responsiveness to drugs. While specific tests for particular polymorphisms will undoubtedly start to be used more and more frequently to inform prescribing decisions, routine genotyping to determine our entire pharmacogenetic profile is still rather a long way off.

FURTHER READING

Pathogen Genome Sequencing: http://www.sanger.ac.uk/Projects/Pathogens/

Pharmacogenetics and Pharmacogenomics Knowledge Base: http://www.pharmgkb.org/

Rang H, Dale M, Ritter J, Flower R 2007 Rang & Dale's pharmacology, 6th edn. Churchill Livingstone: Edinburgh.

Royal Society 2005 Personalised medicines: hopes and realities: http://www.royalsoc.ac.uk/document.asp?id=3780

SNP Consortium and HapMap Projects: http://snp.cshl.org/

10

Gene therapy
M. Keen

One of the most alluring aspects of the genomic revolution is the promise of gene therapy; if faulty genes are at the root of a disease, then surely the most logical approach to the treatment of that disease is the replacement or repair of those faulty genes?

What is gene therapy?

Gene therapy is a technique for 'correcting' defective genes responsible for disease development. Several different approaches are being developed to achieve this goal (see below).

However, despite the apparent simplicity of the gene therapy approach, and the many millions of pounds that have been poured into gene therapy research over the last 25 years, gene therapy remains experimental. No therapies are yet licensed in Europe or the USA for general use, and the only access to this technology is via participation in a clinical trial.

Clinical experiences with gene therapy

Among the first diseases to be treated using gene therapy were two severe combined immunodeficiencies:

- adenosine deaminase deficiency combined immunodeficiency disorder (ADA-SCID)
- X-linked immunodeficiency disorder (X-SCID).

Both of these are extremely debilitating, single-gene disorders, which are difficult to treat by other means. In both disorders, the defective genes are expressed in blood cells. This makes it possible to obtain haematopoietic stem cells from the patient's blood or bone marrow, transfect these cells with the desired gene in the test tube, and then reintroduce the cells to the patient. There is a reasonable expectation that the transfected cells will become re-established and start producing genetically modified blood cells. Such ex vivo treatment of cells is summarized in Figure 10.1. It avoids any risk of insertion of the gene into the wrong cells or tissues (see below) and is one of the key reasons why these diseases were chosen for the first clinical trials of gene therapy.

In 1990, two ADA-SCID patients had T cells removed, purified and amplified in culture. These cells were then transfected in culture with the adenosine deaminase gene (*ADA*) in a retroviral vector (see below) and reintroduced into the patients. The trial was a success in that the patients were unharmed, and the 'new' gene was expressed in their bodies for at least 12 years. Sadly, however, these patients were not cured; the level of expression of the gene was simply insufficient to alleviate the disease, and the patients had to be maintained on the standard treatment: regular injections of adenosine deaminase conjugated with polyethylene glycol (PEG-ADA). Indeed, it may have been the concurrent treatment of these patients with PEG-ADA that contributed to the lack of success of the gene therapy; ADA-PEG improves survival of adenosine deaminase-deficient T cells, and thus may reduce the selection pressure in favour of the survival and proliferation of the genetically modified cells. More recent studies, in which PEG-ADA treatment has been withheld, have been more successful. Nevertheless, the lesson is clear. Expression of the gene is not enough; it has to be expressed in sufficient quantities for it to be clinically useful.

The first human disease to be successfully treated entirely by gene therapy was X-SCID. This is an extremely severe form of immunodeficiency, which is also known as 'bubble baby syndrome', as sufferers lack any functional white blood cells and must be completely isolated in order to avoid the risk of infection. It is due to a loss of function of the gene *IL2RG*, which codes for the common γ-chain forming part of the receptors for several of the interleukins (IL-2, IL-4, IL-7, IL-9, IL-15 and IL-21). Ten infants had bone marrow cells transfected ex vivo with *IL2RG* in a murine leukaemia virus-derived retroviral vector. Following reinfusion of the treated cells, 9 of the 10 patients developed apparently normal T cells, B cells and natural killer cells expressing *IL2RG*. They did well clinically, were able to go home, developed normal antibody responses to childhood vaccines and did not require any other therapy: a resounding success.

Unfortunately, 30 and 34 months after treatment, the two youngest patients both developed leukaemia-like illnesses, with proliferation of particular T-cell clones. These cases did not appear to be a coincidence; in both cases it was found that the retroviral vector had inserted itself close to the 5' end of the gene for a transcription factor (LMO-2), and this appeared to have led to the inappropriate expression of LMO-2, and thus dysregulation of T-cell proliferation.

Insertion of a retrovirus itself into another gene is called insertional mutagenesis (Fig. 10.2); it is a known risk associated with retroviral vectors. Until this time, it was thought that the insertion of retroviruses into the genome was a random process. It has since become clear that insertion of retroviruses is not as random as we first

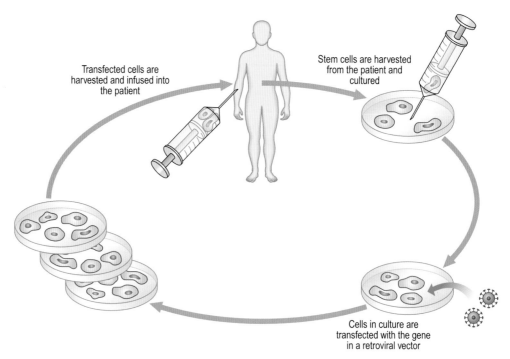

Figure 10.1
Ex-vivo transfection of stem cells. Stem cells are harvested from the blood or bone marrow of the patient. They are transfected in culture, using a retroviral vector. Finally the transformed cells are administered to the patient.

thought and the identification of possible integration sites for retroviruses is becoming possible. Different retroviruses also have different preferences. The murine leukaemia virus, used here, seems particularly likely to insert itself near the beginning of a gene, leading to inappropriate expression. On the other hand, HIV-derived vectors seem more likely to land in the middle of a gene and thus prevent its expression. Nevertheless, the risk of carcinogenesis with retroviral vectors appears to be very low in animal experiments and in other clinical trials; so what had gone so wrong here? The answer is still unclear, but it seems likely that the extreme selective advantage gained by the gene-corrected cells, and the higher proliferation rate of cells in the younger patients, may well have contributed. Clearly, the use of retroviral vectors has come under considerable scrutiny.

Prerequisites for successful gene therapy

Successful gene therapy requires the following:

- a candidate gene to be replaced, or a strategy for repairing or silencing a faulty gene
- a delivery mechanism for getting the new gene into the correct tissue, so that it will be expressed in the correct amounts and for a sufficient period of time

- beneficial expression of the new gene
- benefits to the new gene that must outweigh any risks of the gene and/or the gene delivery system.

An obvious requirement for gene therapy is that the genetic basis for any particular disease must have been identified (see Ch. 2). Perhaps the most obvious candidate diseases for treatment with gene therapy are the single-gene disorders, such as haemophilia, cystic fibrosis or the severe combined immunodeficiencies, and indeed these disorders have been the subject of much research. However, while in many cases devastating, these single-gene disorders are comparatively rare. There are far more lives to be saved (and much more money to be made!) targeting common diseases such as cancer or ischaemic heart disease, and it is not surprising that various strategies are being developed to exploit gene therapy in the treatment of these conditions. As an example, Table 10.1 shows some of the various gene therapy approaches which have been used in clinical trials for the treatment of prostate cancer.

The main approaches used to correct a faulty gene

Having identified a target gene, a strategy must be developed by which the function of that gene can be repaired.

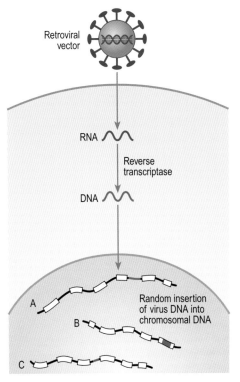

RNA

Reverse
transcriptase

DNA

Retroviral
vector

A

B

C

Random insertion
of virus DNA into
chromosomal DNA

Figure 10.2

Insertional mutagenesis. DNA encoded by a retrovirus inserts itself randomly into chromosomal DNA. If the insertion occurs between genes (A), there is likely to be no disruption of function. However, if the insertion occurs in the middle of a gene (B), it is likely to disrupt production of that protein. If insertion occurs into the control region of a gene (C), it may lead to over-expression of that gene.

Replacement

For diseases caused by 'loss-of-function' mutations or gene deletions, it may be sufficient to simply 'add in' a functional version of the gene, such as the gene for the appropriate clotting factor in haemophilia, or for the chloride transporter in cystic fibrosis. In these cases, there is little control over where in the genome the new gene will become inserted, but in many cases this may well not matter.

Repair

A more subtle approach is to attempt to repair a faulty gene. In Duchenne muscular dystrophy, a wide variety of mutations of the dystrophin gene lead to a reading frame shift that produces a premature stop codon in the mature mRNA. The single most common mutation in Duchenne's is deletion of exon 45. Interestingly, in the much milder Becker-type muscular dystrophy, deletions of exons 45–54 can occur; so long as the mutation does not cause a reading frame shift, some function of dystrophin seems to be preserved. Antisense oligonucleotides have been engineered which bind to the splice sequences of exon 46 and result in this exon also being omitted from the mRNA. In this case, the frame shift does not occur, a premature stop sequence is not encountered and a functional dystrophin protein is produced (Fig. 10.3).

Another approach to gene repair could exploit the phenomenon of homologous recombination. Homologous recombination is a natural repair mechanism that can occur during cell division; if the DNA strands in one chromosome break, it can be repaired using the

Table 10.1
Examples of some of the gene therapy approaches that have reached clinical trials for the treatment of prostate cancer

Therapeutic strategy	Gene	Vector	Route of administration
Stimulation of an immune response to eradicate tumour	Granulocyte macrophage-colony stimulating factor (GM-CSF)	Retrovirus	Subcutaneous
Stimulation of an immune response to eradicate tumour	Interleukin-2 (IL-2)	Cationic liposome	Intradermal; intratumoral
Tumour vaccine	Prostate-specific antigen (PSA)	Vaccinia	Intradermal
Vector-directed cell lysis	Prostate-specific antigen (PSA)	Adenovirus	Intratumoral
'Suicide gene': transfection of an enzyme which will activate a pro-drug to kill transfected cells	Herpes simplex virus thymidine kinase (HSV-tk) activates ganciclovir	Adenovirus	Intratumoral; intraprostatic
Inhibition of an oncogene	Antisense c-myc	Retrovirus	Intraprostatic
Addition of a tumour suppressor gene	p53	Adenovirus	Intraprostatic; intratumoral
Addition of a tumour suppressor gene	Breast cancer 1 (BRCA1)	Retrovirus	Intraprostatic

A Becker-type muscular dystrophy

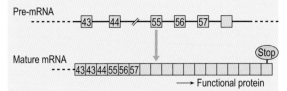

B Duchenne-type muscular dystrophy

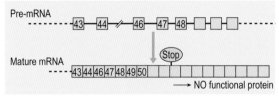

C Treated Duchenne-type muscular dystrophy

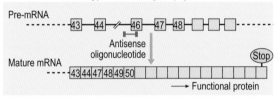

Figure 10.3
'Exon skipping' strategy for the treatment of Duchenne muscular dystrophy. (A) In Becker-type muscular dystrophy there may be deletion of multiple exons (45–54 inclusive in this example). However, there is no frame shift mutation and the mRNA can be used to synthesize a protein that retains some function. (B) In Duchenne-type muscular dystrophy, deletion of a single exon (45) leads to a shift in the reading frame, so that a premature stop codon is encountered. This mRNA cannot produce functional protein. (C) Use of an antisense oligonucleotide to induce the 'skipping' of exon 46. When both exons 45 and 46 are excluded from the mRNA there is no frame shift and no premature stop codon, and the mRNA can encode a 'Becker-type' protein with some function.

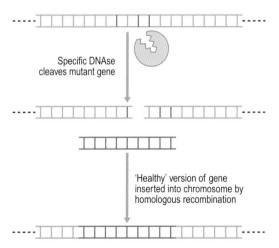

Figure 10.4
Homologous recombination. Homologous recombination is a mechanism for the repair of double-stranded, chromosomal DNA in which both strands have broken. This figure shows how it can be exploited in gene therapy. The DNA encoding the mutant gene is first cleaved by a specifically engineered DNAse. This broken strand is repaired by homologous recombination with a copy of the 'healthy' gene, which has also been introduced into the cell.

corresponding DNA from the other chromosome as a template. One potential treatment for X-SCID involves the introduction of an engineered DNAse into the bone marrow cells along with a healthy copy of the *IL-2R* gene. The enzyme specifically cleaves the DNA of the mutant *IL-2R* gene and the healthy gene acts as a template for its repair (Fig. 10.4).

Gene silencing

In other situations it might be necessary to 'silence' expression of a particular gene, using antisense or siRNA. For example, an antisense oligonucleotide against the androgen receptor and an siRNA against the type 1 insulin-like growth factor receptor have both been shown to inhibit cell proliferation in human prostate cancer cells *in vitro*.

Gene therapy vectors

Having decided on the genetic material that you would like to introduce into cells, the next challenge is to find a suitable vector that will deliver the genetic material safely into the right cells, so that the gene can be expressed in appropriate amounts and for long enough to cure the disease or to alleviate its symptoms. It is undoubtedly this aspect of gene therapy that has proved to be the most problematic in clinical practice.

At present there is no ideal vector and so a variety of approaches are being used, some of which involve viral vectors and some non-viral vectors. Each vector system has its own advantages and disadvantages, and these are summarized below.

Viral vectors

In many ways, viruses are the ideal gene therapy vectors. Viruses have evolved extremely efficient mechanisms for inserting their 'foreign' genetic material into the host cell and for persuading the host cell to express that genetic material; as Figure 10.5 shows, this is how viral replication works!

In order to exploit viruses as gene therapy vectors, however, a number of precautions must be taken.

- The virus must be rendered replication-deficient, to prevent its uncontrolled proliferation, which would result in infection of the human host.
- Similarly, the virus should not provoke an immune response from the host, as this in itself can cause tissue damage (see below).

Importantly, there is a limit to the amount of genetic material that any virus particle can physically contain, and there is also a limit to the amount of the viral genome that can be deleted while still allowing the virus to function as a vector. There are thus stringent size restrictions on the genes that can be delivered using viral vectors.

Most retroviruses will only infect dividing cells and this property has been exploited in an experimental treatment for brain tumours, in which retroviruses have also been used to deliver 'suicide genes' to kill the tumour cells. As normal brain tissue is mostly non-dividing tissue, the retroviral vector infected only the tumour.

Lentiviruses

A special type of retroviral vector has now been developed as a gene delivery vehicle for non-dividing cells: the lentiviral vectors. These vectors will deliver genetic material into non-dividing cells and integrate into the genome. However, as lentiviral vectors are developed from the highly pathogenic HIV virus, which causes AIDS, widespread clinical application of such vectors will only be allowed after rigorous safety testing.

Adenoviral vectors

Adenoviruses are DNA parvoviruses, best known as being one of the viruses associated with the common cold. They are able to infect both dividing and non-dividing cells. There are many different adenoviruses but type 5 is the one that has been most commonly used in clinical trials. These viruses are maintained transiently within cells because they do not integrate into the genome. They therefore pose no risk of insertional mutagenesis but do not give rise to prolonged expression of the therapeutic gene. The adenoviruses are attractive gene therapy vectors, as they can accommodate relatively large gene inserts (up to 30 kb), replicate well within cells to give high copy numbers and can be readily purified from culture. However, adenoviruses have a major drawback — their immunogenicity (see below). This problem is compounded by the fact that treatment may well require repeated administration of the transiently expressed gene.

Pox viruses

Pox viruses, such as vaccinia, the cow pox virus, are also being tried as gene therapy vectors. Their properties are generally very similar to those of the adenoviruses.

Adeno-associated virus (AAV)

AAV is another member of the parvovirus family which is infectious to humans. However, infection has not so far been associated with any known disease. AAV can replicate both with and without incorporation into the host cell genome, and thus shares some of the retroviruses' advantages and risks. Despite these risks, the AAV vectors currently have the best safety profile of the various viral vectors. Unfortunately, they are rather small viruses, with a single-stranded DNA genome of about 5 kb; this limits the maximum size of transgene that can be incorporated to about 4.5 kb, which precludes the insertion of long regulatory sequences or large genes.

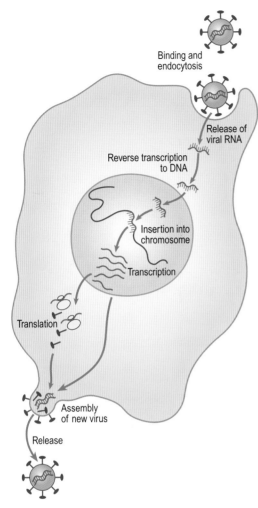

Figure 10.5
The life cycle of a retrovirus. The virus enters the host cell by endocytosis, following binding of the virus to specific cell surface proteins. Once inside the cell, the viral RNA is released and copied into a DNA transcript by reverse transcriptase. This DNA then inserts itself into the host cell's chromosomes. The host cell then transcribes multiple copies of the virally encoded RNA and translates the appropriate sequences into protein. Viral protein and RNA are assembled into new virus particles and released from the host cell by exocytosis.

Retroviral vectors

In a retrovirus, such as murine leukaemia virus, the genetic information is in the form of RNA, which must be transcribed into DNA by reverse transcriptase and then inserted into the chromosomal DNA of the host cell, prior to replication (Fig. 10.5). When retroviruses are used as gene therapy vectors, this insertion into chromosomal DNA is both a blessing and a curse. It leads to the risk of insertional mutagenesis but it also means that genes carried on a retroviral vector become part of the chromosome, and are thus likely to persist in the cell for a long time and even be inherited by any daughter cells following cell division. This makes retroviruses particularly appropriate for the insertion of genes into stem cells, as was required by both of the SCID trials.

Herpes simplex virus

The herpes virus has a natural ability to travel into the central nervous system along peripheral nerves, and this property makes it ideal for delivering genes into, for example, sensory nerve cells for the treatment of neuropathic pain. The virus also has a tendency to lie dormant in infected nerves for long periods, and it may well be possible to exploit this characteristic to obtain fairly stable expression of a therapeutic gene. Naturally, herpes simplex viral vectors have to be rendered non-pathogenic by deletion of a number of viral genes, but this provides room for the insertion of a relatively large transgene of up to 30 kb.

Non-viral vectors

It is not essential to use viruses as vectors for gene therapy. There are several non-viral options for gene delivery and currently over 25% of gene therapy trials are using non-viral vectors. The advantages of this approach are:

- There is no risk of infection by the vector.
- Generally, much larger DNA sequences can be incorporated.

However, the efficiency of delivery of DNA to cells is usually much lower than with a virus.

Naked DNA

The simplest method is to administer the therapeutic DNA and hope that some of it is taken up into target cells. Surprisingly, perhaps, some does, but the efficiency of this method is extremely low and it requires large amounts of DNA. There are many reasons why we might expect DNA uptake into cells to be poor:

- DNA molecules are large in comparison with the cell.
- Both DNA and the cell membrane are negatively charged, posing a substantial electrostatic barrier to their interaction.
- They are rapidly broken down by DNAses in the blood and tissues.

Despite this low efficiency, naked DNA may potentially be of use for the delivery of 'genetic vaccines', which would only require the expression of relatively low amounts of protein (see Ch. 7). Naked DNA appears to have low immunogenicity, but there is at least a theoretical risk of developing anti-DNA antibodies, which are associated with the development of the severe autoimmune disease, systemic lupus erythematosus.

Particle guns

Particle guns have been used in an attempt to improve cellular uptake of DNA. In this approach, microparticles of tungsten or gold are coated with DNA and then fired at the target tissue at high velocity. This technique has been successfully used to deliver genes into the liver.

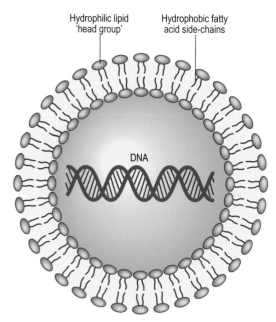

Figure 10.6
The structure of a simple liposome containing DNA for gene therapy.

Liposomes

In their simplest form, liposomes are artificial lipid spheres with an aqueous core, formed by sonicating a mixture of water, lipid and (in this case) DNA (Fig. 10.6). The liposome encapsulates the therapeutic DNA, protecting it from breakdown by DNAses. Furthermore, if the liposome is made with cationic lipids, its net positive charge overcomes the electrostatic barrier of the cell membrane and the liposome is capable of passing the DNA into the target cell. A further advantage of using cationic lipids is that these help to condense the long DNA molecule into a more compact form, which further protects it from metabolism and improves delivery to cells.

The use of lipids to condense and encapsulate DNA for cell delivery is becoming extremely sophisticated. Different lipids, possessing head groups with a variety of desirable properties, can be used to optimize the properties of the vector. For example, spermine head groups are very efficient at condensing DNA, while specific peptide or saccharide groups could be added to confer cell selectivity by binding to specific cell-surface receptors; fusogenic peptides (such as N-t-HA) could improve endocytosis of the vector and NLS-SV40 could optimize uptake into the nucleus.

Chimeric proteins

Therapeutic DNA can also be induced to enter target cells by chemically linking the DNA to a genetically engineered bifunctional protein. These chimeric proteins are essentially two proteins linked together:

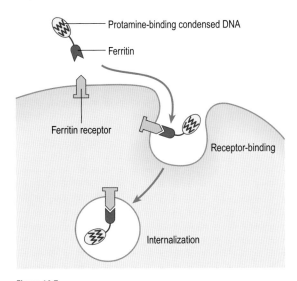

Figure 10.7
A chimeric protein vector for gene therapy. This chimeric protein is made up of a protamine moiety, which binds and condenses DNA, and a ferritin moiety, which binds to the ferritin receptor on the surface of cells and is endocytosed. This combination, therefore, provides a sophisticated mechanism for getting DNA into cells.

- a DNA-binding protein, such as protamine, to bind and condense the DNA
- a protein, such as ferritin, that will bind to specific receptors on the target cell membrane and facilitate entry into the cell (Fig. 10.7).

Although sophisticated, these delivery systems tend to be less effective than other options.

Artificial chromosomes

Researchers also are experimenting with introducing a 47th chromosome into target cells. This chromosome would exist autonomously alongside the standard 46 — not affecting their function or causing any mutations. It would be a very large vector capable of carrying substantial amounts of genetic code, and it is hoped that the body's immune systems would not attack it. However, a problem with this potential method is the enormous difficulty in delivering such a large molecule to the nucleus of a target cell.

The various vectors and their properties are summarized in Table 10.2.

Targeting genes to particular cells

In most cases of gene therapy it is important to get the therapeutic gene expressed in the correct cells. Thus, while it may not be critical which type of cell expresses a protein that is to act as a vaccine or manufactures a missing clotting factor, it is clearly essential that genes designed to kill cancer cells are expressed in the right place. There are broadly two ways of targeting gene therapy:

- anatomically, via the route of administration
- molecularly, using the molecular properties of the target cells and/or the vector.

Routes of administration

As with conventional drug therapy, the route by which a gene therapy vector is administered will have an impact both on the tissues that the therapy can access and on the potential risks and acceptability of that therapy. Vectors for gene therapy in clinical trials have been delivered by intratumoral, subcutaneous, intravenous, intramuscular or intradermal injections, as well as by bone marrow transplantation and aerosol inhaled into the lungs (Fig. 10.8). Some techniques are clearly more suitable for a particular disease. Bone marrow transplantation works well for SCID and inhalation of an aerosol is an ideal way of delivering a gene to the lungs in the treatment of cystic fibrosis. Intratumoral injection is most efficient for cancers, but this is an invasive technique and only possible when the location of the cancer is known and reasonably accessible; under these circumstances, it seems likely that the tumour could be removed surgically, obviating the need for gene therapy entirely.

It is not only the nature of the disease that is a factor in the choice of route of administration; the type of gene, amount of DNA to be delivered and type of vector to be used are also important factors. For example, a gene that causes programmed cell death (apoptosis), in a non-selective vector, has to be administered straight into a tumour; however, if the same gene could be delivered in a vector which specifically targeted the tumour cells, it could be administered intravenously.

Molecular targeting

The ideal vector would be one that acted as a 'magic bullet', only transmitting genes to the desired cell type, and much work is being done to try to develop such selective vectors. An alternative approach is to control the expression of the therapeutic gene in a cell type-specific fashion; it does not really matter which cells take up the therapeutic gene, if it is only expressed in the desired target cells.

Cell type-specific vectors

Many viruses are, in fact, very selective in the types of cell that they will infect. They can only be taken up into cells that they bind to, and this binding depends on a specific interaction between molecules on the virus particle and the surface of the target cell. Furthermore, it is possible to engineer viruses to modify their interaction

Table 10.2
Advantages and disadvantages of various vectors for gene therapy

Vector	Advantages	Disadvantages
Viral vectors		
Retroviruses, e.g. murine leukaemia virus	Non-pathogenic in humans, much prior experience, efficient transfection, stable gene expression	Risk of insertional mutagenesis, only targets dividing cells, small insert size
Lentiviruses, e.g. HIV	Stable gene expression, will target non-dividing cells	Risk of insertional mutagenesis, risk of virulent reversion
Adenovirus	Much prior experience, easy to grow, targets both dividing and non-dividing cells, inserts up to 30 kb	Transient gene expression, immunogenic, risk of virulent reversion
Adeno-associated virus	Non-pathogenic in humans, stable gene expression, will target non-dividing cells	Risk of insertional mutagenesis, immunogenic (but less than adenovirus), small insert size (< 4.5 kb)
Herpes simplex virus (HSV)	Readily enters CNS, inserts up to 30 kb	Risk of virulent reversion
Non-viral vectors		
Naked DNA	No size limitation, very simple to produce	Poor stability *in vivo*, very inefficient transfection, risk of anti-DNA antibodies
Liposomes	No size limitation, simple to produce, improved stability and transfection efficiency, properties can be modified to improve cell selectivity, for example	Low transfection efficiency
Chimeric proteins	Can be designed to target particular cell types	Very ineffective in studies to date
Artificial chromosome	No size limitation, well tolerated within cells, stable gene expression	Difficult to make, very difficult to get into cells

with a particular cell type. As an example, the murine leukaemia virus, an important retroviral vector, has been genetically modified to include an envelope protein from the human vesicular stomatitis virus, which enables the virus to target epithelial cells selectively (Fig. 10.9). Similar approaches can also be used with non-viral vectors to try to improve their cell-type selectivity (see above).

Tissue-specific control of gene expression

Several approaches have been used in an attempt to achieve tissue-specific transgene expression. Eukaryotic genes include complex regulatory sequences which in turn include promoters, located adjacent to transcription start sites. These promoters can include sequences which restrict transcription of a gene to specific tissues. If these tissue-specific gene promoters are used, the expression of the therapeutic gene can be restricted to the target tissue. Development of such promoters is not easy, as tissue specificity has to be preserved while still achieving high promoter activity and consequently high levels of

expression of the transgene. Nevertheless, several such promoters have been developed for use in the treatment of prostate cancer, which can distinguish between prostate and bladder tissue, and even between benign and malignant prostate tissue. Similarly, the SM22a promoter seems able to restrict gene expression to smooth muscle cells, which could prove to be of enormous use in the therapy of cardiovascular or respiratory disorders.

Gene 'silencing' or repair

Despite these advances, it seems unlikely that the cell specificity of gene delivery or expression will ever be absolute. What is more, even if a gene is expressed in exactly the right tissue, expression of too much (or too little) of the gene, or expression at the wrong times, may well still lead to problems. Approaches aimed at repairing or silencing a faulty gene would seem to be ideal ways of avoiding this; these interventions would clearly only have an effect when the faulty gene was being expressed. Examples of these approaches — the use of antisense or siRNA technology in the treatment of Duchenne muscular dystrophy and prostate cancer — have been previously outlined (see above).

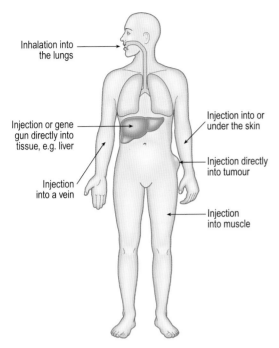

Inhalation into
the lungs

Injection or gene
gun directly into
tissue, e.g. liver

Injection
into a vein

Injection into or
under the skin

Injection directly
into tumour

Injection
into muscle

Figure 10.8
Some of the ways in which gene therapy vectors can be administered.

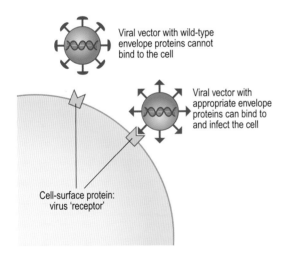

Viral vector with wild-type
envelope proteins cannot
bind to the cell

Viral vector with
appropriate envelope
proteins can bind to
and infect the cell

Cell-surface protein:
virus 'receptor'

Figure 10.9
Modification of a viral vector to alter its cell-type selectivity. As viruses have to bind to specific cell surface proteins before they can enter a cell, they can be very selective about the type of cell that they can infect. This selectivity can be altered by engineering the vector virus to express envelope proteins, which bind to the appropriate cell surface receptors, from another virus.

Problems with gene therapy

At the moment gene therapy remains experimental and has not really proven very successful in clinical trials. What factors have kept gene therapy from becoming an effective treatment?

Insertional mutagenesis

As considered in more detail above, insertion of therapeutic genes into the genome can present considerable problems; the insertion of the gene may well disrupt normal gene function and has led to death from cancer in at least two patients. Thus at present it seems (at best) unwise to attempt to achieve long-term expression of a therapeutic gene via incorporation of that gene into the cell's genome.

Short-lived nature of gene therapy

Before gene therapy can become a permanent cure for any condition, the therapeutic DNA introduced into target cells must remain functional, and the cells containing the therapeutic DNA must be long-lived and stable. Problems with integrating therapeutic DNA into the genome and the rapidly dividing nature of many cells prevent gene therapy from achieving any long-term benefits. Patients have to undergo multiple rounds of gene therapy.

Infection

The ability of a virus to mutate is well known, and viruses can also exchange genetic material with different viruses infecting the same cell, in a process known as recombination. Thus even with genetically engineered, replication-deficient viral vectors, there is always the fear that the viral vector, once inside the patient, may undergo 'virulent reversion' and recover its ability to cause disease.

Immune response

Whenever a foreign object is introduced into human tissues, the immune system is likely to attack the invader. The risk of stimulating the immune system in a way that reduces gene therapy effectiveness is always a potential risk. For example, in a trial of adenovirus-mediated gene therapy for cystic fibrosis, patients treated with a low concentration of vector were not helped because the efficiency of gene transfer was too low. However, when patients were treated with larger amounts of vector, although the chloride transporter gene was expressed, there was a marked immune response to the vector and the expression of the therapeutic gene was very short-lived, because the immune system killed off the 'infected' cells. Clearly, nobody had told the immune system that this particular virus had been modified to make it non-pathogenic!

Furthermore, the immune response alone can cause toxicity. In 1999, gene therapy suffered a major setback with the death of 18-year-old Jesse Gelsinger. Jesse was participating in a gene therapy trial for the treatment of ornithine transcarboxylase deficiency (OTCD). He died from multiple organ failure, 4 days after starting the dose-escalating study. His death is believed to have been triggered by a severe immune response to the large amounts of adenovirus vector administered.

Difficulty in controlling levels of expression

Current technology allows therapeutic genes to be expressed in a variety of cells, but the amount of gene product that is produced is still fairly hit and miss. This means that at present the effectiveness of gene therapy is at best unpredictable, and renders gene therapy useless for the treatment of conditions such as the haemoglobinopathies, where the relative amounts of particular gene products are of paramount importance.

Gene toxicity

While too little gene expression will render the treatment ineffective, too much can lead to toxicity. The nature of the toxicity will clearly depend on the individual gene. For example, over-expression of erythropoietin will lead to polycythaemia, whereas over-expression of insulin will produce hypoglycaemia.

Ethical implications

The debate over genetically modified organisms and food reveals how sensitive we are about the idea of 'messing about' with genes. It is likely that public pressure may demand an almost impossible level of proof of the safety of gene therapy before it becomes widely acceptable. The potential power of gene therapy also raises the issue of 'when to stop'. It may well be desirable to use gene therapy to reduce the risk of someone developing breast cancer or cardiovascular disease, but what about using it to prevent alcoholism or aggression? There is currently a moratorium on any research into germline therapy, in which any modifications would be inherited by the patient's children. However, is it really best to avoid a treatment that would wipe out, for example, cystic fibrosis in future generations?

Expense

Preliminary attempts at gene therapy have been exorbitantly expensive, which raises questions of who will have access to these therapies and who will pay for their use.

Prospects for gene therapy

Despite the difficulties, there is enormous research and commercial interest in gene therapy; the number of companies actively involved in developing gene therapies has quadrupled in the last 10 years, rising from fewer than 50 in 1995 to nearly 200 in 2005. Most commercial research is concentrating not on the single-gene disorders, such as cystic fibrosis, but on multigene disorders and even on conditions which do not seem to be due to any particular gene defect. Thus there is interest in developing gene therapy with *AC6*, an adenylate cyclase gene that increases the contractility of cardiac muscle, for the treatment of chronic heart failure, and the vascular endothelial growth factor, VEGF, which promotes formation of new blood vessels, for the treatment of peripheral vascular disease.

The area in which gene therapy seems likely to first make an impact is in the treatment of cancer, and indeed Gendicine®, the tumour protein *p53* gene in an adenoviral vector, was licensed for the treatment of head and neck squamous cell carcinoma in China in 2004. There is considerable interest in the use of *p53* in cancer (see Table 10.1), as many cancer cells lack *p53*, which enables their uncontrolled proliferation.

Clearly, gene therapy holds very real promise for the treatment of a whole range of human diseases. However, it also presents very real risks. It is clear that any developments must involve rigorous and appropriately controlled trials of both efficacy and safety.

FURTHER READING

Nowroozi MR, Pisters LL (no date) The current status of gene therapy for prostate cancer. Cancer Control Journal: http://moffitt.org/moffittapps/ccj/v5n6/article5.html.

Online Mendelian Inheritance in Man (OMIM) Johns Hopkins University (Baltimore, MD) and National Center for Biotechnology Information, National Library of Medicine (Bethesda, MD): http://www.ncbi.nlm.nih.gov/omim/

van Deutecom JCT, van Ommen G-JB 2003 Advances in Duchenne muscular dystrophy gene therapy. Nat Rev Genet 4:774–783.

11

Biopharmaceuticals
M. Keen

One of the most obvious (and profitable!) contributions of biotechnology to medicine is in the area of biopharmaceuticals: drugs manufactured using biotechnology. There has been a veritable explosion of such drugs on to the market in recent years, and this rate of innovation seems likely to carry on for some time; more than a third of new drugs in the development 'pipeline' are biopharmaceuticals.

What are biopharmaceuticals?

A biopharmaceutical is a protein or nucleic acid, used as a drug, which has been produced by living organisms as a result of biotechnology. Thus, the term encompasses monoclonal antibodies, recombinant proteins or oligonucleotides used as vaccines (see Ch. 7), the nucleotide sequences and vectors used in gene therapy (see Ch. 10), and a wide range of recombinant proteins used as drugs, which will be the main focus of this chapter.

Excluded from this strict definition are proteins and nucleic acids extracted from sources that have not been manipulated using biotechnology. Thus, while recombinant human growth hormone qualifies as a biopharmaceutical, human growth hormone extracted from human pituitary gland does not. Also excluded are products of genetically modified organisms which are not proteins or nucleic acids.

Many of the biopharmaceuticals considered in this chapter can also be described as 'biological response modifiers' or simply 'biologics', which are defined as natural body substances, or drugs made from natural body substances, that modify the body's normal (often immune) response. This term is probably more widely used than the more general term 'biopharmaceutical' but is, if anything, even harder to define precisely; surely the vast majority of drugs work by modifying the body's normal response!

In some cases, biopharmaceuticals provide the first and only effective treatment for a particular condition, such as some of the lysosomal storage disorders (Box 11.1). Biopharmaceuticals are also making a big impact in the treatment of autoimmune conditions such as rheumatoid arthritis (Box 11.2), psoriasis and Crohn's disease. The majority of products under development, however, are targeted at cancer. Cancer is a serious condition, with many sufferers, for which current therapies are generally inadequate. Furthermore, the rapid advance in our understanding of the development of

tumour cells provides a wealth of knowledge regarding potential targets (see Ch. 6). An example of a biopharmaceutical effective in the treatment of breast cancer is trastuzumab (Herceptin®): a monoclonal antibody against the Her2 tyrosine kinase receptor which is over-expressed in about a third of breast tumours (see also Chs 3 and 9).

The range of biopharmaceuticals

It was in the 1970s that the first human recombinant protein was produced, when somatostatin was expressed in *E. coli*. This technology has proved to be extremely lucrative; in 2003, the global sales of somatostatin were worth approximately $1.4 million.

The first true biopharmaceutical was produced in 1982, with the production of recombinant human insulin for the treatment of diabetes mellitus, and the first therapeutic use of a monoclonal antibody was in 1986.

A wide range of biopharmaceuticals are now available. Many of these are substances produced by the human body, such as hormones, clotting factors, cytokines, growth factors, thrombolytic agents and enzymes. Other biopharmaceuticals are designed to reduce the activity of endogenous substances; many of these are monoclonal antibodies, but other strategies are also used such as 'decoy' receptors and even endogenous antagonists (see Box 11.2).

Table 11.1 shows some of the variety of biopharmaceuticals currently licensed for use in the UK. The extraordinary growth in the number of biopharmaceuticals available seems to be due a combination of:

- the rapid increase in our understanding of disease processes which has been made possible by the use of biotechnology
- the relative ease with which the same techniques can be used to produce biologically active molecules, at least in the laboratory.

Biopharmaceuticals are becoming established as part of the pharmacological armoury of treatment, and this has important implications for the manufacture, design and testing of these substances. If a new biopharmaceutical provides the only effective treatment for a rare condition, it will only be required in small quantities. Furthermore, as no competing treatments are available, both high costs and high risks of the biopharmaceutical may well

Box 11.1

Lysosomal storage disorders

The lysosomal storage disorders are a group of inherited conditions associated with impaired lysosomal function. Due to an inherited enzyme deficiency, various macromolecules are not broken down and therefore accumulate in the lysosomes. This leads to an increase in the size and the number of lysosomes found in the cells, which causes problems with normal cell function. All cell types may be affected by these conditions, but neurons and macrophages appear to be especially vulnerable: macrophages because they are particularly rich in lysosomes, and neurons because they cannot divide and so accumulate large amounts of macromolecules that cannot be metabolized. The severity of the disorders can vary enormously; some individuals may be virtually asymptomatic, whereas the same condition may be fatal in others.

There are about 40 distinct lysosomal storage disorders, characterized according to the type of macromolecule that accumulates and the enzymes that are affected. The total incidence is about 1 in 5000 live births, so each individual condition is reasonably rare, and the development of effective therapies has not been a priority for the pharmaceutical industry. However, biotechnology now provides a relatively straightforward (albeit expensive) way of producing recombinant enzymes for replacement therapy, and treatments for three lysosomal storage disorders (Gaucher's disease, Fabry disease and the Hurler–Scheie syndromes) are now licensed in the UK (see Table 11.1 below). These drugs appear to be extremely effective in treating many cases of these disorders.

Box 11.2

Biopharmaceuticals in chronic inflammatory disorders

One area in which biopharmaceuticals are making a big impact is in chronic inflammatory conditions such as rheumatoid arthritis.

It is not clear what initiates the inappropriate inflammatory response in the joints of someone with rheumatoid arthritis. What has become clear, however, is that two chemical mediators — tumour necrosis factor α (TNF) and interleukin 1 (IL-1) — are important in maintaining the chronic inflammatory response. TNF and IL-1 act synergistically to promote the inflammatory response, with each mediator greatly enhancing the response to the other. There is some evidence that suggests, while TNF is particularly important in maintaining inflammation, IL-1 may be primarily responsible for the damage to cartilage and bone resorption that is so disabling in rheumatoid arthritis.

Monoclonal antibodies that bind to TNF and thus inactivate it were used as an experimental tool to demonstrate the role of TNF in inflammation. The use of anti-TNF antibodies in therapy was simply a logical extension of this work, and a number of anti-TNF monoclonals are now available for the treatment of

rheumatoid arthritis and some other chronic inflammatory conditions. One of these anti inflammatory antibodies is Adalimumab (Humira), a fully humanized monoclonal antibody with TNFα binding specificity (for further antibodies used in therapy see Table 11.1 below). Another strategy that is used clinically to bind and inactivate TNF is the use of a 'decoy receptor', etanercept. Etanercept is a soluble fusion protein formed from two human p75 TNF receptors linked to the Fc region of an IgG molecule.

Anakinra is a biopharmaceutical that targets the actions of IL-1. It is produced in *E. coli* and is a recombinant version of the human protein, IL-1ra. IL-1ra is a naturally occurring analogue of IL-1, produced from a member of the IL-1 gene family; it binds to the IL-1 receptor but does not activate it, thus acting as an endogenous antagonist. Anakinra thus mimics this effect and blocks the effect of endogenous IL-1.

These approaches are summarized in Figure 11.1. They are proving to be very useful in the treatment of rheumatoid arthritis, where they represent the first rational treatments of the underlying cause of the disease. They are also useful in other conditions associated with chronic inflammation, such as Crohn's disease, multiple sclerosis and ankylosing spondylitis.

be acceptable. However, when biopharmaceuticals are marketed for the treatment of common conditions, such as asthma, for which there are many established drug therapies, the relative effectiveness, cost and safety of biopharmaceuticals become of overwhelming importance. Moreover, simply producing sufficient of the molecule to meet potential demand can represent a considerable challenge for the manufacturing process (see below).

Biopharmaceuticals compared with conventional drugs

While there are, of course, many differences between individual biopharmaceuticals, there are a number of general ways in which these drugs differ from more conventional, small-molecule drugs. These can be summarized as a number of advantages and disadvantages of the biopharmaceuticals.

Advantages

- Biopharmaceuticals can be engineered to be identical to human proteins, thus avoiding problems of allergy, etc. Perhaps the best example of this is the use of recombinant human insulin for the treatment of diabetes mellitus, which was the first therapeutic use of a biopharmaceutical.
- Molecularly engineered biopharmaceuticals avoid the need to extract important proteins from human tissue. Thus it is now possible to avoid the risk of infection with AIDS, which was a big problem when haemophiliacs were treated with clotting factors extracted from blood, or Creutzfeldt–Jakob disease, which was transmitted to children by contaminating prions in growth hormone extracted from the pituitary of cadavers.
- Biopharmaceuticals are relatively easy to produce (at least in the laboratory; see below) and these drugs typically have a shorter development time than conventional 'new chemical entities'.
- The ease of production means that many small companies have been able to launch products on their own; some have even made a profit with a single product.
- Many of these drugs have a very high degree of specificity, producing effects only on a single type of molecule, in one particular species. However, while this high degree of selectivity should reduce the likelihood of unwanted side-effects, it can bring about considerable problems of its own when it comes to determining the likely safety of a new biopharmaceutical (see below).

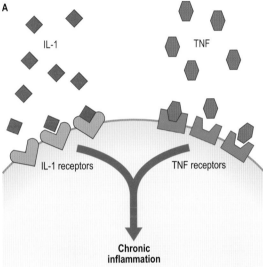

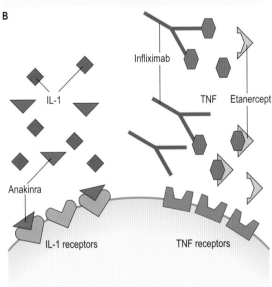

Figure 11.1
Inhibitors of interleukin-1 (IL-1) and tumour necrosis factor (TNF) in chronic inflammation. (A) There is an established role for the activation of both IL-1 and TNF receptors in the maintenance of chronic inflammation. (B) How various biopharmaceuticals interfere with this process. Anakinra binds to the IL-1 receptor and prevents IL-1 binding and therefore receptor activation. Infliximab (a monoclonal antibody against TNF) and etanercept (a 'decoy receptor' for TNF) both bind to TNF, which reduces the concentration of free TNF available to bind to and activate its receptor.

Disadvantages

- Despite being easy to produce at the laboratory scale, the large-scale production of biopharmaceuticals is complex and extremely costly. Thus these drugs tend to be extremely expensive.
- With new conventional drugs, most of the cost lies in developing and testing the new compound. When the patent for the drug expires, other companies can usually manufacture and market the generic drug much more cheaply, reducing the cost of treatment. For biopharmaceuticals, production is so expensive that generic products may not offer much, if anything, in the way of cost savings.
- There is a risk of contamination from infectious agents or other components of the host cells, the medium or by-products of the production process. Moreover, very small changes in the production process can produce significant changes in the product (see below). Thus, quality control, process validation and purification of the final product are of the utmost importance.
- In terms of marketability, the 'ideal' drug is one which can be given orally, as a single daily dose. Most of the biopharmaceuticals have very unconventional dosing regimes. For example, etanercept (see Box 11.2 above) has to be administered by subcutaneous injection once or twice a week. Similarly, the anti-TNF antibody, infliximab (see Box 11.2), is given by slow intravenous infusion; after the first dose, the second

Table 11.1
Examples of some of the biopharmaceuticals currently licensed for clinical use in the UK

Example	Mechanism of action	Indications
Monoclonal antibodies		
Infliximab Adalimumab	Monoclonal antibodies against TNF	Rheumatoid arthritis, ankylosing spondylitis, Crohn's disease
Rituximab	Monoclonal antibody against CD20	Non-Hodgkin's lymphoma, rheumatoid arthritis
Alemtuzumab	Monoclonal antibody against CD52	Chronic lymphocytic leukaemia
Trastuzumab	Monoclonal antibody against Her2	Her2-positive breast cancers
Omalizumab	Monoclonal antibody against IgE	Asthma
Palivizumab	Monoclonal antibody against respiratory syncytial virus A and B	Respiratory syncytial virus
Recombinant hormones		
Follitropin α and β	Recombinant follicle-stimulating hormone	Infertility
Somatropin	Recombinant human growth hormone	Growth hormone deficiency
Apidra®, Humalog®, Levemir®, etc.	Recombinant human insulin analogues	Diabetes mellitus
Teriparatide	Recombinant parathyroid hormone fragment	Osteoporosis
Salcatonin	Recombinant salmon calcitonin (not all biopharmaceuticals have to be of human origin!)	Paget's disease, osteoporosis
Thyrotropin α	Recombinant thyroid-stimulating hormone	Diagnosis of hypothyroidism
Recombinant enzymes for lysosomal storage disorders		
Laronidase	Recombinant alpha-L-iduronidase	Hurler–Scheie syndrome and other mucopolysaccharidosis type 1 conditions
Agalsidase α and β	Recombinant galactosidase enzymes	Fabry's disease
Imiglucerase	Recombinant glucocerebrosidase enzyme	Gaucher's disease
Other recombinant enzymes		
Dornase α	Recombinant deoxyribonuclease	Mucolytic in cystic fibrosis
Rasburicase	Recombinant urate oxidase	Cytotoxic drug associated hyperuricaemia
Recombinant cytokines, etc.		
Drotrecogin α (activated)	Recombinant activated protein C	Sepsis with multiple organ failure
Filgrastim Lenograstim Pegfilgrastim	Recombinant granulocyte colony stimulating factors	Neutropenia
Epoetin	Recombinant human erythropoietin	Various anaemias
Interferon α Peginterferon α-2a Peginterferon α-2b	Recombinant human α interferons	Chronic hepatitis

Table 11.1
Examples of some of the biopharmaceuticals currently licensed for clinical use in the UK—cont'd

Example	Mechanism of action	Indications
Interferon β-1a Interferon β-1b	Recombinant human β interferons	Multiple sclerosis
Interferon γ-1b	Recombinant human γ interferon	Reduction of infections in chronic granulomatous disease
Lutropin α	Recombinant human luteinizing hormone	
Becaplermin	Recombinant human platelet-derived growth factor	Chronic leg ulcers in diabetics
Anakinra	Recombinant IL-1ra	Rheumatoid arthritis
Aldesleukin	Recombinant IL-2	Metastatic renal carcinoma
Substances affecting blood clotting		
Lepirudin	Recombinant hirudin (from the medicinal leech)	Heparin-induced thrombocytopenia
Clotting factors	Recombinant human clotting factors VIIa, VIII and IX	Haemophilia
Alteplase, etc.	Recombinant tissue plasminogen activators	Myocardial infarction, stroke (?)
Urokinase	Cultured human kidney cells	Myocardial infarction, stroke (?)
Vaccines		
Cholera vaccine	Recombinant cholera toxin B subunit	Prevention of cholera
Hepatitis B vaccine	Recombinant hepatitis B surface antigens	Prevention of hepatitis B
Other		
Etanercept	Recombinant TNF 'decoy receptor'	Rheumatoid arthritis

dose is administered after 2 weeks and the third after another 4 weeks, with subsequent doses then administered at 8-week intervals.

- Despite the often extreme selectivity of these drugs, they do still produce side-effects. For example, omalizumab is a highly specific monoclonal antibody against IgE, which is licensed for the treatment of severe and persistent allergic asthma. The *British National Formulary* lists an impressive range of side-effects that have been associated with this drug, which include nausea, diarrhoea, dizziness, fatigue, paraesthesias, weight gain and flu-like symptoms.

Large-scale production of biopharmaceuticals

Small-scale production of particular nucleic acids or recombinant proteins is much easier than the production of a bespoke small molecule by conventional chemical techniques. Standard transfection and culture techniques can be used to produce any number of natural or engineered products. However, the reverse is true when the time comes to scale up manufacture for large-scale testing or marketing. The production of biopharmaceuticals tends to be much more problematic, and consequently much more expensive, than the commercial production of conventional small-molecule drugs.

Most commercial production of biopharmaceuticals uses cultured mammalian cells; however, other expression systems can also be used.

Other expression systems

Bacteria

Bacteria such as *E. coli* and *Bacillus subtilis* are widely used as expression systems, both commercially and in the laboratory. They have simple physiology, grow rapidly and can produce large product yields — sometimes up to 10% of the bacterial mass. Many bacteria can be made to secrete the product into the culture medium, which helps in product recovery and purification.

However, bacteria are not always suitable for the production of mammalian proteins, as these may be inactive due to incorrect folding. Moreover, bacteria do not perform post-translational modifications, such as glycosylation, and so are unsuitable for the production of proteins, such as luteinizing hormone, in which such modification is important for function. Bacteria are used, however, in the commercial manufacture of, for example, insulin, growth hormone and Anakinra (see Box 11.2).

Yeasts

Yeasts are widely used in the biotechnological industry and are occasionally used for the production of biopharmaceuticals. They are simple eukaryotes and perform post-translational modification of proteins, although this is not necessarily identical to the processing that would occur in mammalian cells. Like bacteria, they can be made to secrete various proteins into growth medium, and this strategy is used in the production of a vaccine against hepatitis B. One disadvantage of yeasts is that they produce active proteases which can degrade protein products; however, various yeast strains have been specifically engineered to lack these proteases.

Insect cells

The use of insect cells is still very much a niche market but its importance is increasing. The baculovirus vector allows expression of very large amounts of protein by insect cells. The risk of infection with the vector, or with other unknown viruses harboured by the insect cells, is considered to be negligible. Protein folding and post-translational modification are similar (but not necessarily identical) to that which occurs in mammalian cells. However, culture of insect cells is more difficult than growing bacteria or yeast, and the growth of the cells is slower. Consequently, insect cells are a more expensive expression system to use than bacteria or yeast, but they are cheaper than mammalian cell culture.

Transgenic animals

The first transgenic mammal, a mouse, was produced at Yale in 1980. In 1996, 'Dolly' the sheep — the first mammal cloned from an adult somatic cell — was successfully cloned at the Roslin Institute, with the express purpose of allowing the reproducible production of therapeutic human proteins in milk. Several companies are now involved in producing recombinant proteins in milk, and recombinant human antithrombin III from the milk of transgenic goats is now licensed in Europe for use as an anticoagulant. In 2007 it was reported that large amounts of therapeutic proteins, such as human interferon β-1a, could be expressed in the eggs of transgenic chickens.

These techniques have several potential advantages over cell culture expression systems. While making the original transgenic animals is undoubtedly complex, subsequent breeding and harvesting involve straightforward and very well-established techniques. Yields can be very good; transgenic goats can produce up to 1 kg of therapeutic protein per year in their milk, so an average-sized dairy herd could produce comparable output to a very large bioreactor. While there is still the potential risk of transmission of animal diseases or oncogenes from these products, presumably the risks are no greater than those involved in consuming milk or eggs for food. The main drawback to the use of transgenic animals would seem to be the issue of animal welfare.

Transgenic plants

There is considerable interest in using transgenic plants to manufacture biopharmaceuticals, and given the number of our current medicines that originated in plants, there is a pleasing symmetry to this endeavour. The technology for producing transgenic plants is well established and a number of therapeutically useful proteins have been expressed in plants such as tobacco and potato.

As with transgenic animals, it is hoped that transgenic plants will provide a much cheaper way of producing large amounts of recombinant protein than cell cultures. However, purification of the product from the plant material is still likely to remain very costly (see below). To avoid this, proteins are being expressed in plants that can be eaten raw, such as lettuce and banana, in the hope that the therapeutic protein could be delivered orally along with the crop! Most of this work is being carried out to produce so-called 'edible vaccines' by engineering plants to express vaccines targeted at the mucosa, which will also stimulate systemic immunity; a rabies vaccine of this type has been successfully produced in tomatoes.

However, while therapeutic proteins obtained in this way may be cheap to produce and administer, this method would not be without problems. It seems inevitable that the concentration of the biopharmaceutical would differ in crops grown under different conditions, and this would lead to problems with determining the appropriate dose. Moreover, even if the product were to be purified after production, transgenic plants are currently meeting with considerable public concern regarding potential problems with cross-contamination of (or by) other crops and wild plants by cross-pollination and plant debris. It is difficult to comply with the strict restraints of Good Manufacturing Practice (see below) when you are working in a field.

Mammalian cell expression systems

Mammalian cell expression systems were first used for the production of inactivated polio virus vaccine. Nowadays, the use of continuous, immortalized cell lines is generally preferred to primary cultures, as these are more consistent, generally easier to culture and faster-growing.

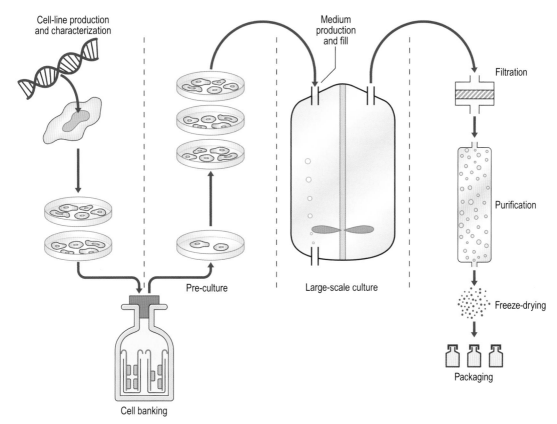

Figure 11.2
The various processes involved in the production of a biopharmaceutical.

However, the use of these immortalized cells for the production of potential biopharmaceuticals was not accepted until the 1980s; there was considerable concern that immortalized cell lines might harbour transmissible oncogenes or viruses which could affect the end user of the product; however good your purification may be, it is extremely hard to be sure that unknown viruses, etc. are being eradicated. Fortunately, these concerns appear to not to have been well founded.

Figure 11.2 illustrates the various phases involved in the production of a biopharmaceutical. The basic process seems fairly straightforward. Cells are transfected with a gene for the desired protein, grown up on a large scale and the target protein is recovered from the resulting 'broth'. However, getting the process right can be extremely difficult. Mammalian cells typically have long generation times and produce relatively low amounts of product. All possible measures must be taken to ensure that the consistency, safety and purity of the product and every stage of the process, from initial production and 'banking' of the cells to purification of the product, complies with Good Manufacturing Practice (see below) as a condition of the licensing of the biopharmaceutical for clinical use. All substances that come into contact with the cells or the product must be well characterized and traceable. Any changes

in the manufacturing process may require a change in the product licence.

Good Manufacturing Practice

Adherence to Good Manufacturing Practice (GMP) is a requirement of the licensing of any drug. This means that all components of the manufacturing process (raw materials, plant, personnel, procedures, etc.) must be strictly defined, to ensure that the product is made to the highest levels of safety and efficacy. As a consequence, any change in the system of manufacture — to increase yields, for example — is likely to necessitate a change in the licence.

Cell characterization and banking

It is essential to validate the nature and source of all cell lines used in the production of biopharmaceuticals, not least because the nature of the cell line used can impact upon the product produced (see below). It is usual practice to maintain several 'banks' of frozen cells in an attempt to ensure the safety and viability of this valuable resource. Typically, there would be:

- two master banks, where the original stocks are stored
- one or more working banks, from which cells are withdrawn for culture and biopharmaceutical production.

Banked cells must be checked regularly to ensure that they are of the right type, that they are genetically stable and that they have not become contaminated with mycoplasma, bacteria, retroviruses or fungi, etc. It is also important to limit the number of times that the cells are subcultured, as even 'immortalized' cell lines cannot be grown indefinitely without changes in their function. The age of the culture can have a number of effects, including effects on post-translational processing of proteins and genetic stability of the cell line itself.

Cell culture

Mammalian cell cultures grow relatively slowly and only produce small amounts of product. Therefore, commercial production of a biopharmaceutical requires very large-scale cell culture. Bigger and bigger bioreactors are being developed and the productivity of individual cell lines is also continually being improved. It is not uncommon to achieve gram per litre output and this is more than 100 times better than the titre that could be achieved for similar processes in the 1980s. It seems likely that further improvements in production systems, coupled with vector and host cell engineering, will increase productivity even further.

The scaling-up of cell culture techniques, from the standard flasks or roller bottles used in a laboratory setting, to the large 'bioreactors' required for the preparation of commercial amounts of product, is one of the most difficult steps in the development of a new biopharmaceutical, and remains largely a process of trial and error. The system that is most widely used for the large-scale culture of mammalian cells is the 'fed batch' approach.

Types of bioreactor

A bioreactor is, in essence, just a large vessel in which cells are grown. The cells need to be maintained at the right temperature and pH, supplied with oxygen and nutrients and have any waste products efficiently removed or neutralized. These basic requirements become more and more difficult to achieve the bigger the bioreactors grow, and the design of bioreactors is complex.

A number of culture systems have been developed. These can be used with both free-floating cells and adherent cells, but for adherent cells there is clearly a need to increase the surface area available for cell growth; this is usually achieved by growing the cells on micro-carrier beads or by using hollow fibre systems (see below).

One of the key factors that differentiates the various systems is the way in which cells are kept in suspension in order to allow efficient mixing. The main techniques used are:

- *Roller bottle*. Cells grow in suspension or on the inside surface of a bottle. The bottle is continuously rolled so that the medium is mixed and suspension cultures can be kept under conditions that closely mimic free fall in zero gravity. This method is widely used for pilot-scale production, but is not suitable for very large-scale production.
- *Air lift*. Cells are kept suspended and the medium mixed by a flow of gas bubbles, which are also used to oxygenate the medium. Some very large bioreactors have been built which utilize this technique, but it is important to limit potential damage to the cells caused by mechanical stresses from the bubbles, particularly when they burst.
- *Stirred tank*. This is probably the most common type of large bioreactor used with mammalian cells. As the name suggests, the cells are kept suspended and the medium is mixed by stirring with one or more impellers. Again, the design of the vessel and the impeller should aim to keep mechanical stresses on the cells to a minimum.
- *Hollow fibre*. In this type of bioreactor, medium is continually perfused through hollow, semi-permeable fibres. The cells grow on the outside of the fibres and exchange nutrients, gases, etc. and (ideally) product with the medium as it passes through. Laboratory-scale hollow fibre bioreactors have been produced using modified kidney dialysis cartridges.

Another key distinction between types of bioreactor is the way the cells are handled.

- *Batch systems*. In the simplest batch systems, cells are grown up in a volume of medium for a period of time, and then all the cells are harvested and the product is extracted from the cells and/or medium. While these systems may seem wasteful in terms of cells, they are the simplest to design and maintain, and are very widely used. The biggest commercial bioreactors are of the modified fed batch type, which is just like the batch system, except that the medium is supplemented one or more times during the growth of the cells.
- *Continuous systems*. Product is continually extracted from the culture either by harvesting a proportion of the cells or simply by taking it from spent medium. While the continuous perfusion systems might seem much more efficient, they are actually more difficult to design and maintain, and tend to be much smaller in scale than the simpler batch systems. They are, however, of use when the product is unstable, such that it would degrade if left in the culture medium for any length of time, or if the product inhibits the growth of the cells, as is the case with β-interferon, for example.

Media

All the chemicals and processes used during production need to be defined for licensing and are potential sources of contamination. This is especially true of the culture media and for the aseptic fill techniques used to add medium to the bioreactors. However, it also applies to other aspects of the process, such as the cleaning and maintenance of the equipment.

The provenance of all chemicals needs to be tracked, and all require validation of their quality and safety. This is rather hard for some components of the culture media. Serum and protein hydrolysates used in cell culture are extracted from blood and are subject to inevitable batch-to-batch variability and potential contamination. The potential risk of infection with bovine spongiform encephalopathy (BSE), coupled with the difficulty in testing for the prion that is the transmissible agent of this disease, has led to abolition of the use of European sera in biopharmaceutical production. It is permissible to use bovine sera from New Zealand, where the risk of BSE is considered negligible.

Because of these problems of batch-to-batch variability and potential disease risk, there is a move towards the use of chemically defined, serum-free (and even protein-free) media for cell culture. However, these are extremely expensive and are not suitable for the growth of all cells.

Purification

Once the culture has been harvested, purification of the therapeutic protein is a major task; even the best mammalian cell culture systems can currently only produce about 7 g of therapeutic protein per litre of culture medium, and for many biopharmaceuticals the yield is much, much less. It is this 'downstream processing' that largely determines the quality and safety of the biopharmaceutical product.

The initial stage in the purification process is the separation of medium from cells and cell debris by centrifugation or microfiltration. The fraction containing the product is then concentrated in preparation for final purification by a variety of chromatographic techniques. Purification adds substantially to the cost of production. The number of purifications steps required and the yield obtained are clearly critical. Also important are the cycle time for a process and the number of times an expensive chromatography resin can be reused.

Purification needs to remove:

- host cell-derived substances (DNA, etc.)
- substances added during processing (lipids, antibiotics, antifoaming agents, cleansing agents, substances added during purification)
- possible infectious agents, such as viruses, bacteria and fungi.

Furthermore the protein of interest has to be separated from many other proteins, including any truncated product, other proteins produced by the cell and constituents of the culture medium (serum is high in protein) using a variety of purification steps. All of this adds considerably to the cost of manufacture.

It is never possible to achieve 100% purification, so acceptable limits have to be determined. The World Health Organization defines the maximal acceptable concentration of DNA, which might harbour harmful genetic material that could be incorporated into human cells, as 100 pg

per single dose of a biopharmaceutical protein. However, how do you know if you have removed something that may or may not have been there to start with, such as a virus or a prion? In order to test for this, cell cultures can be 'spiked' with model viruses, etc. However, this is usually done in small-scale test systems, to avoid contaminating whole plant; it would clearly be unfortunate to add a virus to the main bioreactor, only to find out that the purification process does not in fact remove it!

Product characterization and validation

Careful characterization of the final product is extremely important, as small changes in the production process can affect the precise nature of the product, and small changes in the product can have profound effects on its biological activity. For example, the tissue plasminogen activators, alteplase and duteplase, differ in just a single amino acid; however, duteplase has only 50% of the fibrinolytic activity possessed by alteplase (Box 11.3).

Perhaps unsurprisingly, the cells used for production can affect the nature of the product. The glycosylation of the soluble immune cell adhesion molecule (sICAM) is different when produced in NSO cells and CHO cells. In NSO cells there is substantially more N-glycolylneuraminic acid glycosylation and less N-acetylneuraminic acid glycosylation than in CHO cells. The significance of this is unclear, but the glycosylation pattern seen in NSO cells does not occur in healthy human cells.

Moreover, changes to the precise conditions under which the cells are cultured can affect the product (see Box 11.3).

Modification of biopharmaceuticals

The original first-generation biopharmaceuticals are simply engineered copies of natural products or antibodies. However, second-generation products are now being produced in which the original compound has been modified in order to improve its characteristics.

One of the best-established modifications is the 'humanization' of monoclonal antibodies to make them less immunogenic in humans. Monoclonal antibodies used as biopharmaceuticals range from those which are 100% murine, through chimeric (30% murine) and humanized (5% murine), to fully human antibodies that are produced using phage display technology. The first monoclonal antibody used in therapy was muromonab-CD3 (Orthoclone®), which is used to prevent rejection following organ transplantation. Perhaps unsurprisingly, muromonab-CD3 is 100% murine. Abciximab (ReoPro®) is an example of a chimeric human:mouse monoclonal; it is

Box 11.3

Tissue plasminogen activators

Tissue plasminogen activator is a key component of the fibrinolytic system, by which plasminogen in the blood is activated to plasmin, which breaks down the insoluble fibrin in a blood clot into soluble fragments (Fig. 11.3). Fibrinolytic drugs, which include alteplase, streptokinase and urokinase, have proved to be extremely useful in improving survival after myocardial infarction, as they allow removal of the clot blocking the coronary vessel.

Tissue plasminogen activator is a serine protease, and like most serine proteases consists of several domains: a fibronectin 'finger', an epidermal growth factor (EGF)-like region, two kringle domains and the catalytic protease domain (Fig. 11.4). The serine proteases are synthesized as inactive zymogen precursors, which are activated by proteolytic cleavage of the original single-chain molecule into two chains; these still interact but in a slightly different conformation, which activates the enzyme activity. Tissue plasminogen activator is somewhat unusual in that both the single-chain and the double-chain forms are active.

The first tissue plasminogen activator to be marketed for the removal of blood clots in acute myocardial infarction was the native human form, alteplase, produced by Genentech. The precise nature of alteplase can be modified by its culture conditions. In pilot-scale production, alteplase was made in roller bottles in serum-containing medium. However, during the scale-up, the manufacturing process was changed to use suspension cultures, grown in serum-free medium. Under these conditions, alteplase is cleaved at a different site (residue 268 instead of the original site, residue 275). Furthermore, less cleavage occurs and more of the single-chain form of alteplase is found in the final product. In addition, an enzyme in serum cleaves off N-acetylneuraminic acid from some or all glycosylated arginine residues; this deglycosylation prolongs the plasma half-life of alteplase, as it prevents binding to asialo receptor in liver. Thus the product produced in serum-free medium is shorter-acting than the original product.

The first 'modified' form produced was duteplase, which differs from alteplase only by a single amino acid in kringle 2. Duteplase was produced by Wellcome, and the substitution of valine 245 in alteplase for methionine in duteplase appears to have occurred as the result of a cloning error. The amino acid substitution reduces the activity of duteplase to about half of that of alteplase. Wellcome did attempt to market duteplase but were successfully sued for patent infringement by Genentech.

More successful deliberate modifications of the structure of native tissue plasminogen activator have now been made, usually with the aim of increasing the plasma half-life, and therefore the duration of action, of the product. Tenecteplase (another Genentech product) differs from alteplase in two amino acid substitutions in the kringle 1 domain (threonine 103 to asparagine, and asparagine 117 to glutamine) and the replacement of amino acids 296–299 in the catalytic domain with a tetra-alanine sequence. Lanoteplase and reteplase are more dramatic deletion mutants of the native protein; lanoteplase lacks the fibronectin finger and the EGF-like domain, while reteplase lacks the finger, the EGF-like domain and also kringle 1 (see Fig. 11.4).

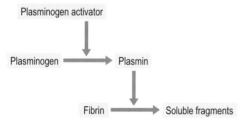

Figure 11.3
The role of plasminogen activators in the fibrinolytic cascade, by which the insoluble fibrin in a blood clot is broken down into soluble fragments.

an antibody against the platelet fibrin receptor and is used to prevent platelet aggregation following cardiac bypass graft surgery. Trastuzumab (Herceptin®; see Chapter 10) is an example of a humanized monoclonal, whereas adalimumab (Humira®; see Box 11.2) is 'fully human'.

Natural products can also be engineered to make them more effective, of higher affinity or longer-acting.

Tenecteplase is a modified tissue plasminogen activator with a longer plasma half-life than the parent molecule. This increase in half-life allows a lower dose to be administered, and also means that tenecteplase can be given as an intravenous bolus, rather than as an intravenous infusion.

Another process which has proved useful for improving the pharmacokinetic properties of a range of substances is pegylation. Pegylation involves the covalent addition of polyethylene glycol (PEG) polymers to a protein or other molecule. PEG is very water-soluble, is devoid of toxicity or immunogenicity, and tends to increase the plasma half-life of proteins to which it is added, usually because it decreases renal elimination. PEG moieties can be added to a number of amino acid residues and/or the N- or C- termini, depending upon the precise chemical processes used. Examples of pegylated biopharmaceuticals are pegfilgrastim (see Table 11.1) and pegvisomant.

Pegvisomant, a growth hormone antagonist, is perhaps an example of a third-generation biopharmaceutical. Its

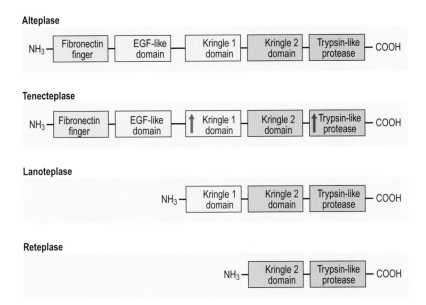

Alteplase

NH₃ — Fibronectin finger — EGF-like domain — Kringle 1 domain — Kringle 2 domain — Trypsin-like protease — COOH

Tenecteplase

NH₃ — Fibronectin finger — EGF-like domain — ↑ Kringle 1 domain — Kringle 2 domain — ↑ Trypsin-like protease — COOH

Lanoteplase

NH₃ — Kringle 1 domain — Kringle 2 domain — Trypsin-like protease — COOH

Reteplase

NH₃ — Kringle 2 domain — Trypsin-like protease — COOH

Figure 11.4
Modifications of natural tissue plasminogen activator (alteplase) to produce 'second-generation' plasminogen activators with increased duration of action. The arrows in the structure of tenecteplase represent the amino acid substitutions by which this protein differs from alteplase.

structure is based on that of human growth hormone but has nine amino acid substitutions. The key substitution (G120K) removes the ability of the molecule to activate the growth hormone receptor, thus converting the agonist hormone into an antagonist. Other substitutions are aimed at increasing binding affinity for the growth hormone receptor or modifying pegylation. The plasma half-life of the modified growth hormone is substantially increased by the addition of 4–6 PEG moieties to lysine residues and the N-terminus. Unfortunately, pegylation substantially decreases the affinity of the antagonist for the receptor, but this is outweighed by the improvement in pharmacokinetics, which allows pegvisomant to be administered by subcutaneous injection once per day.

How safe are biopharmaceuticals?

There seems to be a tendency to view 'natural' products as potentially less damaging than other types of drug and this is sometimes exploited in the marketing of biopharmaceuticals. Moreover, these drugs can be extraordinarily selective, which might also be expected to reduce the risk of unwanted 'side-effects' associated with their use.

The fact that many biopharmaceuticals are produced naturally by the body, coupled with their excellent selectivity, does not make them safe, however. Most biopharmaceuticals have the potential for producing serious and even life-threatening side-effects, which can limit their clinical usefulness (Table 11.2).

In many cases, the potential adverse effects can be predicted from the substance's mechanism of action. For example, many of the new drugs recently introduced for the treatment of rheumatoid arthritis work by inhibiting the activity of TNF. TNF has a large number of actions in the body, so inhibition of the activity of this molecule, however selectively, would be expected to produce an equally wide range of effects. One important effect of TNF is suppression of infection with tuberculosis and other serious infections. A number of people treated with TNF inhibitors have succumbed to active tuberculosis and it is now considered essential to test for subclinical tuberculosis infection before commencing treatment.

The problem of safety is compounded by problems inherent in the testing of these drugs. If a drug is only effective in humans, how can you test its potential toxicity before you give it to humans for the first time? This problem was brought into sharp focus in March 2006 with the disastrous phase 1 trial of TGN1412.

TGN1412

TGN1412 is fully humanized monoclonal antibody against human CD28. It is one of several so-called 'superagonistic' antibodies developed by TeGenero which are capable of activating T cells without the requirement for simultaneous activation of the T-cell receptor. Early studies suggested that TGN1412 selectively increased the proliferation of regulatory T cells, which suppress the activity of autoreactive T cells, thus reducing the likelihood of autoimmunity and inflammation. It was proposed as a potential treatment for rheumatoid

Table 11.2
Some of the adverse effects reported with a variety of biopharmaceuticals

Biopharmaceutical	Adverse effects
Anakinra	Headache, severe infections, neutropenia
Laronidase	Vomiting, diarrhoea, tachycardia, angioedema, blood pressure changes, headache, fever, musculoskeletal pain, rash, respiratory arrest
Lutropin α	Nausea, vomiting, abdominal pain, headache, drowsiness, ovarian hyperstimulation syndrome, ovarian cyst, breast pain, ectopic pregnancy, thromboembolism
Omalizumab	Headache, nausea, diarrhoea, dyspepsia, postural hypotension, flushing, pharyngitis, cough, fatigue, dizziness, drowsiness, paraesthesia, weight gain, influenza-like symptoms, rash, pruritus, photosensitivity
Teriparatide	Nausea, gastro-oesophageal reflux, haemorrhoids, palpitations, fatigue, depression, dizziness, anaemia, increased sweating, muscle cramps, sciatica, muscle and joint pain
Trastuzumab	Gastrointestinal symptoms, cardiotoxicity, chest pain, hypotension, headache, taste disturbance, anxiety, malaise, depression, insomnia, drowsiness, dizziness, paraesthesia, tremor, peripheral neuropathy, hypertonia, mastitis, urinary tract infection, leucopenia, oedema, weight loss, muscle and joint pain, bone pain, leg cramps, rash, pruritus, sweating, dry skin, alopecia, acne, nail disorders

arthritis, B-cell chronic lymphocytic leukaemia and even some cancers. Unfortunately, when TGN1412 was administered for the first time to humans, all six of the healthy volunteers who received the drug became extremely ill. TGN1412 activated the immune system to such an extent that the volunteers suffered a 'cytokine storm' or 'cytokine release syndrome', which resulted in multiple organ failure.

So why did this happen? There was nothing wrong with the drug preparation used, the trial was conducted according to the protocol agreed with the Medicines and Healthcare Products Regulatory Authority, and preclinical testing of the compound had not suggested any untoward toxicity.

Of course, it is not unprecedented for drugs that look promising in preclinical studies to fail following their first administration to man. Some side-effects, such as hallucinations or headache, are notoriously difficult to detect in animal studies. Furthermore, there are many differences between species which make any extrapolation of findings in animals to man rather unreliable. However, the magnitude of the adverse reaction to TGN1412 was unprecedented.

Drug trials and safety testing procedures have developed from the experience of pharmaceutical companies and regulatory authorities with traditional small-molecule drugs. There are a number of characteristics possessed by the biopharmaceuticals which make them inherently more difficult to test using these established procedures, or potentially more dangerous should an adverse reaction occur.

Specificity

The big advantage of monoclonal antibodies is that they can be extraordinarily specific. The precise epitope recognized by TGN1412 is thought to be a stretch of six amino acids in the extracellular region of human CD28. In rodent CD28, all six of these amino acid residues are different from the human sequence and TGN1412 is therefore ineffective. Thus, all initial safety testing in rodents was performed using an entirely different antibody, JJ316, which binds to the analogous sequence on the rodent protein. No significant toxicity was detected in rodents, but these data were obtained not only in a different species, but using a different drug.

Even if different species have precisely the same epitope, the binding affinity of the antibody will be affected by the precise 3D shape of the epitope, which will be modified by the overall conformation of the protein, and thus by differences in amino acid sequence which may be quite distant from the epitope itself. As a consequence, the same antibody, binding to the same epitope on the same molecule, may do so with different affinities in different species. As binding affinity determines the likelihood that a particular concentration of antibody will interact with its target, these differences can be critical in determining the appropriate dose to use in man compared with animal studies.

Immunogenicity

Like most biopharmaceuticals, TGN1412 is a protein and, as such, is potentially immunogenic. It has been humanized to render it non-immunogenic to humans, but it will provoke an immune response, with the generation of antidrug antibodies, in other species. This potentially makes testing difficult. A lack of effect in a test species may reflect inactivation of the drug, rather than a genuine lack of efficacy. Fortunately, immunity does not develop immediately. However, when TGN1412 was tested in monkeys, some did develop antibodies to the drug during a 28-day trial.

Unusual dose–response characteristics

In common with many biopharmaceuticals, TGN1412 does not appear to exhibit the 'normal' relationship between dose and response that is found with traditional drugs. The very high affinity of many of the biopharmaceuticals can produce an extremely steep relationship between an increase in dose and size of the response, such that the drug appears to have an almost 'all or nothing' effect. Moreover, many of these substances have markedly 'bell-shaped' dose–response curves; depending on the initial dose, reducing the dose will not necessarily reduce the effect produced — it may indeed increase it.

Duration of action

Many biopharmaceuticals are very long-acting and the plasma half-life of TGN1412 is about 8 days. As a consequence, toxic levels of the drug will persist in the body for a long time, increasing the effects produced.

Prospects for the future

In many cases biopharmaceutical products are making a significant impact in the treatment of disease and there is no doubt that these drugs will become a bigger and bigger part of the available formulary.

However, it is important to realize that biopharmaceuticals are not 'magic bullets', able to treat disease without producing unwanted side-effects. Safety testing of biopharmaceuticals is at least as important as for conventional drugs, and is likely to require the development of new testing methods, including the use of engineered human tissues (see Ch. 12).

The extreme expense of these products is largely accounted for by the way in which they are manufactured, and the cost seems unlikely to decrease significantly in the short term. This means that a biopharmaceutical needs to produce an impressive benefit to health in order to outweigh its cost, particularly as health economics plays an ever-increasing role in drug evaluation. As an example, in 2006 and 2007 the Scottish Medicines Commission did not recommend the use of omalizumab (see above) in severe asthma, as the economic case for its use had not been proven.

Thus, while biopharmaceuticals will remain a significant growth area in the development of new pharmaceutical products, bringing these products to market will not always be straightforward.

FURTHER READING

Bhogal N, Combes R 2006 TGN1412: time to change the paradigm for the testing of new pharmaceuticals. Altern Lab Anim 34:225–239.

Daniell H, Streatfield SJ, Wycoff K 2001 Medical molecular farming: production of antibodies, biopharmaceuticals and edible vaccines in plants. Trends Plant Sci 6:219–226.

Longstaff C, Thelwell C 2005 Understanding the enzymology of fibrinolysis and improving thrombolytic therapy. FEBS Lett 579:3303–3309.

Werner RG 2004 Economic aspects of commercial manufacture of biopharmaceuticals. J Biotechnol 30:171–182.

Stem cells and tissue engineering

L. Buttery, F. Rose and K. Shakesheff

Regenerative medicine aims to use biomedical and engineering expertise and techniques to restore a fully functional tissue that has been lost or damaged within the human body. Virtually all the tissues of the body are under investigation as potential targets for regenerative medicine, and major breakthroughs are already entering into the clinic in the repair of bone, liver, cartilage, heart, brain, pancreas and other tissues.

There are four major reasons why a patient may need to have tissue restored within his or her body:

- *Injury* — for example, as can happen to bone (and cartilage) in a physical injury, where the volume of tissue damaged or lost is too large to be repaired by normal mechanisms.
- *Congenital defects* — for example, heart valves that do not fully form within the fetus
- *Degenerative and autoimmune diseases* — for example, type 1 diabetes, which is caused by an autoimmune attack on the islets of Langerhans
- *Surgical removal* — in some cancer treatments, the surgical removal of the cancer also removes substantial amounts of normal tissue from the patient.

Cells, scaffolds and signals

This chapter explores the various components that contribute to the development of a regenerative medicine product. As shown in Figure 12.1, there are, broadly speaking, three starting components to a regenerative medicine therapy: cells, scaffolds and signals. These can be applied singly and in various combinations.

- *Cells* must be able to form the desired tissue and this is ultimately dependent on the type and source of the cells. This is discussed in more detail in later sections of this chapter.
- *Scaffolds* play an important role in creating an environment, which is compatible with supporting the growth of the cells leading to development of the mature tissue and also interacting and integrating with the surrounding tissues after implantation.
- *Signals* are delivered by molecules such as growth factors or extracellular matrix components (ECM), which need to be present at the site to stimulate the correct response from the cells.

The simplest forms of regenerative medicine treatments use just one of the three components; for example, the cell therapies used in the treatment of cartilage injuries involve injecting a cell population (usually isolated from a normal piece of tissue from the patient and grown in culture for several weeks to obtain sufficient cell numbers) into the site of the body at which tissue is required; the tissues then self-assemble to the required state. Scaffold-only therapies may be used in tissues where the patient has a native cell population that can migrate from a site outside of the injured area into the scaffold and form new tissue. These types of scaffold are used in the field of orthopaedics to help repair bone tissue. Signalling molecules, such as growth factors, can be also used as a drug treatment. For example, bone morphogenic proteins are used to promote the formation of bone tissue as part of spinal fusion surgery for treating damaged or degenerating vertebrae.

In many cases, the use of just one of the three key components is not sufficient to encourage tissue to regenerate fully and a combination approach is required. Cells, scaffolds and signals can be combined in various ways and implanted into the patient directly, requiring the body to help coordinate and sustain the interactions between the various components and promote tissue growth, repair or regeneration *in situ*. Alternatively, the tissue can be fully formed within the laboratory and supplied as a ready-for-use product. The best example of this approach is tissue-engineered skin, e.g. Apligraf®, a living skin substitute comprising skin cells (keratinocytes and fibroblasts) within a natural scaffold (collagen type 1), used clinically to treat burns and non-healing ulcers. A further example of where such an approach would be essential is the growth of living heart valves, which would need to be fully functional at the point of implantation.

Finally, the field of regenerative medicine introduces ethical, legal and social issues that must be addressed in parallel with the scientific developments and these will be explored at the end of the chapter.

Scaffolds

The physical properties of scaffolds

There is a large and often somewhat confusing range of scaffolds that have been reported as potential templates for cell and tissue growth. However, while the chemical composition of different scaffolds can be highly varied, most share a number of common basic physical properties that are fundamental to their purpose (Box 12.1).

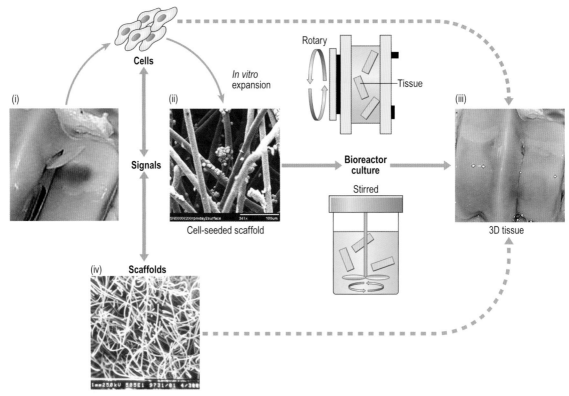

Figure 12.1

The concept of tissue engineering. The premise of tissue engineering/regenerative medicine is centred around three core elements — cells, signals and scaffolds — and the various ways in which they can be combined and controlled to grow functional tissues. There are several possible sources of cells: (1) primary cells isolated from tissues, e.g. cartilage; (2) adult stem cells isolated from sites like the bone marrow; (3) in the longer term, possibly embryonic stem cells. Cells are grown in *in vitro* culture for several days/weeks to expand numbers sufficiently for the intended use. Cells can be also combined with a scaffold. Scaffold format — e.g. chemistry, size, shape, porosity, strength, elasticity, inclusion of growth factors, etc. — can be designed to complement the biology of the cells and the tissue. Bioreactor culture serves to improve supply of nutrients to cells and is especially useful for growing cells seeded on a scaffold or 3D cell aggregates. There are many types of bioreactor (rotary and stirred are shown here) that have the advantage that nutrients can be constantly replenished and also monitored to assess the function of the cells/tissue. Cells/tissues can be readily maintained for several weeks, allowing them to mature and grow sufficiently for implantation. Alternatively, for some tissues, cells and/or scaffold can be implanted with minimal *in vitro* culture (dashed arrows), allowing the body to serve as a 'natural bioreactor'.

Porosity

A scaffold must comprise sufficient free space for cells to migrate into the 3D structure and form tissue. Therefore, most scaffolds are highly porous materials with free space occupying 50–90% of the volume of the scaffold. The size of the pores and whether the pores are interconnected are also very important parameters affecting the rate of diffusion and fluid flow across and through the scaffold. In addition, the size of the pore has an effect on the immediate environment in which a cell finds itself.

- If the pore size is large (> 400 microns in diameter), the cell could find itself within a large community of cells occupying the pores.
- If pore size is reduced to < 100 microns, cells may be clustered with just a few neighbours and separated from other populations.

Such physical features can produce marked effects on cell growth and differentiation. Porosity is also important in

permitting in-growth of surrounding cells and tissues, especially blood vessels.

Biodegradability

Once the scaffold has served its function, such as physical delivery of cells and/or signals, it is often desirable for the scaffold to be naturally removed or degraded to leave the newly grown tissue as the only remaining component. The biodegradable properties of a scaffold, including its rate of degradation, can be controlled largely using its chemistry, and breakdown can be mediated by chemical hydrolysis or via the action of endogenous enzymes. Ideally, the degradation products of the scaffold should be biologically inert or non-toxic.

Mechanical properties

The mechanical properties of a scaffold very much depend on its intended application and are also linked to its chemical composition. If the scaffold is to be used in an orthopaedic application, where it will have to withstand substantial mechanical loading forces within

Box 12.1

Features of an 'ideal' scaffold

- Promote cellular interaction and tissue development
- Provide suitable mechanical support
- Provide an environment for the appropriate regulation of cell behaviour
- Should have a degradation profile that supports the construct until neotissue is formed
- Produce degradation products that are non-toxic and easily eliminated
- Promote vascularization and enable transport of nutrients by having an appropriate network of interconnected pores
- Have a suitable surface chemistry to enable the adhesion of proteins and lipids to mediate the cellular response
- Have suitable properties to maintain a normal physiological pH and osmolarity

a patient, then the mechanical properties must meet this challenging environment. In contrast, for many other tissues — for example, the liver — the mechanical properties are not particularly important and the scaffold may be required simply to hold its own shape within this soft-tissue environment.

Surface characteristics

The surface of the scaffold is the part that interacts directly with the cell and also with the local environment into which it is implanted. Random features, such as surface roughness or inclusion of engineered micro- and nano-topographical features (aligned grooves, etc.), can significantly influence cell adherence, spreading and orientation on, and within, the scaffold. Such surface features can also influence adsorption of proteins and other molecules from tissue culture medium or from the local environment within the patient. This in turn influences how cells interact with the scaffold.

The chemical compositions of scaffolds

There are two major classes of material that have been used to form scaffolds for tissue engineering.

- The majority of scaffolds are formed from both natural and synthetic polymers and these will be described in detail in later sections of this chapter.
- The other major class of materials is the ceramics. These are inorganic, non-metallic materials that are most commonly used for orthopaedic applications, because their composition and structural characteristics can be made to mimic that of skeletal tissues. Ceramic materials have proved to be very successful in promoting the adhesion of bone cells and supporting the regeneration of bone tissue. It is also possible to blend together different types of

polymer or polymers with ceramics and these blends often yield scaffolds with physical properties that are distinct from the parent polymers or ceramics, such as changes in degradation rates or mechanical strength.

Synthetic polymers and ceramic scaffolds routinely use solvents or high temperatures (up to 500°C) as part of their production and for many applications this does not present any problem. However, as discussed below, it is often desirable to introduce biological molecules, such as a growth factor, into the scaffold to help improve its function. This has required the development of alternative methods of processing scaffolds, which do not destroy the activity of the growth factor. An example of such an alternative method is processing synthetic polymers in an environment of gaseous carbon dioxide at high pressure (e.g. ~74 Bar) and temperatures below 40°C; this technique is also called supercritical carbon dioxide. Under these conditions the carbon dioxide behaves as a solvent and is also non-toxic, enabling growth factors to be mixed with the polymer without loss of bioactivity. The carbon dioxide is then vented and, as the pressure returns to normal atmospheric levels, the scaffold forms with the growth factor distributed through its structure.

Polymers and ceramics can be produced in various sizes, shapes and structures ranging from porous blocks, through meshes and fibres, to micro-scale particles. Prior to use in cell culture or clinical applications, the scaffold needs to be sterilized and various methods are used, including ultraviolet irradiation, soaking in a solution of ethanol or exposure to ethylene oxide gas. Whichever sterilization method is chosen, care needs to be taken to check that it does not alter the chemistry or bioactivity of the scaffold, and it is routine to subject batches of each scaffold to various biological and physical assays to confirm the quality of the scaffolds.

It is important to note that the scaffold materials used in regenerative medicine and tissue engineering are distinct from the scaffold materials used for prosthetic devices, such as those used in a replacement hip. Although prosthetic devices help to support normal body functions, they are almost entirely inert, with minimal or no degradation, and are not designed to promote growth of tissues.

The use of polymers in scaffold formation

Polymers are long-chain molecules which have useful properties in terms of their ability to be manufactured into the type of high-porosity scaffolds that are required in tissue engineering. Our own cells synthesize and secrete polymeric materials to form the natural scaffolding that holds our tissues together. This natural scaffolding is called the extracellular matrix (ECM) and there is a range of different molecules that contribute to the ECM. Of these, collagen is the most abundant and is used in various biomedical applications. Natural polymers, such as collagen, can be readily purified from animal tissues, such as from the skins and bones of cows and pigs. As an alternative, entirely synthetic polymers can be prepared and can be designed to mimic natural polymers.

Natural polymers

The advantage in using a natural polymer like collagen is that it has been designed by nature to function as a natural scaffold. Such natural polymers already have the structural and mechanical features to match the function of the tissue, and also incorporate specific signals into their structure that promote adhesion of cells and can stimulate cell proliferation and differentiation. An example of such a signal is the 'RGD motif', which is a sequence of amino acids that may vary in length but includes arginine (R), glycine (G) and aspartate (D); these sequences may be repeated. This motif interacts specifically with a particular class of adhesion molecule (the integrins) that is expressed on the surface of a cell.

In the laboratory, collagen will self-assemble into a gel-like material, which contains small pores allowing a certain amount of fluid flow and exchange of nutrients across the scaffold. Being a natural material, cells are also able to remodel the collagen scaffold, which means that they are able to break down the structure using enzymes that they secrete to create their own space or microenvironment within the scaffold. Natural scaffolds are also very responsive to mechanical signals, such as the micromechanical forces exerted by individual cells as they explore and adhere to the surface of a scaffold, through to larger-scale forces applied across the whole of the scaffold structure, such as stretching. These forces are important in stimulating biological responses in the cells and can also encourage the cells to organize themselves into defined orientations and alignments. This approach has been useful in engineering tissues like tendons, where the cells are aligned along the axis of the force applied to the tissue.

There are a number of other natural, non-animal polymers that are used for tissue engineering. While these may lack the ability to mimic the ECM, they have other beneficial properties that derive from their natural biological function. For example, alginate materials, which are derived from seaweeds, are widely used in tissue engineering applications to form hydrogels. These gels are formed rapidly from a solution by simply increasing the concentration of calcium ions. This makes the formation of the scaffold from alginate materials very rapid and convenient: for example, allowing cells to be encapsulated within alginate structures. To achieve this, the gel solution plus cells is added drop-wise into a calcium-containing buffer, where it polymerizes into a bead on contact. The size of the bead can be controlled by controlling the size of the drops.

Synthetic polymers

The major advantage of synthetic polymers is that they can be mass-produced to a very high quality whenever they are required. This is in contrast to some of the natural polymers, which are dependent on animal sources and can suffer from high batch-to-batch variability, affecting both their physical and biological properties. However, synthetic polymers do suffer from a major

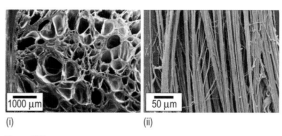

disadvantage, which is that they invariably lack any degree of specific interaction with the cells that we wish to grow on their surfaces. To a large extent, this disadvantage can be overcome by surface or chemical engineering to introduce biological functionality and in many ways mimic natural polymers.

To date, the major class of polymers used in tissue engineering has been the polyesters (Fig. 12.2). These polyester materials have been used for many decades as the component of synthetic sutures that can be used within the body and which slowly degrades over time. Synthetic polymers usually degrade by the process of hydrolysis, where water permeates through the polymer structure and cleaves ester bonds. The rate of degradation can be controlled, ranging from weeks to months or years, and potentially this can be matched to the rate of new tissue growth. Synthetic polymers degrade to yield products that are generally non-toxic and which can be metabolized or excreted from the body. However, products from synthetic polymers are often acidic and can potentially lead to local acidification. It is not clear if such effects occurring within a highly porous scaffold are sufficient to cause significant effects on cell viability and to inhibit tissue formation.

Figure 12.2
Synthetic polymers used for tissue engineering scaffolds. Examples of synthetic polymers used routinely in biomedical and tissue engineering applications. The varied chemical properties and degradation rates can be used to control a variety of structural features (e.g. porous scaffolds and fibres) and tuned to a specific cell or tissue type.

Adding signals to scaffolds

Surface signals

As discussed above, a cell population that is seeded on to a scaffold will interact with it via the surface. In order to prompt cell adhesion and growth, it is often desirable to mimic the interaction that occurs between the body's natural scaffolds (the ECM) and the cell. For scaffolds that lack natural ECM properties, such as synthetic polymers, it is possible to add ECM molecules to the surface and thus engineer bioactivity into the scaffold. A large number of ECM components are readily available as recombinant proteins or synthetic peptides and they can also be purified from animal tissues. Examples of ECM proteins that are commonly used for coating scaffolds include fibronectin, laminin and collagen. They can be prepared at different concentrations and adsorbed on to the surface of the scaffold by simple soaking or by using techniques such as plasma polymerization, which energizes deposition of molecules on to a surface. It is also possible to physically trap or tether ECM molecules directly into the surface of the scaffold. In all examples, ECM proteins can be deposited in defined patterns, encouraging cells to grow in specific orientations or regions of the scaffold.

Controlled-release signals

In addition to interactions with the ECM, various secreted growth factors and cytokines are important in controlling cell proliferation, differentiation and tissue formation. Growth factors are also required to encourage in-growth of new blood vessels, which is essential for sustaining the growth of most tissues. As we have already discussed, it is possible to incorporate biologically active growth factors directly into the structure of the scaffold. This, combined with the ability to control scaffold degradation rates, allows scaffolds to be used as controlled-release and delivery systems for biological molecules and also drugs.

The concept of controlled drug delivery is well established within the pharmaceutical industry; for example, therapies such as Zoladex® LA use a biodegradable polyester that is implanted under the skin to release a hormone slowly over several weeks for the treatment of prostate and breast cancers. This principle can be readily applied to scaffolds for tissue engineering, although the difference in scale — particularly the very high surface area presented by porous scaffolds — can make the controlled release of growth factors quite challenging. Some of these challenges are being met by using microparticles to deliver growth factors, and these microparticles can be distributed within specific regions or zones within a bulk scaffold. Zonal release systems can combine more than one type of growth factor and this sort of approach has been used experimentally for bone tissue engineering; bone morphogenetic protein (BMP) is released from one zone of the scaffold to stimulate bone tissue formation, and release of vascular endothelial growth factor (VEGF) from another zone to stimulate in-growth of blood vessels.

Incorporating cells on to and into scaffolds

Both scaffold porosity and the inclusion of ECM and growth signals are designed to encourage cells to adhere to, and grow on and within, the scaffold. While such features are important, more fundamental physical methods are often required to augment this process of cell recruitment and colonization (also called 'seeding' or uptake). Simply soaking the scaffold in a solution containing the cells will result in some cells occupying the scaffold, but most will 'prefer' to grow on the simple flat surface of the culture plate, rather than the complex porous structure presented by the scaffold. Getting the cells on to the scaffold thus presents a significant problem. This is made more challenging, as it is often necessary to know how many cells are being delivered on the scaffold to assess subsequent function. Delivering cells in a small volume of liquid and dropping this directly on to the scaffold, via a syringe or hypodermic needle, can improve uptake of cells. Similarly, agitating the solution of cells can also improve uptake of cells on to the scaffold. Whatever the method, it is important to determine percentage uptake, and this is done by collecting the solution in which the cells were mixed before and after seeding on to the scaffold. Cell counts can then be performed and seeding efficiency determined.

Bioreactors

For long-term culture of a cell/scaffold construct and growth of tissues that will be functional at the time of implantation, a bioreactor is usually required (Fig. 12.1). There are many designs of bioreactor, but a feature common to all is improving supply of nutrients to the growing tissue and removing waste products. By improving transport and exchange of nutrients, tissues can be grown larger and maintained for longer than in conventional static culture.

- Some of the more basic systems, such as stirred bioreactors, simply use some sort of electronically or magnetically controlled propeller to stir the culture medium. The rate of stirring can be controlled and the growing tissue is usually supported on a fixed needle just above the propeller to prevent the tissue being struck and damaged.
- A more elaborate system is the rotary bioreactor where the tissue is freely suspended in the culture medium and is uniformly rotated at defined rates. This type of bioreactor is sometimes called the NASA-type bioreactor, as it was originally developed as part of the space programme; rotating an object in a liquid at a defined rate can simulate the effects of reduced or zero gravity. It also simulates the neutral buoyancy our body experiences when immersed in water, which is similar to the environment created within the pregnant uterus to support growth of the fetus. Scientists found that this system is also conducive to supporting growth of tissues.
- Other systems include perfusion bioreactors, where culture medium is pumped over or across growing cells and tissues. This is particularly useful for those cells and tissues that experience fluid flow within the body, such as endothelial cells and blood vessels.

In all systems, culture medium can usually be readily replenished and sampled, to assess viability and function of the growing cells and tissues. In the most elaborate systems, all parameters can be controlled automatically and may also include in-line monitoring.

Cells and tissue engineering

Many tissue engineering and regenerative medicine strategies are dependent on cells supplied from an exogenous source. For these cells to contribute to achieving effective, long-lasting and stable repair of damaged or diseased tissues there are a number of important criteria that ideally should be met. These include:

- Obtaining sufficient numbers of cells to be able to achieve the repair; even small amounts of tissue may require tens of millions of cells.
- Ensuring accessibility. How easy is it to take samples of the relevant tissue from which to isolate cells?
- Differentiating the cells to the correct cell type and ensuring that the cells perform the necessary functions, such as secreting molecules like ECM proteins, hormones and cytokines.
- Ensuring that the cells adopt the appropriate 2D or 3D organization and tissue architecture and that they are structurally and mechanically compliant with the normal demands of native tissue.
- Integrating with the native cells and tissues (including vascularization and innervation, if required), and overcoming or minimizing the risk of immune rejection.

To some extent the ability to satisfy these criteria is dependent on the qualities and sources of the cells. There are a number of different sources of cells that are or possibly can be used for tissue repair and regeneration. These are summarized in Box 12.2 and include:

- mature differentiated cells isolated from the patient's own tissues, e.g. skin
- 'adult' stem cells isolated from specific tissue sites or compartments within the patient, e.g. haematopoietic stem cells (HSCs) from the bone marrow

Box 12.2

Examples of current sources of adult stem cells

- Ectoderm tissues: skin, eyes and brain
- Endoderm tissues: gastrointestinal tract, lungs, liver and pancreas
- Mesoderm tissues: bone marrow, skeletal muscle, fat, heart and kidneys

- cells isolated from aborted fetuses, e.g. embryonic germ (EG) cells derived from the developing gonad region
- cells isolated from the very early stages of the developing embryo, e.g. embryonic stem (ES) cells derived from the pre-implantation blastocyst.

Mature differentiated cells and 'adult' stem cells are integral components of our bodies, and are also often referred to as somatic cells and somatic stem cells, respectively. Conversely, ES cells are derived from small clusters of cells that exist only transiently during the very early stages of development, and in some respects they can be regarded as being 'man-made'.

Mature cells isolated from tissue biopsies could potentially be used for reimplantation into the same donor or an immunologically matched recipient. This would limit problems of immunocompatibility, but this is probably not the best source of cells for tissue repair. Such cells usually comprise differentiated and/or differentiating cells that inherently have a low potential to proliferate. This makes generating sufficient cells to promote tissue repair potentially difficult. Moreover, these cells are usually committed to a particular cell type that is restricted to the type of tissue from where they were harvested. This therefore raises issues of accessibility of tissue sites from which cells can be harvested. For example, while skin tissues can be readily harvested with minimal risk to the patient, harvesting tissues like heart and brain is more challenging and poses a far greater risk to the patient.

Stem cells can potentially overcome many of the limitations of mature cells and consequently there is currently much interest in the use of stem cells for tissue repair. In the following sections, some of the characteristics of stem cells, their basic biology, sources and applications in tissue repair and regeneration are discussed.

Stem cells

A stem cell can be described as an immature, primal or undifferentiated cell that is capable of dividing to produce at least one daughter cell that is identical to the mother cell: a process called self-renewal. This may be perpetuated over a number of cell divisions or even indefinitely. Figure 12.3 illustrates some of the general concepts of self-renewal.

All three mechanisms illustrated in Figure 12.3 may be relevant and may, to some extent, occur in the same stem cell population. However, overall asymmetric division, contributing to both self-renewal and differentiation, is probably the predominant mechanism. Evidence for symmetric differentiating division, where a stem cell population is reduced and eventually exhausted, is supplied by the fact that, as our bodies age, our capacity to repair stem cell-containing tissues like bone and skin also diminishes. Evidence for symmetric, replicating division, where a stem population expands and potentially overgrows the tissue, is somewhat more controversial. However, there is evidence to suggest that some cancers may be the result of stem cell self-renewal.

Stem cells can be isolated from various tissues and grown in the culture dish. In this environment, self-renewal of stem cells can often be readily stimulated and maintained for several weeks, months or even years, resulting in considerable amplification of stem cell numbers. In terms of cell therapy and tissue engineering, this can be extremely useful. In the body, however, stem cells

A Asymmetric, replicating and differentiating division – maintenance of the stem cell population with differentiation

B Symmetric differentiating division – depletion of the stem cell population without self-renewal

C Symmetric replicating division – expansion of the stem cell population without or limited differentiation

D Asymmetric division – amplification of cell numbers and differentiation via progenitor cells

- Stem cell
- Progenitor transit-amplifying cell
- Differentiated cell

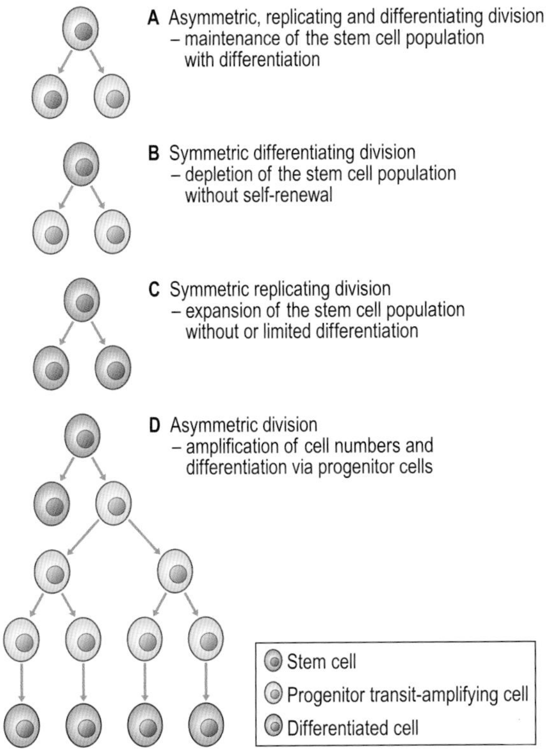

Figure 12.3

Basic concept of stem cell self-renewal and differentiation. The purpose of a stem cell is to give rise to specific differentiated cell types, enabling our bodies to grow and function normally. Since, over our lifetime, which may be several decades, our body is required constantly to replenish and repair its tissues, it is also incumbent on the stem cell to remain responsive and active for many years. With only relatively small numbers of stem cells present in our body, it meets these demands through the process of self-renewal. Possible basic mechanisms of stem cell self-renewal are represented in Figures A–C. Of these, asymmetric replicating and differentiating division (A) is the classic self-renewal process, with the stem cell dividing to give rise to two daughter cells, one remaining identical to itself (i.e. self-renewal) and the other responding to subtle changes in the local environment and going on to differentiate. However, the fact that our bodies age, marked by a decreasing capacity to repair our tissues, and the fact that we are also prone to developing tumours indicate that processes B and C are also important. In effect, stem cell division is likely to be a mosaic of several processes. Differentiation is also a complex process, but that depicted in D, involving generation of progenitor/transit-amplifying cells, is one likely mechanism. The role of progenitors is to enter into several rounds of division, increasing cell numbers. With each division the progenitor may become progressively more differentiated and eventually stops dividing, having acquired the characteristics of a specific differentiated cell type. The activity of progenitors, such as number and rate of cell divisions and range of differentiated cell types formed, varies within different tissues.

may divide relatively infrequently, remaining dormant or quiescent for prolonged periods until they receive the appropriate set of signals to start (and then stop) dividing. This tight control of stem cell self-renewal *in vivo* is necessary to ensure that these cells do not divide indeterminately and potentially overgrow the tissue: in effect, to prevent them from becoming a cancer. For these reasons stems cells are also usually quite rare, with only small numbers being found at defined locations within our tissues: for example, within the bone marrow.

Another important concept is stem cell potency – the range of cell types to which it can give rise. There are three basic measures of stem cell potency:

- *totipotent* – can form all cell types that contribute to the formation of an organism. This is restricted to the fertilized egg or zygote.
- *pluripotent* – can form most cell types of an organism, including germ cells, but not the placental tissues (e.g. ES cells and EG cells)
- *multipotent* – can form most cells in a particular tissue or tissues (e.g. 'adult' stem cells, or HSCs).

What determines stem cell potency is dependent to a large extent on the programming epigenetic regulation of gene expression (see Ch. 4). The environment in which the stem cell is located or placed is also significant. For example, changes in local gradients of growth factors, etc. and cell–cell and cell–matrix contacts are important in the switching 'on' and 'off' (and possibly even the reprogramming) of genes and gene pathways, thereby changing the type and range of cells that can be generated. It is becoming evident that the distinction between pluripotent and multipotent is becoming increasingly more blurred, with some cells seemingly having greater plasticity than previously realized (Table 12.1).

The process of differentiation, in which a cell acquires a particular set of characteristics enabling it to perform a specific function (such as insulin production by pancreatic β cells, dopamine production by neural cells or bone formation by osteoblasts), usually involves formation of an intermediate progenitor cell, sometimes called a transit-amplifying cell. To some extent, progenitor cells are similar to stem cells, particularly 'adult' stem cells. They can divide a number of times and may even have a very limited capacity for self-renewal. However, with each successive division, the cells usually become progressively more differentiated.

The main function of progenitor cells is to increase cell numbers (often exponentially), allowing the formation of tissue and organs with the appropriate size, shape and mass. Progenitor cells may also exhibit a degree of plasticity, ranging from being unipotent and restricted to differentiating to one specific cell type, through to being bi- or tripotent and giving rise to several differentiated cell types. For example, in skeletal tissue, cartilage cells (chondrocytes), fat cells (adipocytes, abundant in the marrow space) and bone forming cells (osteoblasts) are believed to arise from a common tripotent progenitor; this progenitor is itself derived from a stem cell located within the bone marrow microenvironment.

Table 12.1
Some comparisons between human embryonic stem (ES) cells and adult stem cells (ASC)

	Human ES cells	Human ASCs
Availability	Initial isolation can be challenging but, once isolated, they can be grown relatively easily. Many cell lines exist	Cells usually quite rare and require invasive procedure for isolation. Culture and *in vitro* expansion of cell numbers can be challenging. No cell lines currently available
Stability	Normal karyotype can be maintained in culture, although abnormalities have been described for some lines and relate to method of passaging. Long-term *in vivo* stability unknown (not tested in humans)	Maintenance of genetic make-up long-term *in vitro* not known but long-term stability shown *in vivo* (e.g. bone marrow transplants). Microenvironmental niche *in vivo* may change with age or disease, affecting differentiation and cell numbers
Differentiation potential	Definitively shown to be pluripotent	Certainly multipotent; some ASCs possibly pluripotent
Ethical issues	Present in many countries and institutions due to religious and moral reasoning	Reduced in comparison to ES cells, as does not involve destruction of embryo
Repair *in vivo*	Yes; shown in a few animal studies. Most existing lines cannot be used in humans	Yes; shown in many animal studies. Also autologous and allogenic transplants in humans
Teratoma risk	Risk of teratoma formation *in vivo* if cells sufficiently purified	Do not form teratomas when transplanted *in vivo*
Telomerase expression	High — cells are able to replicate indefinitely	Low — undergo senescence, proliferation limited

Sources of stem cells

Adult (somatic) stem cells (ASCs)

ASCs are found in many tissues throughout the body. These cells divide and differentiate, either to replenish the supply of differentiated cells that die as part of the natural 'life cycle' of the tissue, or to repair damaged tissue. Tissues like the blood, skin, liver, gut and bone are replenished and repaired almost constantly, and while the ability to maintain and repair our tissues diminishes as we get older, the fact that we can live for several decades clearly demonstrates the capacity of ASCs for self-renewal.

In the body, ASCs usually differentiate to a particular cell type or range of cell types and these are usually associated with the tissue in which they are located. In this regard, ASCs are considered to be multipotent cells. However, evidence is accumulating to suggest that ASCs might in fact have pluripotency, and this theory is supported by several lines of experimental investigation:

- Stem cells from the bone marrow have been differentiated into neural cells, and likewise stem cells from the brain have been differentiated into blood cells.
- Studies on bone marrow transplantation in rodents and humans have demonstrated that small numbers of marrow-derived stem cells can migrate to various tissues and organs around the body. This may simply represent colonization, but it is possible that the cells can stimulate cells in the tissues or possibly even differentiate into the same cell type.
- Bone marrow stem cells have been used successfully in clinical trials to help promote repair of heart tissue damaged after a heart attack.
- The expression of genes and proteins associated with pluripotency (e.g. those expressed by ES cells) has been detected in some ASCs.

The adult stem cell niche

The capacity of ASCs to self-renew and to differentiate into mature cell types is a tightly regulated process. In order to maintain tissue homeostasis, these cells often reside in what is referred to as a 'stem cell niche'. This 'niche' is essentially a microenvironment that limits the exposure of stem cells to differentiation, apoptotic and other signalling events that would otherwise deplete stem-cell reserves. In addition, the 'niche' tightly controls stem-cell division, to avoid over-population of a tissue with these cell types. When required, stem cells can be activated to produce transit-amplifying or progenitor cells that are at that point committed to producing the mature cell types of that tissue. Hence, the dynamic interplay between stem cells and their niche is essential in the maintenance of healthy tissues, and so it is important to understand these relationships, in order to utilize these cell types effectively for therapeutic applications.

In mammals, the bone marrow niche is probably the best studied of these niches, although the marrow is a fairly diffuse tissue and involves very complex interactions between cells and signalling molecules. Possibly one of the best examples of a niche that is well defined in terms of morphology and basic function is that of the intestinal crypt, which regulates differentiation of intestinal epithelial cells (Fig. 12.4).

Bone marrow stem cells

The bone marrow is one of the most abundant sites for ASCs and cells from this location are also probably the most studied and best understood of all ASC types. Part of the reason why marrow stem cells have been studied so extensively is that they are accessible; samples can be collected relatively easily by introducing a needle directly into the bone marrow, usually at the iliac crest, and aspirating marrow tissue. The marrow tissue can then be cultured for further investigation. Stem cells from the bone marrow also often enter the circulation and can be found in peripheral blood samples.

There are in fact two distinct types of ASC within the bone marrow:

- *the haematopoietic stem cell* (HSC), that classically gives rise to the entire blood cell lineage
- *the bone marrow stromal stem cell* (BMSC), also called the mesenchymal stem cell (MSC), that classically gives rise to various connective tissues, notably bone, cartilage and adipose tissue.

Other cell types are also found in bone marrow aspirates, notably red blood cells, endothelial cells, fibroblasts, adipocytes and osteoblasts. There is also evidence for distinct subpopulations of stem cells within the marrow environment: notably, multipotent adult progenitor cells. With such a heterogeneous mix of cells it is necessary to apply specific methods to isolate and characterize the stem cells. Such methods are considered in Figure 12.5 and include:

- centrifugation on a Ficoll® density gradient
- cell-sorting methods, such as fluorescence activated cell sorting (FACS) or magnetic activated cell sorting (MACS).

Ficoll is a high molecular weight sugar polymer, which works as a 'cellular sieve', sorting cells into distinct fractions based on their density; these fractions can be visualized as distinct layers in the gradient. Red blood cells can be easily recognized at the bottom of the gradient; plasma and fat collect at the top. A whitish, narrow band of cells is usually seen below the plasma fraction; this is described as the mononuclear cell fraction and contains the marrow stem cells. These cells can be aspirated from the gradient and used in subsequent experiments.

The mononuclear cell fraction will contain various cell types, including the marrow stem cells. Two principal types of experiment are performed to characterize and purify the stem cells.

- *Colony-forming unit (CFU) assay.* This is the classic experiment in terms of characterization; the cell fraction is diluted to specific densities or number of cells, right down to a single cell. The cells are cultured for several days and then observations are made regarding the growth of distinctive colonies of differentiating cells, which are the progeny of any stem cells present in the culture. The colonies can be characterized by morphology and also by more detailed molecular and biochemical assays. The colonies can also be counted and these data can be used, collectively with data from the other assays, to assess the relative abundance or frequency of a particular stem cell type within the bone marrow.
- *Differential adhesion assay.* There are also some more rudimentary differences between the HSCs and BMSCs. HSCs tend not to adhere directly to cell culture plates, requiring co-culture or a semi-solid matrix (see below); BMSCs will, in general, adhere to cell culture plates. Thus, a simple adhesion assay performed over an hour or so can be used initially to differentiate between the HSC and BMSC fractions.

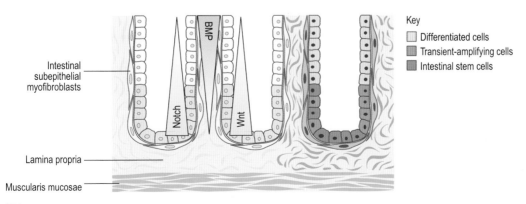

Figure 12.4
The gut stem cell niche. Anatomy of the intestinal epithelium illustrating the location of intestinal stem cells (dark pink), transient-amplifying cells (pink) and differentiated epithelial cells (light pink). Signalling events (simplified) from the lamina propria generate gradients of signalling factors (wedges) that maintain the stem cell niche and stimulate differentiation.

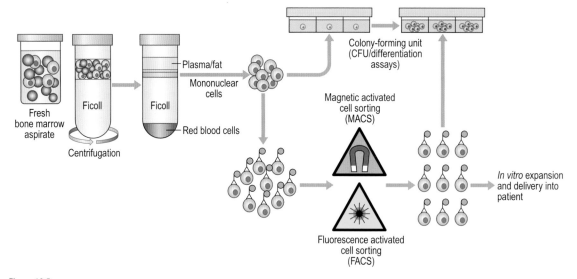

Figure 12.5

Steps to isolate and characterize bone marrow stem cells. Freshly isolated bone marrow tissue contains a mixture of cells, including blood cells, stromal cells, adipocytes, osteoblasts and stem cells. Centrifugation on a density gradient (Ficoll) separates out various cell fractions, with the stem cells being present in the mononuclear layer. The stem cells are characterized by colony-forming unit (CFU) assays and/or cell sorting methods like fluorescence activated cell sorting and magnetic activated cell sorting (FACS and MACS). Stem cells (e.g. HSCs and BMSCs) can initially be characterized based on differential adhesion assays (HSCs will only adhere to stromal cell co-cultures or methylcellulose). Cells are seeded at defined densities, including single cells, and after several days of culture any colonies that have formed are characterized by morphological and molecular and biochemical methods. Cells can also be stimulated with growth factors to encourage differentiation of specific cell types. Methods such as FACS and MACS use antibodies to target specific cell surface antigens or 'markers' that are specific to a particular stem-cell type. The selected cell populations can then be used for *in vitro* CFU and differentiation assays or culture expanded for clinical application.

The other experimental approach is use to cell-sorting methods, such as fluorescence-activated cell sorting (FACS) or magnetic-activated cell sorting (MACS). Both FACS and MACS are very sensitive, efficient and rapid methods for quantitatively characterizing specific cell types (e.g. stem cells) within mixed cell populations. They can be also performed under sterile conditions to sort and collect specific cell types for further culture.

Both of these methods are similar and are based on using antibodies tagged with either a fluorescent label or a magnetic microparticle. The antibodies are directed against specific antigens or 'markers', such as a receptor expressed on the surface of a cell, and ideally this should be 'unique' to the target cell type, e.g. HSCs. If necessary, it is possible to use a combination of different antibodies to increase selectivity. These methods can be used to assess number or frequency of cells expressing a particular 'marker', together with CFU assays (described above); it is believed that the stem cell population within the marrow is somewhere between 1 in 10 000 and 1 in 100 000 cells.

Haematopoietic stem cells (HSCs)

Of all the different types of stem cell, HSCs are the best studied. They are also an example of a very successful stem-cell therapy, forming the basis of bone marrow transplantation to treat various types of leukaemia.

Within the body, HSCs are found mainly in the bone marrow, although they may also be found circulating in the blood and in other tissues, such as the spleen. They function to generate the entire blood cell lineage, including red blood cells, leucocytes and lymphocytes.

Although the marrow is a diffuse tissue, the proliferation and differentiation of HSCs are tightly controlled within microenvironments or niches. The exact nature of the HSC niche is not known (see above), but physical contact with stromal cells (including BMSCs) and osteoblasts is important, as is the presence of various growth factors, in particular stem cell factor (SCF) and also a number of specific cytokines, the colony-stimulating factors (CSFs).

One of the most common methods for selecting HSCs is FACS or MACS (see above), usually performed after density gradient separation of the mononuclear cell fraction. There are a number of 'markers' expressed on the surface of HSCs, notably CD34. (The term 'CD' refers to a 'cluster of differentiation antigens'; a large number of CD antigens have been identified and are associated with specific cell types and stages of differentiation.) CD34 is known to be a glycoprotein that functions in cell–cell and cell–matrix interactions.

Once collected, the HSCs (CD34-positive population) can be cultured and stimulated with various growth factors to study mechanisms of differentiation. They can also be grown on to increase the number of HSCs available for clinical applications.

As we have already discussed, HSCs do not generally adhere to cell culture plates, so are co-cultured either on a feeder layer of growth-arrested stromal cells or fibroblasts (see also p. 161), or on a semi-solid support matrix such as methylcellulose, a gel-like material. In both cases biochemicals such as SCFs and CSFs need to be added to the culture medium to help stimulate and maintain HSC proliferation.

Since only small numbers of HSCs are usually present in the body, it is possible to treat a patient with CSFs, which stimulate and mobilize HSCs within the body and can potentially increase the 'yield' of stem cells from bone marrow biopsies.

Bone marrow stromal stem cells (BMSCs)/mesenchymal stem cells (MSCs)

This stem-cell type 'shares' the marrow environment with HSCs and several other cell types. As indicated above, there is a certain amount of interaction between the different cell populations. Again, the exact nature of the microenvironment or niche in which the BMSCs reside is not known, but the marrow and the bone tissue that confine it are dynamic environments and the key function of BMSCs is to help maintain these environments, differentiating into cells such as osteoblasts, adipocytes and stromal cells/fibroblasts. Throughout our life, bone is constantly being resorbed by osteoclasts (derived from HSCs) and replaced by osteoblasts, in response to normal physiological demands, such as the mechanical loading associated with walking and metabolic turnover. Bone tissue serves as a reservoir of essential mineral ions and cytokines. Our ability to repair fractured or broken bones serves as a powerful illustration of the function of BMSCs.

Selection of BMSCs from marrow aspirates is probably less efficient than that of HSCs, because fewer specific markers exist for BMSCs. Initial isolation can be achieved by differential adhesion assays, which will remove the HSC fraction. However, other cells present in the marrow, like adipocytes and stromal cells/fibroblasts, will also adhere to cell culture plates. There are some markers that are useful for selection of BMSCs. These include:

- Stro-1, an as yet uncharacterized cell-surface antigen
- CD44, a glycoprotein that binds hyaluronan, a component of the extracellular matrix
- CD105, also called endoglin, a receptor for the cytokine transforming growth factor beta.

Both CD44 and CD105 can be also used for selecting HSCs, and some distinction can be achieved by subsequent adhesion of the selected cells.

The BMSCs can, in general, be maintained and expanded in culture quite easily, without the need for specific growth factors, such as those required by HSCs. Some of the basics of cell culture are described in Box 12.3.

The differentiation potentials of BMSCs can be assessed by CFU assays and also by adding specific growth factors to stimulate differentiation into a particular cell type. Such experiments reveal that BMSCs can be readily differentiated *in vitro* to osteoblasts, chondrocytes, adipocytes, stromal cells, tendon cells, muscle cells and possibly several other cell types. BMSCs have therefore been used in a number of tissue engineering studies, including the repair of damaged bones and joints in both animal models and humans.

Although bone tissue can, under most circumstances repair itself, there are cases, such as the removal of a bone tumour, where the injury is so extensive that the defect is too large to be repaired naturally. A number of studies have shown that various natural and synthetic polymer and ceramic scaffolds, or demineralized bone tissue seeded with BMSCs, can be implanted into such bone defects and can promote full repair. Such scaffolds can also be used to deliver specific growth factors, such as BMPs, which can stimulate local recruitment of BMSCs and bone tissue formation. Similar approaches

---

 Box 12.3

The basics of cell culture

All cell types are cultured in a defined 'base' medium containing various amino acids and salts; the formulation can be precisely varied to suit a particular cell type. The medium is usually supplemented with 10–15% (v/v) serum (e.g. fetal bovine serum; FBS), which is used as a source of growth factors and other biochemicals needed to help the cells grow. The composition of the serum is completely undefined and, in the same way as the composition of our blood and serum varies between individuals, so does FBS. However, to minimize these effects, the serum from a number of animals is usually pooled into batches. Batches of serum will vary in their composition and this can affect the growth and differentiation of the cultured cells. Therefore, when performing any culture experiment, it is important to test a number of different batches of FBS to determine which 'best suits' the growth of the cells being studied. Once the most suitable batch has been identified, a reserve can be made with the supplier, but once that batch has been exhausted the process of batch testing needs to be repeated.

The reasons for using an undefined component, such as FBS, to culture cells are based on the fact that it works and it is also relatively cheap! While there are some completely defined compositions of growth factors and biochemicals to replace FBS, which is obviously desirable, they are often very expensive. More significantly, they may only work for one, or at best a few different, cell types and they often involve a lot of time-consuming trial and error experiments as part of their development (see also Ch. 11).

have been applied to help repair damaged cartilage and tendons, which have a much more limited capacity for natural repair.

There are also a few clinical examples of where BMSCs have been used to help treat genetic diseases of the bone, such as osteogenesis imperfecta, where the osteoblasts have an impaired capacity to synthesize bone matrix protein (collagen type 1), which results in brittle bones. Implantation of donor BMSCs can help restore differentiation of normal osteoblasts, leading to synthesis of normal bone tissue.

Multipotent adult progenitor cells (MAPCs)

Multipotent adult stem cells, MAPCs, are isolated as a subset of BMSCs/MSCs and as such are extremely rare cells. They express cell surface markers that are distinct from those of BMSCs and also express markers associated with ES cells and pluripotency. Relatively few experiments have been performed to date to explore and confirm the biology of these cells.

ASCs from other tissues

Many tissues have now been shown to contain a population of stem cells, or cells with stem cell-like characteristics. These serve to replace or repair cells that are lost due to normal wear and tear or injury. Notable examples of such tissue include skin, gut and liver, which as part of their normal function have high cell attrition rates. However, many other tissues, which appear to have a much more limited capacity for normal repair, such as cartilage, heart, teeth and brain, have also been shown to contain stem cells or putative stem cells. Given the presence of these stem cells, it is not known why these tissues are unable to effect self-repair as efficiently as other tissues, such as the skin.

Clearly, the isolation and therapeutic application of ASCs from some tissues is going to be challenging. Nevertheless, their study using animal models or human surgical and post-mortem samples is still important for understanding their biology and designing methods to stimulate these cells in the body.

Cord blood stem cells and fetal stem cells

Blood collected from the umbilical cords of newborn babies has been shown to contain populations of stem cells with characteristics similar to both HSCs and BMSCs; these could potentially be useful in allogenic transplants. There is also much interest in cryo-preserving cord blood stem cells for future therapeutic use: for example, to treat the child, should he or she develop a disease like leukaemia. However, the clinical value of such long-term storage of cord blood remains largely unproven.

Stem cells have also been isolated from the cord blood during early pregnancy, using a needle guided by ultrasound. Again, these stem cells have characteristics similar to both HSCs and BMSCs, but unlike cord blood collected from term pregnancies, these fetal stem cells appear to be less developed immunologically, and potentially could cause fewer problems with immune rejection. More controversially, fetal stem cells can also be isolated from elective abortions.

Embryonic stem cells

Embryonic stem (ES) cells are derived from the inner cell mass of the pre-implantation blastocyst and have been obtained from a number of different species, including mice, non-human primates and humans (Fig. 12.6). The small cluster of cells that forms the inner cell mass is in fact the developing embryo. As mentioned earlier, ES cells are in many respects 'man-made', as these cells exist only fleetingly during normal development.

To produce ES cells, the inner cell mass is teased away from the surrounding trophectoderm cells, which will eventually form the placenta, by physical and enzymatic methods resulting in the destruction of the developing embryo. In humans, strict ethical and legal measures have been implemented and only embryos that are surplus to *in vitro* fertilization and fertility studies can be used for generating ES cells. Manipulation of the human embryo is also restricted to within the first 14 days of its creation. This time point marks a specific stage in embryonic development, with the onset of organogenesis and, in particular, the formation of the primitive streak, which is the rudimentary central nervous system. ES cells are usually isolated before day 5, when the entire embryo is comprised of a few hundred cells.

Experiments *in vitro* and *in vivo* show that, while ES cells retain the capacity to form any and all fetal and adult cell types, including the germ cells, they seem unable to form tissues like the placenta. For this reason, ES cells are described as being pluripotent; they are not totipotent.

When implanted into immunodeficient mice, a single undifferentiated ES cell has the capacity to form a teratoma (also known as a germ cell tumour, normally affecting the testis). This type of tumour is comprised of ectodermal, mesodermal and endodermal cells; classic examples can have perfectly formed teeth, hair or kidney tubules, etc. inside the tumour. The ability to induce formation of a teratoma is often used as a measure of stem cell pluripotency. Further evidence of pluripotency is provided by injecting ES cells into a fresh blastocyst, implanting the blastocyst into a surrogate mother and allowing the embryo to develop naturally. The resulting chimera demonstrates the ability of the injected ES cells to contribute to normal development (see Ch. 8). If the ES cell has been genetically manipulated either to overexpress or lack a specific gene, or to express a fluorescent 'marker' like green fluorescent protein (GFP), then specific developmental processes can be investigated and observed in the resulting chimera.

Maintaining ES cells in an undifferentiated pluripotent state *in vitro* has required the development of a number of specific cell culture techniques. Most ES cell

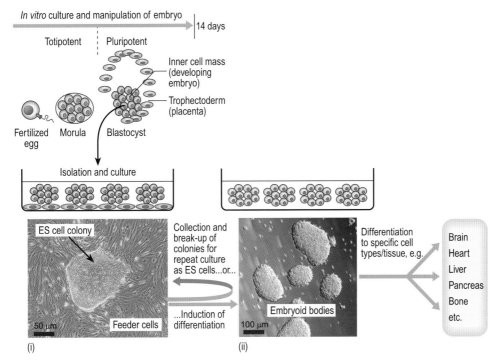

Figure 12.6

Derivation and propagation of ES cells. ES cells are derived from the inner cell mass of the pre-implantation blastocyst, which develops a few days after fertilization. The inner cell mass cells are dissected away from the trophectoderm, which will form tissues like the placenta. At this stage the cells are pluripotent. The inner cell mass cells are cultured (now ES cells) under specific conditions, such as on growth-arrested fibroblasts, together with certain cytokines, which work as a 'brake' on differentiation to help maintain ES cell pluripotency. ES cells grow as distinct colonies, which, once they have reached a certain size/density, can be collected, dispersed into small clusters and either recultured (on fresh plates) as ES cells or, in the absence of feeders and cytokines, induced to differentiate. ES cells usually differentiate via formation of 3D aggregates called embryoid bodies, which can be left intact or dispersed and stimulated with specific growth factors to encourage differentiation of particular cell types.

lines have been derived by co-culture with mouse embryonic fibroblasts (MEFs) and require specific cytokines to be added to the culture medium.

Mouse ES cells require leukaemia inhibitory factor (LIF), whereas human ES cells appear to be unresponsive to LIF and instead require basic fibroblast growth factor (bFGF). While LIF and bFGF are the predominant cytokines used in culture of ES cells, others, such as BMP-4 and noggin, have also been shown to be useful in maintaining pluripotency.

Some ES cell lines are amenable to culture in the absence of a fibroblast feeder layer and this has the advantage that the ES cells can be more easily cultured and manipulated. Few, if any, ES cell lines can be grown directly on tissue culture plastic and most require a thin coating (probably a few nanometres' thickness) of protein. They still require tissue culture medium to be supplemented with cytokines like LIF and bFGF and usually at higher concentrations compared to co-culture with fibroblasts.

Mouse ES cells can be readily maintained on tissue culture plastic coated with a dilute solution of purified bovine gelatin. Human ES cells, however, seem somewhat more fastidious in their requirements and are often maintained on tissue culture plastic coated with Matrigel®, a commercial product that is an extract from a mouse sarcoma cell line and is composed of a number of extracellular matrix proteins, including collagens,

laminin and proteoglycans. While being free from direct contact with feeder cells, human ES cells may still require a certain amount of feeder cell-conditioned medium to be added to the culture. This conditioned medium is collected from culture plates on which fibroblasts have been grown for 1–2 days and contains soluble factors secreted by the fibroblasts, which, in combination with the Matrigel and bFGF, help to maintain pluripotency.

While these co-culture and surface coating methods generally work well, the mechanisms by which they help to maintain ES cell pluripotency remain largely unknown. A number of studies are therefore in progress to investigate these mechanisms and potentially to develop defined surfaces for ES cell culture. Such studies include microarray techniques, where a variety of specific proteins, peptide fragments or synthetic polymers, etc. are spotted on to a glass side and then used for ES cell culture to determine if specific spots are able to support ES cell attachment, promote growth and maintain pluripotency.

General morphology and characteristics of ES cells

ES cells are usually rounded cells with a relatively large nucleus (Box 12.4). When cultured on feeder cells, they proliferate as distinct colonies, with well-demarcated boundaries. In feeder-free culture, the cells may initially form similar colonies, but can also form a continuous monolayer, often with a cobblestone appearance.

Box 12.4

General requirements for classification of human ES cells

- Immortality and telomerase expression
- Pluripotency and teratoma formation
- Maintenance of a normal euploid karyotype over extended culture (formation of abnormal karyotypes such as trisomy 12 and 17 have been reported in some human ES cells but it is thought that this is due to the method of passaging)
- Clonality
- Expression of high levels of the transcription factor octamer-binding protein 4 (Oct-4), Nanog and other markers of pluripotency such as the stage-specific embryonic antigens 3 and 4 (SSEA 3 + 4), tumour-rejection antigen (TRA) 1-60 and 1-81, and alkaline phosphatase, as well as surface antigens CD9, CD24 and
- The ability to contribute to chimera formation through blastocyst injection (although this has not been exploited for ethical reasons in humans)

Observation of morphology is a good guide to confirm the undifferentiated characteristics of ES cells, but when conducting any experiment with ES cells it is also important to confirm their pluripotency, usually by molecular or biochemical analysis. Undifferentiated ES cells express specific transcription factors, such as octamer-binding protein 4 (Oct-4) and Nanog, and cell surface markers called stage-specific embryonic antigen (SSEA1–4). These characteristics are common to both mouse and human ES cells, although they vary slightly in their expression of SSEA.

ES cells normally express the enzyme telomerase, which maintains specific cap regions (telomeres) on the chromosomes and functions to prevent mutations or damage when the chromosomes are segregated during normal division. Telomerase is therefore associated with the capacity for a cell to divide. Most somatic cells do not express telomerase; with cell division, the telomeres progressively shorten and the cell stops dividing when the telomeres research a certain minimum length.

Chromosome integrity is reflected by the cell karyotype. With stem cells, in particular, it is necessary to perform regular karyotype analyses to confirm a normal complement of chromosomes. Any change in chromosome number (aneuploidy) can have deleterious effects on cell behaviour and function. Such changes have been reported in some human ES cell lines.

Differentiation of ES cells

Differentiation of ES cells is induced almost immediately when they are removed from contact with feeder cells and the cytokines LIF or bFGF. The ES cells can be removed from the feeders or culture plates either by physical scraping methods or by enzymatic procedures with collagenase or trypsin. The dispersed ES cells (now differentiating cells) are usually maintained in suspension culture, where they proliferate and differentiate to form distinctive cellular aggregates or 'embryoid bodies'. These contain differentiating cells of ectodermal, endodermal and mesodermal lineage.

Other methods for forming embryoid bodies include culturing a single or small number of ES cells in a small droplet of culture medium suspended from the lid of the culture plate (hanging drop) or similarly in a small tube (pellet culture). Both the hanging drop and pellet methods produce single embryoid bodies; while being much more labour-intensive than suspension culture, these methods offer better control over embryoid body growth and size, and this can potentially improve subsequent control of differentiation. Another method that combines elements of the hanging drop and suspension methods is the encapsulation of single or small numbers of ES cells within alginate beads, which are then cultured in a bioreactor.

To some extent embryoid bodies mimic the process of gastrulation seen in early development. Embryoid bodies can be left intact, or dispersed by mechanical and/or enzymatic methods to single cells, and then used in a variety of culture experiments. These include CFU assays or stimulation with specific growth factors, in order to study and control differentiation to particular cell types. Although stimulation with specific growth factors is a useful approach for directing differentiation of ES cells, it is rarely, if ever, 100% effective, with some cells differentiating to other (unwanted) cell types. This random differentiation also occurs with ASCs and, in terms of studying mechanisms of differentiation and/or the potential clinical applications of stem cells, where a pure cell population is required or desirable, the unwanted/contaminating cell types need to be eliminated.

As we have already discussed for HSC, methods like FACS or MACS are extremely useful for sorting a particular cell type, and this approach can be readily applied to ES cell differentiation, provided that the cell type of interest expresses a suitable cell surface marker.

Stem cells (both ES cells and adult stem cells) are also particularly amenable to gene manipulation techniques, which can be used to generate cultures that are near 100% pure for the desired cell type. Such techniques can result in a target gene being inactivated or over-expressed. The most common approach, known as gene transfection or transduction, involves introducing a gene into a population of cells, e.g. ES cells, and then selecting the cells that over-express the gene. The gene is usually packaged in an engineered construct and delivered across the cell membrane, into the cell, by one of several methods. These methods include:

- electroporation, which punches transient small holes in the cell membrane, allowing the gene construct to enter the cell
- use of liposome carriers such as Lipofectamine®, which encapsulates the gene construct; the chemistry

of the liposome enables it both to interact with and to traverse the cell membrane

- use of viral vectors, which exploits the natural ability of a virus to infect our cells but usually involves an attenuated form of the virus, so it is only able to infect the cultured cells and not escape into the environment.

The gene construct is engineered to carry one of several drug resistance genes or fluorescent tags, such as green fluorescent protein, which allow for preferential selection of cells expressing the construct. Such methods have been used to select neural and cardiomyocyte phenotypes from ES cells; in the latter example, the selected cardiomyocytes were subsequently implanted into the damaged hearts of mice and shown to form stable grafts.

Somatic cell nuclear transfer (SCNT)

In light of the success of cloning Dolly the sheep and the various other animals that have followed, much interest has been generated in understanding the mechanisms of nuclear cloning/reprogramming and potentially harnessing them for tissue repair strategies. In SCNT, the genetic material of an oocyte is first removed and the nucleus from a somatic cell is then injected into the enucleated oocyte (Fig. 12.7).

Under appropriate conditions, the oocyte–somatic nucleus 'hybrid' can be stimulated to start dividing and has the potential to generate an intact embryo and produce a viable organism that is genetically identical to the donor of the somatic nucleus. The mechanisms that

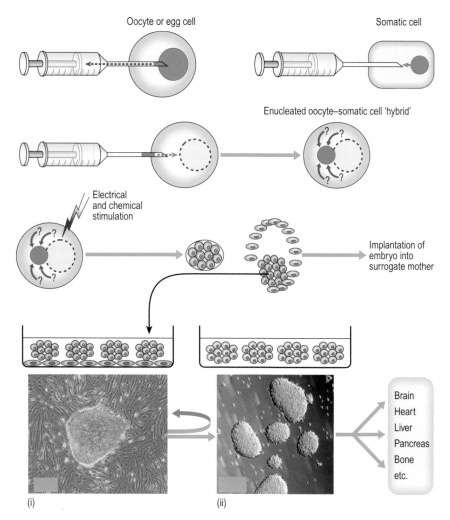

Figure 12.7
Basic concepts of somatic cell nuclear transfer (SCNT). The chromosomes/DNA are removed from the oocyte and discarded. Similarly, the intact nucleus of a somatic cell is removed. The somatic cell nucleus is injected into the enucleated oocyte where various factors present in the cytoplasm help to 're-program' its DNA. After stimulation, the oocyte–somatic cell nucleus 'hybrid' begins to divide and appears to follow the normal developmental process to generate a viable embryo; if implanted into a surrogate mother, this can develop into an intact offspring that will be a clone of the donor of the somatic cell. This is reproductive cloning, e.g. 'Dolly' the sheep. Alternatively, cells from the developing blastocyst can be used to create embryonic stem cells, which can then be differentiated into specific cell types that will be genetically identical to the donor of the somatic cell and therefore immunologically compatible with that donor. This is therapeutic cloning.

induce such a remarkable transformation are not fully understood, but it seems likely that factors present in the enucleated oocyte can initiate reprogramming of the somatic nucleus to generate a totipotent cell, with the capacity to form a viable embryo.

Although controversial, such experiments are important in helping us to understand the mechanisms of development and the basis of genetic diseases. They could also be helpful in enabling the cloning of endangered animal species. Such studies also have significant therapeutic applications. For example, goats have been engineered to make large amounts of human factor VIII (a clotting factor used in the treatment of haemophilia) in their milk, which can then be readily purified (see Ch. 11). Pigs have been engineered so that their organs express human antigens, raising the possibility that these humanized organs could be used in human transplants; many pig organs are similar in size to those of humans.

In several countries, the cloning of an embryo (for up to 14 days) is currently allowed. It is hoped that this can be used to generate cloned human ES cells, which could then be used to generate cells and tissues matched to a specific patient: therapeutic cloning. However, success has so far been very limited due, in part, to the technical challenges of cloning and also to our incomplete understanding of the mechanisms involved. The efficiency of cloning is often very low (requiring large numbers of oocytes), and in the case of animal cloning, developmental abnormalities are also very common; Dolly the sheep was the product of hundreds of experimental attempts.

To overcome some of the technical challenges — in particular, the demand for large numbers of donor oocytes — studies are being performed on analysing and using oocyte extracts, to try to identify the factors and mechanisms that stimulate reprogramming of a somatic nucleus. It is hoped that such factors could be used to reprogram a somatic cell to become pluripotent, without the need to create or destroy an embryo.

Oocytes from cows and rabbits are also being used to clone human ES cells; remember that the genetic material is removed from the oocyte and it is the implanted somatic nucleus that determines the genetic identity of the cloned cells. Thus, while the oocyte may be from a cow or a rabbit, the cloned cell should be almost entirely human.

Regulatory issues

Research and clinical application of tissue engineering and stem cells are subjected to a number of ethical, moral and societal rules and regulations. It is not the intention to debate those rules and regulations here, but simply to present some of the key issues.

Work on virtually any human cell, especially if it involves a patient, requires ethical approval. This involves writing a detailed description of how the cells will be collected and for what experiments they will be used. Justification for the number of subjects to be involved and a description of the potential biomedical or therapeutic applications, and of the potential outcomes and risks are also required. This information is debated by the ethics panel, which will normally include some experts in the field, together with lay members.

If the cells are going to be transplanted into a patient, it is important to demonstrate aseptic, clean processing of the cells to avoid any risk of transferring infections. These are described as Good Laboratory Practice (GLP) and Good Manufacturing Practice (GMP) and usually require laboratories dedicated solely to the clinical applications of the cells; this is very expensive to implement and maintain.

Use of ES cells and SCNT is particularly emotive since their derivation involves destruction of an embryo. The debate on the use of these cells and techniques involves an ethics review process conducted at governmental level. Issues surrounding permission to use human ES cells vary in different countries around the world (Table 12.2). The UK has some of the most liberal laws

Table 12.2
Current legal position of various countries on use of human ES cells and SCNT*

Country	Position
Ireland, Poland, Lithuania, Austria	Forbid generation and research
Germany, Italy	Forbid generation of hESC but permit work on imported and existing cell lines for research only
France, Brazil, Australia, Canada, Japan, Netherlands	Permit derivation of stem cells only from donated embryos; forbid SCNT
Belgium, China, India, Israel, Singapore, South Korea, Sweden, UK	Permit SCNT (with some restrictions), generation and use of hESC. Enjoy generous government support
USA	No national regulations. Federal funds can only be used for cell lines created before August 2001. Private research allowed under licensed protocol

*N.B. These are subject to change.

and currently permits work on human ES cells, including derivation of new lines and also SCNT. It is also one of the first countries to establish a human stem cell bank, which includes ASCs and ES cells. Samples of human stem cells that have been isolated or derived by researchers in the UK must be sent to this central facility, which not only banks the stem cells, but also performs quality assurance tests in line with GMP and develops standardized protocols to expand these cell lines and distribute them to other researchers. In order to receive stem cells from the UK Stem Cell Bank, a researcher must make a request that is processed in manner similar to ethical review.

FURTHER READING

Gehron Robey P 2000 Stem cells near the century mark. J Clin Invest 105:1489–1491.

Kemp P 2006 History of regenerative medicine: looking backwards to move forwards. Regen Med 1:653–669.

Stock UA, Vacanti JP 2001 Tissue engineering: current state and prospects. Annu Rev Med 52:443–451.

Watt FM, Hogan BLM 2000 Out of Eden: stem cells and their niches. Science 287:1427–1430.

Appendix 1
Perspectives — future developments

M. Keen and J. Pongracz

Medical biotechnology is still at a very early stage of development but is already making a major impact. It is difficult to foresee the advances that may be possible over the next 20 years.

There is a growing hope that, as we understand more about the full complement of genes and proteins in particular cells and tissues, and the way in which they interact, we may be able to model entire cells, tissues and indeed organisms in the computer. It may be possible then to do complex experiments 'in silico', testing the effects of novel drugs — for example, on computer models of human beings. Computer models are already being used to predict antigenic sites in proteins and computer models of organs such as the heart have been developed. The growing field of systems biology aims to incorporate our growing body of knowledge of the various '-omes' (genome, proteome, interactome, etc.) into a detailed understanding of physiology in order to develop such models. Nevertheless, however sophisticated these models become, they will remain only models; their predictions will still need to be tested in real human beings, and real human beings will still require treatment to cure or prevent disease.

There is a growing tendency to avoid the use of animals in the testing of new drugs. This is driven by several factors, including concerns regarding animal welfare, the marked species differences that make the use of animals to predict effects in humans difficult, and the unsuitability of conventional animal models for testing 'human-specific' biopharmaceuticals (see Ch. 11). Human receptors expressed in cell lines and even transgenic animals are already being extensively used in drug development, and a number of in vitro systems for toxicity testing have been developed. However, traditional tissue culture techniques are not ideal for drug testing, as normal cell-to-cell interactions do not occur. To overcome this, mixed cultures mimicking the shape and organization of real tissues are being developed for use as model systems for drug testing.

Apart from understanding 'omics', the ability to replicate entire organs in culture, for drug testing or for transplantation, also requires an understanding of the biophysics of tissue development (Forgacs and Newman, 2005). Veins have already been 'grown' using a 'tissue printing' technique, in which small groups of cells are 'printed' in a defined pattern on to a suitable substrate. The first tissue printer was in fact a modified ink jet printer. At the current rate of technological development, it may not be very long before replacement organs can be custom-grown to order.

Biopharmaceuticals are already making a big impact on therapy. In the medium term, it seems likely that more and more biopharmaceuticals will be introduced. However, in the longer term, the development of successful gene therapies may obviate the need for many drugs.

Nanotechnology promises the development of nanomachines that could perhaps be injected into the body to repair damaged organs. This is reminiscent of the shrunken submarine used to remove a blood clot in the film *Fantastic Voyage*!

When diseases can be cured by gene therapy or nanomachines, how will they be diagnosed? Advances in the identification of metabolomic markers may well mean that one day a definitive diagnosis will be possible from a single blood test or saliva sample. The development of the type of electronic scanners used on *Star Trek* may take a little longer!

FURTHER READING

Forgacs G, Newman SA 2005 Biological physics of the developing embryo. Cambridge University Press: Cambridge.

Appendix 2
Glossary of experimental techniques

T. Czompoly and K. Kvell

Antibodies

Following activation of the immune system, antigen-specific B cells differentiate into plasma cells which produce antibodies. In medical research, diagnostics and therapy two types of antibody are used:

- polyclonal antibodies
- monoclonal antibodies.

Polyclonal antibodies

During the specific immune response, each plasma cell produces only one type of specific antibody. Antibodies produced by different plasma cells recognize different parts (epitopes) of the antigen; an epitope is the part of the antigen molecule that evokes the immune response. Since each antigen induces activation and differentiation of many individual B cells, the serum of the immunized animal will contain a mixture of antibodies produced against the given antigen. This mixture of antigen-specific immunoglobulin molecules is called a polyclonal antibody.

To generate polyclonal antibodies, an animal is injected with the antigen of interest and then, following a period of time to allow activation of the immune system and antibody generation, serum containing the antibodies is collected. Polyclonal antibodies are prepared most frequently using rabbits, although pigs, goats, sheep, horses, guinea pigs, hamsters, mice and rats can also be used. The aim of immunization is to achieve antibodies with high affinity for the antigen in a high 'titre' (a high concentration). Adjuvants and repeated immunization are often used to enhance the immune response. Adjuvants form an antigen depot and slowly release the antigen, which allows time for the immune cells to become activated. In addition, some adjuvants contain immunostimulatory molecules that enhance the immune response. Once a good serum titre is achieved, antibodies against the antigen can be purified relatively easily from serum by affinity chromatography if required.

Monoclonal antibodies

A monoclonal antibody is produced by a single clone of B lymphocytes (Fig. A.1), such that monoclonal antibodies recognize a single epitope of the antigen.

The first step in monoclonal antibody production is the establishment of a cell line that is derived from a single antibody-producing plasma cell (Fig. A.1). This process is called hybridoma technology and was described by Georges JF Köhler and Cesar Milstein in 1975. Köhler and Milstein shared the Nobel Prize for the hybridoma technology with Niels K Jerne in 1984.

Generation of a hybridoma involves the fusion of antibody-producing plasma cells with myeloma tumour cells; the myeloma cells have lost their capability for antibody secretion but have acquired the ability to grow indefinitely in culture. Plasma cells are isolated from the spleen, lymph node or bone marrow of a repeatedly immunized animal (mouse, rat or hamster). The two cell types are induced to fuse, by permeabilizing the cell membranes with polyethylene glycol or electroporation. The resulting plasma cell–myeloma hybrid cells are called hybridoma cells.

Fusion is an inefficient process and so a selection step is required to eliminate the non-fused myeloma cells. The myeloma cells used do not possess hypoxanthine-guanine phosphoribosyltransferase HGPRT, an enzyme involved in the salvage pathway of nucleotide synthesis. In order to select out the unfused myeloma cells, the cell mixture fusion is cultured in medium containing hypoxanthine, aminopterin and thymidine (HAT). Aminopterin blocks the de novo synthesis of GTP and TTP; therefore cells defective for the salvage pathway enzyme HGPRT (non-fused myeloma cells) die in this medium. The fused hybridoma cells survive, as plasma cells express the functional HGPRT enzyme. Non-fused plasma cells have a short lifespan *in vitro* and they will also die eventually.

After selection, hybridoma cells are diluted and plated at very low density, so that each resulting colony will have come from a single cell and thus be 'monoclonal'. The individual clones are tested for antibody production against the specific antigen. Once the ability of the hybridoma cell line to produce high-specificity monoclonal antibody is established, the antibody production can be scaled up using *in vitro* cell culture, and the antibody purified using liquid chromatography techniques.

Polyclonal and monoclonal antibodies are used in virtually all areas of human medical research and diagnostics. The various techniques of antigen–antibody interaction include ELISA, immunohistochemistry, Western blotting, etc. In order to make the antigen–antibody interaction more easily detectable, antibodies are often conjugated with different fluorescent (e.g. fluorescein

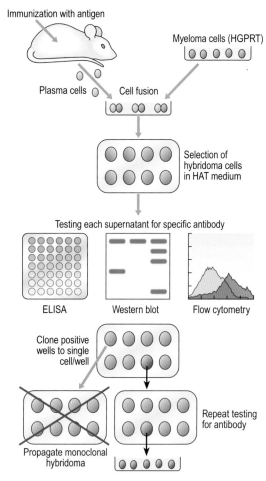

Figure A.1
Monoclonal antibody production. Monoclonal antibodies are produced by immortalization of plasma cells obtained from an animal immunized with the antigen. Plasma cells are fused with a myeloma cell line and the hybrid cells (hybridoma cells) are selected. The resulting hybridoma cells are tested for antibody production and diluted to a single cell/well. Daughter cells producing the antibody originate from a single cell; thus antibodies produced in this way are called monoclonal antibodies.

isothiocyanate) or non-fluorescent (e.g. biotin or horse-radish peroxidase enzyme) molecules.

Several monoclonal antibodies are also used in human therapy (see also Ch. 11).

FURTHER READING

Köhler G, Milstein C 1975 Continuous cultures of fused cells secreting antibody of predefined specificity. Nature 256:495–497.

Ritter MA, Ladyman HM (eds) 1995 Monoclonal antibodies. Cambridge University Press: Cambridge.

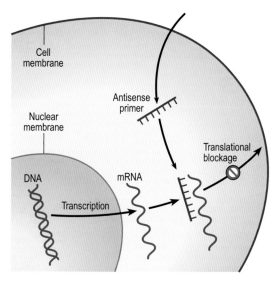

Figure A.2
Antisense technique. Antisense DNA oligonucleotides are similar to primers used for PCR. They identify and anneal to target mRNA sequence according to rules of base-pairing. Hybridization to specific mRNA sequences results in specific blockade of translation into amino-acid and protein sequence.

Antisense

Antisense is a technique that blocks the translation of mRNA into protein. When ribosome complexes move along single-stranded mRNA sequences during translation, the process can be blocked by complementary oligonucleotides that hybridize to the specific mRNA sequence (Fig. A.2). Such complementary oligonucleotides resemble PCR primers (see ' PCR' below).

As RNA is very sensitive to degradation, these complementary oligonucleotides are often engineered to be nuclease-resistant, and therefore more stable, by linking the nucleotides with phosphorothioate bonds. The efficiency of antisense techniques is variable, the outcome difficult to predict and the choice of appropriate controls problematic. Therefore, the recently discovered, more robust and reliable RNA interference technique is taking over in gene-silencing studies (see 'siRNA' below).

FURTHER READING

Stein CA, Krieg AM 1998 Applied antisense oligonucleotide technology. Wiley-Liss: New York.

Blotting techniques

The main principle in all blotting techniques is that biological material (DNA, RNA or protein) is transferred ('blotted') to an adsorbent solid surface such as nitrocellulose or nylon (Fig. A.3). This 'blotting' step usually follows electrophoretic separation of the nucleic acid or protein on an agarose or acrylamide gel. The transferred material is then detected by hybridization to a specific probe.

There are three main types of blotting techniques:

- Southern blotting — for DNA detection
- Northern blotting — for RNA detection
- Western blotting — for protein detection.

Southern blotting

Invented by and named after Sir Edwin Mellor Southern in 1975, this technique is used for the detection of specific DNA sequences. Firstly, DNA strands are separated on the basis of size by agarose gel electrophoresis. Then the DNA from the gel is transferred to a solid surface, usually nitrocellulose or nylon, by capillary action. The transferred DNA is fixed to the surface by ultraviolet irradiation or heating. Pre-synthesized DNA probes will hybridize with the DNA bound to the surface according to the rules of base-pairing. Depending on the way in which the probes are labelled, visualization may be radiographic, fluorescent, luminescent or chromogenic.

Northern blotting

Developed by James Alwine, David Kemp and George Stark in 1977, this is used for the detection of specific RNA sequences. Similarly to Southern blotting, samples

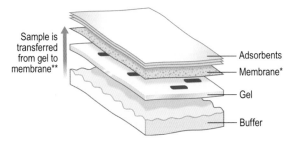

Sample is transferred from gel to membrane**

— Adsorbents
— Membrane*
— Gel
— Buffer

* May be different for various blotting methods
** Transfer is accomplished by capillary or electric force, depending on blotting methods

Figure A.3
Blotting techniques. This involves transfer of DNA, RNA or proteins to a nitrocellulose or nylon membrane, prior to detection of specific nucleic acid sequences or proteins with oligonucleotide probes or antibodies respectively. Nucleic acids can be transferred from the gel to the membrane by capillary action, whereas the transfer of proteins requires the application of an electrical current.

of RNA are separated by electrophoresis, transferred to a solid phase by capillary action and then hybridized by base-pairing to DNA or RNA probes. By definition this method detects gene expression. The basic principle of Northern blotting has been revolutionized by microarray technology.

Western blotting

Originating from the laboratory of George Stark, this is used for the detection of specific amino-acid sequences in denatured proteins. In Western blotting, protein samples are separated by polyacrylamide gel electrophoresis, usually under denaturing conditions. The proteins are then transferred onto a nitrocellulose membrane using an electric current ('electro-blotting'). Specific proteins can then be identified using antibodies which bind to specific short amino-acid sequences within the denatured proteins. The protein band is usually visualized using a labelled 'second antibody', which binds to the primary antibody bound to the protein of interest.

FURTHER READING

Darling DC, Brickell PM 1994 Nucleic acid blotting (basics). BIOS Scientific: New York.

Dunbar BS 1994 Protein blotting: a practical approach (The Practical Approach Series 140). Oxford University Press: New York.

Cell culture

Cell culture methods were developed to keep cells of various origin under suitable *in vitro* conditions for laboratory testing and experimentation. The basic equipment required in a standard cell culture laboratory is shown in Figure A.4. Several different types of cell culture system are used in medical biotechnology. The most frequently used are:

- Mammalian cultures
  Mammalian cell lines
  Mammalian primary cell cultures
    Mammalian stem cell cultures
    Mammalian 3D cultures
  Recombinant viral packaging cultures
- Bacterial cultures

Mammalian cultures

Most mammalian cell-culture systems share some basic characteristics. Cells are grown in suitable culture media in incubators with a stable temperature of 37°C, saturated humidity and at 5% (v/v) CO_2 content. Some cells grow attached to a substrate (adherent cells), whereas

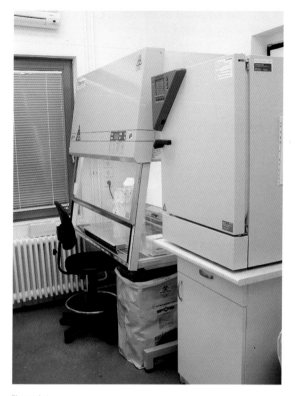

Figure A.4
A typical cell culture laboratory. All manipulations are performed in a laminar flow cabinet (shown on the left of the image) equipped with ultraviolet lamps to maintain a germ-free environment. Most cell types require an elevated CO_2 level and saturated humidity at a constant 37°C temperature. These ambient conditions are maintained in a cell incubator, shown on the right of the image. Labware contaminated with cells is considered biologically hazardous and must be collected separately following safety protocols; this is the purpose of the yellow box in the middle of the bottom of the image.

A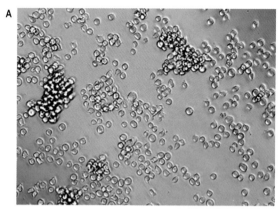

B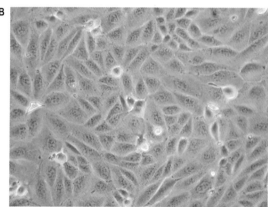

Figure A.5
Cell line cultures. (A) Suspension cells do not adhere to glass or plastic surfaces used for their cultures. Therefore these cells remain spherical and move freely as the culture flask is moved. However, they may adhere to each other following cell division, creating larger balls. (B) Adherent cells make up the other major cell type based on microscope morphology. These cells adhere to the hydrophilic glass or plastic surfaces and therefore have an irregular polygonal shape. Flattening of the cells on the substrate reduces their thickness and makes them easier to view using phase-contrast microscopy. If the cells exhibit contact inhibition, cells only grow in monolayer and then growth halts.

others will grow in suspension in medium (non-adherent cells); examples of adherent and non-adherent cells can be seen in Figure A.5.

- *Mammalian cell 'lines'.* 'Immortal' cell lines originate from malignant tumour cells. They proliferate fast and may be subcultured many times in standard cell-culture media. Although these are the simplest mammalian cells to maintain in culture, they may be quite different from their *in vivo* counterparts; most cell lines exhibit extensive genetic mobility and alterations.
- *Mammalian primary cell cultures.* More 'life-like' models than immortal cell lines can be achieved using primary cultures. For a primary culture, 'normal' cells are removed from an organism and grown in culture, usually for a limited time. However, maintaining these cells ex vivo is generally much more demanding than growing immortalized cell lines. Primary cultures are more dependent on specific activation signals and growth factors and their capacity for proliferation is usually limited.

In some cases it may be possible to preserve basic cellular interconnections in tissue or organ culture systems. This is often achieved by supplying primary cells by artificial tissue scaffolds that mimic the environment that supports them (see below).

- *Mammalian stem cell cultures.* By definition, stem cells are 'uncommitted' cells that may be induced to differentiate into various cell lineages depending on the specific culture conditions, such as the presence of particular growth factors, cytokines, cell membrane-bound signals, etc. In stem cell culture systems it often seems to be the case that true stem cells can either remain multipotent (able to give rise to a great variety of different cell types) but quiescent, or divide and then become committed into progenitor cells, which can only give rise to a more limited number of potential cell types. The daughter progenitor cells have an immense capacity for proliferation. Therefore these cells have the potential to be cultured for a long period of time. Such stable and long-term stem cell cultures appear to require an increased CO_2 level and also a decreased O_2 level, resembling their natural niche in the bone marrow.

— *Mammalian 3D cultures.* Going beyond primary cell mono(layer) cultures, in certain cases it is possible to preserve or reconstruct basic cellular interactions in tissue or organ culture systems. This may be achieved in several ways. In certain cases it is possible to remove pieces of solid tissue (e.g. a whole mouse thymus), and culture the whole organ. Using this method, the original tissue structure can be preserved in an ex vivo organ culture system, provided that the basic structure is sufficiently thin that all the cells in these tissue communities can have their metabolic demands satisfied by diffusion. Alternatively, tissue models can be created first by purification of all the cell types of the organ (e.g. mouse thymus, cartilage, liver, etc.) using cell surface markers; intercellular connections are then recreated in a 're-aggregate' organ culture, usually formed by centrifugation of the mixed cells. This approach has the advantage that particular cell types can be genetically modified before creation of the re-aggregate culture. Another possibility is to seed primary cells on to an artificial 'scaffold' that mimics the natural tissue environment. Contemporary scaffold systems are highly sophisticated in terms of delicate 3D structure and chemical composition (see Ch. 12). Scaffolds may even be biodegradable, so that as they are colonized with cells, the synthetic 3D backbone is replaced by a biological structure, ready for implantation, etc.

• *Recombinant viral packaging cell cultures.* Certain pathogenic retroviruses have been 'domesticated' for research purposes. These include the murine leukaemia retrovirus (MLV) and the human lentivirus (HIV). 'Domestication' means that most genetic elements responsible for pathogenesis have been removed to yield viral vectors. By having the vast majority of wild-type genetic material removed, these viral vectors become much less hazardous and provide sophisticated delivery tools for a variety of genetic elements. The vectors can be used to produce stable transgenic cell lines, primary cells or animals and have a potential use as vectors in gene therapy. These viral vectors have to be grown in mammalian cell culture systems. The genetic information necessary for the recombination of viral vectors is further grouped and divided into plasmids, because of safety and practical considerations. These plasmids are co-transfected into a mammalian cell line (e.g. the human kidney epithelial cell line, HEK293, or its daughter cell line, PHX (Phenix)), which is therefore transiently turned into a vector-producing cell line (Fig. A.6). Recombination of

genetic information, integration of RNA and protein yields viral vectors secreted into the cell supernatant that is harvested and purified before subsequent transfection procedures.

Bacterial cell cultures

Prokaryotic cells are far less sensitive than eukaryotic cells in terms of culture conditions. For highest efficiency they are also cultured at 37°C in standard bacterial media; in return they proliferate extremely quickly by dividing every 20 minutes or so, and provide a sufficient platform for numerous applications. There are commercially available bacterial strains which have been engineered with specific genetic features that allow them to be robust fermentation organisms for the rapid production of high quantities of various proteins, plasmids, etc. Antibiotic selection permits the maintenance of high-purity bacterial cultures. Although prokaryotic post-transcriptional modifications can limit utilization in eukaryotic organisms, the economy, robustness and pace of bacterial platforms often outweigh this disadvantage.

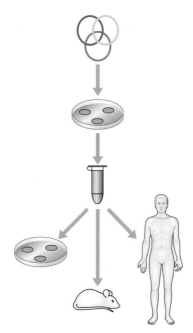

Figure A.6
Recombinant viral packaging cell cultures. Modern biotechnology allowed for the domestication of certain pathogenic retroviruses (i.e. M-MLV, HIV) into viral vectors used for gene delivery. Following the deletion of sequences responsible for pathogenicity, the remaining genetic information is further split into several plasmids (typically three). These are transiently transfected into cell lines that in turn become virus-producer cells; these are often marked by reporter genes, such as green fluorescent protein. The supernatant of virus-producer cells can then be harvested, purified and concentrated for subsequent use for *in vitro* experiments and even *in vivo* gene delivery.

FURTHER READING

Bacakova L, Filova E, Rypacek F et al. 2004 Cell adhesion on artificial materials for tissue engineering. Physiol Res 53(Suppl 1):S35–45. Review.

Hadjantonakis AK, Papaioannou VE 2002 Can mammalian cloning combined with embryonic stem cell technologies be used to treat human diseases? Genome Biol 30:3(8): REVIEWS1023. Epub 30 Jul 2002. Review.

Kurian KM, Watson CJ, Wyllie AH 2000 Retroviral vectors. Mol Pathol 53(4):173–176. Review.

Schmeichel KL, Bissell MJ 2003 Modelling tissue-specific signalling and organ function in three dimensions. J Cell Sci 116(Pt 12):2377–2388. Review.

Trono D 2000 Lentiviral vectors: turning a deadly foe into a therapeutic agent. Gene Ther 7(1):20–23. Review.

Vogel HC, Todaro CC 1996 Fermentation and biochemical engineering handbook. Principles, process design, and equipment. Noyes: Westwood, NJ.

Chemical synthesis of biomolecules

The biomolecules synthesized most frequently in biotechnical methods are:

- nucleic acids
- peptides.

Nucleic acids

Synthetic nucleic acids have a fundamental role in recombinant DNA technology. Numerous techniques rely on the use of chemically synthesized DNA or RNA molecules, including polymerase chain reaction (PCR), real-time PCR, site-directed mutagenesis, DNA sequencing, genotyping assays and RNA interference.

Oligonucleotides are synthesized in 3' to 5' direction by phosphoramidite chemistry utilizing glass beads with controlled pore size as solid support. Nucleotides are incorporated consecutively, one at a time, in cycles of four repeatedly performed steps, until the 5'-most nucleotide is attached. The steps in each synthesis cycle are as follows:

- *deprotection*, which generates a reactive hydroxyl group on the recipient nucleotide which is already attached to the glass bead
- *coupling*, the formation of a new chemical bond between the activated nucleotide and the next nucleotide to be attached
- *capping*, which inactivates the free hydroxyl groups of those nucleotides which failed to couple

- *stabilization* of the phosphate linkage between the growing oligonucleotide and the most recently added base.

Once the synthesis is completed, the oligonucleotide is cleaved from the glass bead, hydroxyl groups are freed at both ends of it and organic salts are removed by desalting. From now, the oligonucleotide exists as a functional, single-stranded DNA molecule. The synthesis process is usually automated. It is possible to link various fluorescent and other (such as biotin) molecules to both the 5' and 3' ends of oligonucleotides.

The need for further purification depends on the length and nature of the oligonucleotide and also on the downstream application. For conventional PCR primers, standard desalting is usually sufficient. However, for long (> 40 base) and for modified (fluorescently or otherwise labelled) oligonucleotides additional purifications are necessary. Polyacrylamide gel electrophoresis and subsequent elution of the oligonucleotide from the gel are used to purify long unmodified oligonucleotides. For purification of modified oligonucleotides, ion-exchange chromatography or reverse-phase high-performance liquid chromatography (HPLC) is used. Capillary electrophoresis or mass spectrometry (matrix-assisted laser desorption ionization time-of-flight, MALDI-TOF) can be used for the analytical testing of the synthesized oligonucleotide.

It is possible to synthesize other molecules which mimic DNA or RNA and are capable of specific base pairing. One of these mimics is 'peptide nucleic acid' (PNA), in which the backbone is built up by pseudo-peptide bonds instead of sugars. PNA has a stronger binding and increased specificity compared to naturally occurring nucleic acids.

Peptide synthesis

Synthetic peptides are used in a variety of applications, including verification of structural data of naturally occurring peptides, structure-activity research, immunization in antibody development, and the synthesis and development of peptides with medical importance, such as hormones, hormone analogues or peptide vaccines.

Currently, peptides are usually synthesized using solid-phase peptide synthesis. This means that the peptide chain is build up on polystyrene or polyamide beads, by incorporating the amino acids one after another. Unlike ribosomal protein synthesis, solid-phase peptide synthesis proceeds in the C to N terminal direction; the first amino acid is linked to the resin through its carboxyl group, and the next amino acid in the sequence is attached through its carboxyl group to the amino group of the preceding amino acid.

To avoid polymerization of identical amino acids, and to keep reactive side-chain groups away from the formation of chemical bonds, the N-terminus and side-chain of the newly added amino acids need to be blocked (protected). The most frequently used protecting group is *fluorenyl-methoxy-carbonyl*; hence this synthesis method is called Fmoc chemistry. In summary, iterative steps of peptide synthesis involve the attachment of the first protected amino acid to the resin, deprotection and coupling of the next protected amino acid. These steps are usually performed with the use of automatic peptide synthesizers. It is possible to incorporate artificial amino acids and D-amino acids into peptides using this technique.

Once the peptide is synthesized, it is cleaved off the resin and purified using ion-exchange chromatography or reverse phase HPLC. Identity of the peptide is confirmed by mass spectrometry. In general, peptides up to 70–100 amino acid residues long can be synthesized; the difficulty of synthesizing a particular peptide depends on its actual amino acid sequence.

FURTHER READING

Benoiton NL 2005 Chemistry of peptide synthesis. CRC: Boca Raton, FL.

Blackburn GM, Gait MJ, Loakes D, Williams DM (eds) 2006 Nucleic acids in chemistry and biology, 3rd edn. RSC: London.

Nielsen PE (ed.) 2004 Peptide nucleic acids: protocols and applications, 2nd edn. Horizon Bioscience: Wymondham, Norfolk.

ELISA

ELISA is the abbreviation for enzyme-linked immunosorbent assay. The first descriptions of the method were published in 1971 by two separate groups. This immunological method utilizes the high specificity of antibody–antigen recognition and binding. ELISA may be used for the detection (qualitative ELISA) or measurement (quantitative ELISA) of a given antigen or antibody in solution. A large number of mass-produced medical diagnostic and quality control kits employ ELISA.

- *Standard ELISA* is used to measure the amount of an antigen (usually a protein) in solution: for example, in blood or urine. The protein solution is applied to the ELISA plate (often a polystyrene microtitre plate) and the proteins non-specifically adhere to its plastic surface; this is known as 'sensitization'. Unbound proteins are washed away and non-specific protein binding sites are blocked, using a protein such as bovine serum albumin (BSA). The antigen to be assayed is then detected by the addition of a specific antibody. The antibody either can be directly labelled with an enzyme or fluorescent probes (direct ELISA), or a second, labelled antibody can be used to bind to the first antibody and amplify the signal (indirect ELISA; Fig. A.7).
- Surplus, unbound antibodies are washed away and then presence of bound antibody is detected by the addition of an enzyme substrate which will produce

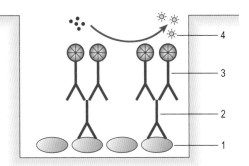

Figure A.7
Enzyme-linked immunosorbent assay (ELISA). The steps involved in a standard indirect ELISA are the following: Firstly, the assayed antigen binds to the polystyrene surface of microtitre plates (1). Then the primary antibody recognizing the antigen is applied (2). If this primary antibody is not labelled (indirect ELISA), then a secondary labelled antibody (usually enzyme-labelled) must also be applied (3). This also provides signal amplification. Finally, a substrate is given to the assay to develop a colour reaction proportional to the original antigen concentration (4).

a coloured product. In the case of fluorescent labels, the plates are exposed to light to excite the fluorescent probes. For *quantitative ELISA*, standard concentrations of the antigen are assayed in parallel with the samples to provide a 'standard curve'.
- A variety of adaptations of the ELISA technique have been developed. In '*sandwich ELISA*' it is not the assessed antigen of the sample that binds to the surface of microtitre plates, but a capture antibody specific to the antigen. This may be exposed to even crude samples, from which antigen is captured at high specificity. Then a second detection antibody is used which, if unlabelled, is followed by a third set of labelled antibodies.
- *Competitive ELISA* works in a similar way to a radioimmunoassay (RIA). In this technique, enzyme-linked antigen is used rather then an enzyme-linked antibody. The labelled antigens and antibody are provided in the ELISA kit; during the assay, the labelled antigen is in competition with unlabelled antigens present in the sample for binding to the antibody, such that the more unlabelled antigen is present, the less labelled antigen can bind and the weaker the signal will be. This competition provides outstanding sensitivity for the assay.

FURTHER READING

Crowther JR 2000 The ELISA guidebook. Methods in Molecular Biology, vol. 149. Humana Press: Totowa, NJ

Voller A, Bartlett A, Bidwell DE 1978 Enzyme immunoassays with special reference to ELISA techniques. J Clin Pathol 31(6):507–520. Review.

FRET

In molecular biology, fluorescent resonance energy transfer (FRET) can be used for the quantification of specific PCR products. Briefly, besides the two regular primers used for PCR (see ' PCR' below), a third oligonucleotide is also used. This probe is labelled with both reporter and quencher fluorescent molecules. Several well-characterized fluorophore molecule pairs are commonly used in this procedure, one such pair being FAM and TAMRA.

During the detection of PCR products in Q-PCR machines (see 'PCR' below), an excitatory light beam forces the reporter molecule to emit light of a particular frequency which can be detected within the machine. However, if the quencher molecule is close enough to the reporter molecule (as it is by default in the probe), the light emitted by the reporter will immediately be absorbed by the quencher. As a consequence, the quencher emits light of a different frequency which is not detectable by Q-PCR machines and no signal is detected. However, if the probe hybridizes to the same sequence that is amplified by, for example, Taq polymerase, the 5' to 3' exonuclease activity of the polymerase will digest the nucleotides of the probe. This allows reporter and quencher molecules to drift apart so that the light emitted by the reporter is no longer quenched and can be detected. The intensity of the light detected is in direct proportion with the amount of probe that has been bound to the specific PCR product being amplified; this provides the basis for the quantitative analysis of template concentration.

FURTHER READING

Didenko VV 2006 Fluorescent energy transfer nucleic acid probes: designs and protocols. Methods in Molecular Biology. Humana Press: Totowa, NJ.

FISH

In fluorescence in situ hybridization (FISH) a short, oligonucleotide DNA or RNA probe hybridizes, through complementary base pairing, to a target sequence in genomic DNA or in mRNA; binding of the probe can be detected because it is fluorescently labelled.

The technique allows for the sensitive detection of specific nucleic acid sequences while preserving morphology of the tissue or cell; hence the attribute 'in situ'. FISH was traditionally used for mapping of genes on chromosomes. It is widely used in diagnostics for testing anomalies and pathological rearrangements of chromosomes. It can also be used for the detection of gene expression in tissues and to correlate it with morphology.

FURTHER READING

Beatty BG, Mai S, Squire JA 2002 FISH (fluorescence *in situ* hybridization). Oxford University Press: Oxford.

Microarrays

In a microarray, specific sequences or probes are arrayed in a specific pattern on a glass, plastic or membrane surface. Arrays can be produced from DNA, RNA or protein. The number of different samples on a microarray (chip) is so high that the size of an individual sample (spot) falls in the micrometre range.

DNA microarrays are used for comparative profiling of gene expression in different samples (e.g. normal and cancerous tissues, cells with differential developmental origin, response to treatment with a compound vs. control). A typical commercially available DNA microarray contains spots of different oligonucleotides (probes), each of them complementary to different cDNAs or different parts of the same cDNA. These microarrays are manufactured with photolithography, ink-jet printing or electrochemistry. For gene expression profiling, total RNA is isolated from tissues or cells of interest, then fluorescently or chemiluminescently labelled cDNA is prepared by reverse transcription and hybridized on the chip. Two methods are used for hybridization. cDNA from two different samples which are to be compared is either labelled by different fluorochromes and hybridized on one microarray in a competitive manner, or labelled with the same fluorochrome or chemiluminescent tag and hybridized on two separate chips. This second method requires sophisticated internal controls in order to generate comparable data.

In addition to gene expression profiling, microarrays are increasingly being used in SNP (single nucleotide polymorphism) genotyping. Microarrays capable of genotyping 1 million SNPs at the same time are soon going to be available. Other lower-density DNA arrays are used for expression profiling of gene families or genes participating in certain biological pathways. Low-density arrays are also used for determining expression of miRNAs.

Low-density arrays of total RNA (dot blots) are used for simultaneous hybridization-based measurement of gene expression. In contrast to microarrays, these systems contain total RNA from different normal or pathological tissues immobilized on nylon or nitrocellulose membranes, and the probe is to be supplied by the user.

Proteins or peptides can also be arrayed on a nitrocellulose surface. Antibody arrays could be considered as multiplex sandwich-type ELISAs; in these systems a capture antibody is immobilized, the unknown sample is applied and binding is subsequently detected by a second antibody, either directly labelled or with secondary detection. Arrays containing full-length proteins are used for profiling the autoantibody repertoire or for searching for protein–protein interactions. Peptide arrays can be used for mapping kinase targets and identifying enzyme targets.

FURTHER READING

Causton H, Quackenbush J, Brazma A 2003 Microarray gene expression data analysis. Blackwell: Oxford.

Knudsen S 2004 Guide to analysis of DNA microarray data, 2nd edn. Wiley: Hoboken, NJ.

PCR

The polymerase chain reaction (PCR) was developed to amplify DNA sequences based on a template. It is a molecular biological method with a wide spectrum of utility. The Nobel Prize for Chemistry was awarded to KB Mullis in 1993 for the discovery of PCR.

The main requirements for a PCR reaction are:

- thermo-stable DNA polymerase
- template
- primers
- nucleotides
- specific buffers
- thermocycler.

This method would not be feasible without the use of thermo-stable DNA polymerase enzymes. The first such enzyme was discovered in the bacterium called *Thermophylus aquaticus* which lives in hot springs; the isolated enzyme is called Taq polymerase. The enzyme has a temperature optimum of 72°C and can maintain its activity at extremely high temperatures (95°C) for prolonged periods.

Taq polymerase elongates primers (single-stranded oligonucleotides of approximately 18–23 bases long) at their 3′ ends following primer hybridization to the template. Two primers are necessary, one complementary with each strand of template DNA. The four nucleotide-triphosphates (dNTPs) are also required at equimolar concentrations for PCR product elongation.

For some PCR applications such as molecular cloning, Taq polymerase is rather error-prone and creates artificial mutations. In these cases other polymerases with higher fidelity (albeit less robustness) may be used, such as the Pfu and Vent polymerases.

During PCR the copy number of a specific DNA sequence is amplified up to a million times. Amplification is achieved by the repetition of thermal cycles (Fig. A.8). Each cycle begins with an initial step of 95°C that denatures the two strands of template DNA sequence to provide accessibility for the two primers. The primers are then allowed to anneal to the DNA strands at temperatures specific to the primer pair (usually ranging from 55°C to 65°C). The last step is the elongation of PCR products at 72°C for a period of time depending

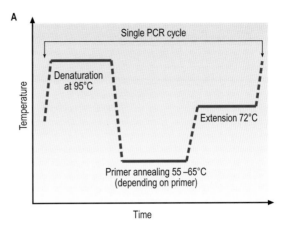

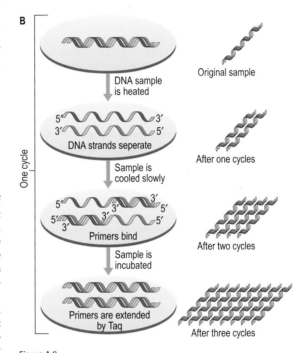

Figure A.8
Polymerase chain reaction (PCR). (A) During PCR a specific DNA sequence is amplified up to approximately a million times. This is achieved through the repetition of thermal cycles up to approximately 38 times. The exact boundaries of the amplified DNA sequence are specified by primer sequences. (B) Briefly, double-stranded DNA is first denatured to single strands by heating to 95°C, then primers anneal at specific temperatures (55–65°C) to locate starting and end-points of DNA synthesis performed at 72°C by special thermo-stable polymerase.

on PCR product size (1000 base pairs normally require 1 minute). Thermal cycles can be repeated up to approximately 38 times for maximum amplification before reaction plateau or non-specific products develop.

Genomic DNA or complementary DNA (cDNA) may be used as templates for PCR. Amplification performed on the former allows for the examination of the genome, while PCR using cDNA templates permits gene-expression analysis. The process that creates cDNA

Ethidium bromide and SYBR Green I in action

A

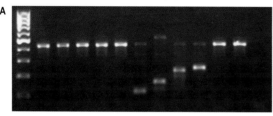

B

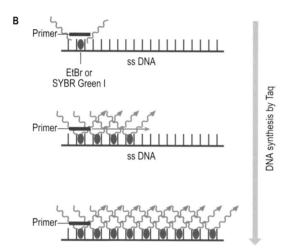

DNA synthesis by Taq

Figure A.9
Detection of PCR products. Ethidium bromide and SYBR Green I are intercalating and cyanine DNA stains, respectively. (A) They both selectively bind double-stranded DNA. (B) Both may be used for end-point analysis of PCR products following gel electrophoresis. SYBR Green I may also be used for real-time detection during Q-PCR, as this latter dye emits fluorescent light.

A

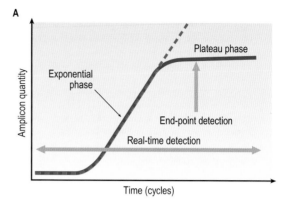

B

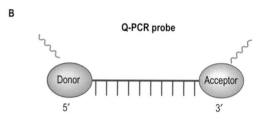

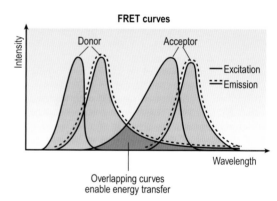

Figure A.10
Real-time quantitative PCR (Q-PCR). (A) During PCR amplification of specific DNA sequence shows a sigmoid curve; an initial phase is followed by an exponential phase, where DNA quantity is doubled in every PCR cycle. Finally, a plateau phase is reached as the reaction exhausts its substrates. PCR products may be visualized at the end of PCR (end-point detection) or throughout the reaction (real-time detection). Real-time detection allows for the quantitation of PCR products. (B) Amplicon-specific Q-PCR probes employ a physical phenomenon known as FRET. Here, a third Q-PCR primer is also used during PCR. This includes a pair of adjacent fluorescent molecules: a donor and an acceptor. These are selected so that donor-emitted light is converted by the acceptor (quenching), unless the two are liberated during PCR by the polymerase. Should this happen, donor-emitted light ceases to be quenched, allowing for sequence-specific real-time detection (see 'FRET' above).

from RNA templates is called reverse transcription (RT and so RT-PCR) and employs RNA-dependent DNA polymerase enzymes of retroviral origin called reverse transcriptases.

Two different types of PCR reaction are end-point analysis and real-time PCR.

- *End-point analysis PCR* is used for the qualitative analysis of PCR products and is often performed in ethidium bromide or SYBR Green-containing agarose gels (Fig. A.9).
- *Real-time PCR* allows for the real-time detection of DNA amplification during PCR and permits quantitative analysis of starting template concentration (Q-PCR). Q-PCR may be performed using SYBR Green or PCR product-specific probes that often utilize a phenomenon known as FRET (see 'FRET' above and Fig. A.10).

FURTHER READING

Baumforth KR, Nelson PN, Digby JE et al. 1999
Demystified … the polymerase chain reaction. Mol Pathol
52(1):1–10. Review.

Persing DH 1991 Polymerase chain reaction: trenches to
benches. Clin Microbiol 29(7):1281–1285. Review.

Valasek MA, Repa JJ 2005 The power of real-time PCR. Adv
Physiol Educ 29(3):151–159. Review.

Phage display

Phage display is a selection technique based on the
display of peptides or proteins on the surface of
bacteriophage particles. This technology physically
links protein-based functions to genetic coding information, allowing high-throughput screening of large
libraries. The selection process is called 'biopanning',
which refers to the repeated affinity selection of the
library leading to the enrichment of clones displaying high-affinity binding molecules (Fig. A.11). After
selection, the DNA encoding the 'high-affinity binders'
can be sequenced and further utilized for downstream
applications, such as production of recombinant antibodies.

The applications of phage display include the display and selection of random peptide libraries, cDNA
libraries, antigen fragment libraries and antibody fragment libraries (single chain fragment (scFv) libraries).
Depending on the application, distinct types of phage
have been found to be optimal vectors for library construction. These different phages differ in a number of
aspects (Table A.1).

Phage display can be used for construction of human
antibody libraries from healthy individuals or from patients with autoimmune diseases or suffering from various types of cancer. It can also be utilized for epitope
mapping of monoclonal or disease-associated antibodies and for identification of ligands for orphan receptors.
Moreover, the selection of phages using intact cells or
in vivo is also possible.

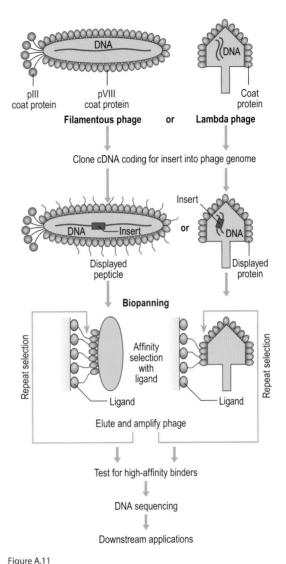

Figure A.11
Phage display. Phage display utilizes bacteriophage particles to display
foreign proteins on the surface of the phage particle. To achieve this,
cDNA coding for the protein or library of proteins is cloned in frame into
the phage genome to the part which codes for a bacteriophage coat
protein. Thus the displayed protein is going to appear on the surface
of the phage particle as a fusion protein with the coat protein. Next,
repeated affinity selection steps are performed with immobilized ligand.
As selection steps are consecutively repeated, phage particles displaying
high-affinity binders are enriched ('biopanning').

Table A.1
Comparison of different vectors used for phage display

	Type of phage		
	Filamentous	**Filamentous**	**Lambda**
Coat protein	pIII	pVIII	D
Life cycle	Continuous production, protrusion through membrane	Continuous production, protrusion through membrane	Sequential, lytic to host cell
Copy number of displayed peptide	~3	~2000	~100–200
Maximal size of displayed peptide (amino acids)	100	15	200–300
Application	Antibody fragment (scFv) libraries	Random peptide libraries	Antigen fragment and cDNA libraries

FURTHER READING

Sidhu SS (ed.) 2005 Phage display in biotechnology and drug discovery. CRC: Boca Raton, FL.

Recombinant proteins

The term recombinant DNA is used to describe artificial DNA constructs in which DNA from at least two biologically different sources is combined into one DNA strand in a vector (e.g. plasmid). If the recombinant DNA contains a sequence which codes for a protein, along with the appropriate regulatory sequences, it will serve as a template for transcription and eventually for synthesis of recombinant protein when it is introduced into bacteria, yeast or mammalian cells.

The first step in recombinant protein production is to obtain (to clone) the nucleic acid sequence coding for the desired protein. To achieve this, RNA is isolated from tissues or cells which are known to express the protein of interest, and cDNA is prepared by reverse transcription. If the sequence of the required cDNA is not known in advance, the traditional approach used to isolate the cDNA is to construct a cDNA library and to screen this library with oligonucleotide or antibody probes. If the cDNA sequence is known, PCR is generally used to amplify the appropriate sequence.

After this, the cDNA is inserted into an expression vector, which is chosen according to the host organism in which the protein is going to be expressed. Bacterial and yeast systems have the advantage of being robust in growth and in the amount of protein produced; however, since post-translational modifications largely differ between these and mammalian cells, mammalian proteins expressed in bacterial or yeast systems often lose their functionality.

Fusion proteins

Once a recombinant protein is expressed, it has to be purified from the cells or culture media. A widely used approach is to construct fusion proteins with molecules (affinity tags), which can be utilized for affinity chromatography. Fusion proteins can also be constructed to combine biologically distinct functions (e.g. ligand binding and effector functions) within a single molecule.

Fusion of the two proteins is achieved at the cDNA level, whereby two originally separate proteins are expressed as a single polypeptide chain. Widely used affinity tags in fusion proteins are those which reversibly bind ligands with high affinity. These include:

- the GST-tag (glutathione S-transferase; ligand: glutathione)
- the MBP-tag (maltose binding protein; ligand: amylose)
- the His-tag (repeat of histidine amino acids; ligand: divalent nickel)
- the Myc-tag (a short part of Myc proto-oncogene; ligand: anti-Myc antibody).

These affinity tags could also be used to detect the fusion protein.

Antibody humanization

Antibody humanization also involves work with recombinant proteins. The therapeutic application of monoclonal antibodies of mouse origin is limited by the inherent immunogenicity of mouse antibodies in humans. To overcome this problem, monoclonal antibodies developed originally in mice need to be engineered in such a way that they contain amino acid sequences of human origin and at the same time retain the antigen specificity. Consequently, these engineered antibodies possess low immunogenicity in humans. One approach is to take cDNAs coding for variable domains of the antibody from the mice and fuse them with human cDNAs coding for constant domains of the antibody. Such an antibody is called a chimeric antibody; about one-third of its sequence is of mouse origin and about two-thirds is human.

To minimize further sequences of murine origin, cDNAs coding for segments of variable domains which determine antigen-binding (CDR: complementarity-determining region) are taken from the mice and grafted into human cDNA sequences of variable domains which show a limited variability (FR: framework region). This process is called antibody humanization. A humanized antibody still contains about 5–10% of sequence of murine origin but this percentage is low enough to avoid immunogenicity in humans. With the use of mice which are knockout for mouse immunoglobulin genes and at the same time transgenic for human immunoglobulin genes, it is possible to produce fully human antibodies.

FURTHER READING

Chamow SM, Ashkenazi A (eds) 1999 Antibody fusion proteins. Wiley: Hoboken, NJ.

Gellissen G (ed.) 2005 Production of recombinant proteins: novel microbial and eukaryotic expression systems. Wiley: Hoboken, NJ.

Kontermann R, Dübel S (eds) 2001 Antibody engineering. Springer: Heidelberg.

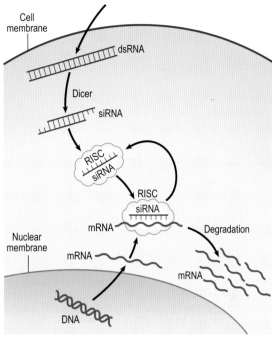

Figure A.12
RNA interference. Double-stranded RNA (dsRNA) enters the cell and undergoes cleavage by Dicer, which tailors small interfering RNAs (siRNAs) based on strict rules. One strand of the siRNA attaches to the RNA-induced silencing complex (RISC) holo-enzyme complex. The RNA-loaded RISC complex identifies target mRNA according to rules of base-pairing and cleaves the specific mRNA sequences, followed by further degradation. As a consequence, protein knockdown is achieved in a specific manner.

RNAi

The RNA interference (RNAi) technique was developed to inhibit the translation of mRNA into protein. The Nobel prize was awarded to AZ Fire and CC Mello for this discovery in 2006.

RNAi (Fig. A.12) is a process that is present in all species of the three phyla of plants, animals and fungi. It is an ancient and well-conserved mechanism used to inhibit the replication of certain viral pathogens, the accumulation of transposable genetic elements, and allows for the precise orchestration of gene expression. Briefly, double-stranded RNA is incorporated into an RISC (RNA-induced silencing complex); it is then cut randomly but precisely into 19 bp-long pieces with 3' overhangs of two bases, by an enzyme called Dicer. Following ATP-mediated activation, an RNA-loaded RISC can target complementary RNA. Depending on the degree of complementarity, the targeted RNA may be cleaved and/or its subsequent translation may be blocked. RNA interference can efficiently decrease the number of cytoplasmic mRNAs and can reduce the expression of the encoded protein, and RNAi may yield a knockout phenotype.

In the experimental use of RNAi, double-stranded RNA complementary with the targeted mRNA sequence is introduced into cells. In vertebrate cells the length of double-stranded RNA should not exceed 30 bp in size; otherwise, apoptosis is triggered. Double-stranded RNA pieces resembling Dicer-digested products are the most convenient to use. These are called small interfering RNAs (siRNAs).

The siRNA pieces may be introduced into target cells by various methods. Direct siRNA transfection techniques employing physicochemical delivery can be used. However, since RNAi operates at the level of RNA, target protein turnover restricts the utility of transient transfection methods. For efficient and long-term results, transient and stable vector constructs are more suitable. In these, siRNA translation is driven by polymerase III promoters and siRNA sequences are encoded in the form of self-folding hairpin structures, known as short hairpin RNA (or shRNA). These constructs can also be introduced into target cells by the above transient transfection methods or via sophisticated viral delivery techniques. Subsequent selection or sorting can yield pure, stable transgenic transfectants.

FURTHER READING

Kurreck J 2003 Antisense technologies. Improvement through novel chemical modifications. Eur J Biochem 270(8):1628–1644. Review.

Sledz CA, Williams BR 2005 RNA interference in biology and disease. Blood 106(3):787–794. Epub 12 Apr 2005. Review.

Tomari Y, Zamore PD 2005 Perspective: machines for RNAi. Genes Dev 19(5):517–529. Review.

SAGE

SAGE is the serial analysis of gene expression; it is used as an alternative to microarray techniques for generating expression profiles. The principle of this technique is to generate small sequences (tags) from cDNA corresponding to the expressed mRNA, subsequently using these tags to identify the expressed mRNA. These tags are ligated to each other, amplified with PCR and then sequenced. The steps involved in SAGE are as follows (Fig. A.13):

- Generation of cDNA from each mRNA expressed in the sample, with the incorporation of biotin at the 3' end of cDNA and subsequent immobilization of cDNA on to streptavidin beads.
- Cleavage of immobilized cDNA with a so-called anchoring restriction endonuclease (NlaIII), which has a short recognition sequence (4 bp) and thus cleaves cDNA molecules often, theoretically resulting in cleavage of all cDNA molecules. This cleavage produces overhanging ends for subsequent linker ligation.
- The immobilized and cut cDNAs are divided into two and ligated to two different linkers. These linkers contain a type IIS restriction endonuclease recognition sequence, and sequences for later PCR amplification.
- Cleavage of linker-containing cDNA with a type IIS restriction endonuclease (also called tagging enzyme; most often BsmFI). Type IIS restriction endonucleases are enzymes which cut the DNA molecule at a defined distance from the recognition sequence. Thus cleavage with tagging enzyme produces tags of uniform size which derive from the individual cDNA molecules.
- The tags are blunt-ended, ligated to each other, and amplified by PCR. Ligation and subsequent PCR amplification produce DNA molecules containing two tags next to each other (ditags).
- Next 'ditags' are digested with the anchoring enzyme to produce overhanging ends for ligation of all 'ditags' into one DNA molecule.
- The DNA molecule containing all of the tags generated is then cloned into a vector and sequenced.

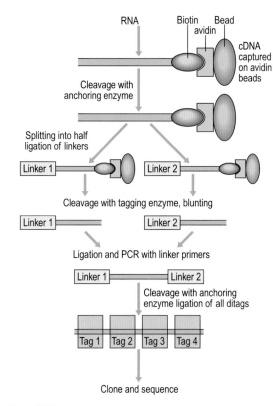

Figure A.13
SAGE. Serial analysis of gene expression (SAGE) is a technique used for generating gene expression profiles. This figure outlines one possible strategy for generating tags from expressed genes. For a detailed explanation of the steps involved, see the text.

FURTHER READING

Nielsen KL 2007 Serial analysis of gene expression (SAGE) Digital gene expression profiling. Humana Press: Totowa, NJ.

Sequencing

Sequencing is used to determine specific nucleic or protein sequences. There are few scientists who have won the Nobel prize twice; Frederic Sanger is one of them. He was awarded the prize first in 1958, for the determination of the amino-acid sequence of human insulin, and then in 1980 for developing the dideoxy method, known as the 'Sanger method', which is still used for nucleic acid sequencing today.

Nucleic acid sequencing

The 'Sanger method' exploits a specific characteristic of dideoxy-nucleotides: namely, chain termination during DNA polymerization. In a currently used version

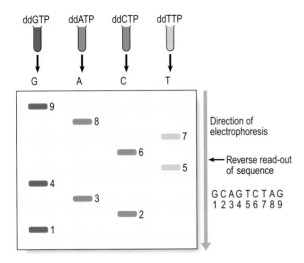

ddGTP　ddATP　ddCTP　ddTTP

G　　A　　C　　T

9
8
7
6
5
4
3
2
1

Direction of electrophoresis

←—Reverse read-out of sequence

G C A G T C T A G
1 2 3 4 5 6 7 8 9

Figure A.14

DNA sequencing: an outline of the Sanger method. In this technique, dideoxy-nucleotides (ddCTP, ddTTP, ddGTP and ddATP) are mixed with regular deoxy-nucleotides (dNTP) at low ratios in separate reactions. Dideoxy-nucleotides result in the termination of chain extension, and if such products are run on a high-resolution gel, DNA sequence may directly be read backwards.

of this method, fluorescent dye-labelled dideoxy-nucleotides are mixed at low ratios (e.g. 1:100) with regular unlabelled deoxy-nucleotides. In this way there is a specific chance that the chain termination will occur at each step of DNA polymerization, leaving a fluorescent dye-labelled nucleotide in the last position. Following

laser-assisted, high-resolution gel analysis, DNA sequence can be directly recorded (Fig. A.14). The method allows for the high-quality sequencing of up to approximately 500 bp per reaction.

Pyrosequencing is a new alternative of the 'Sanger method' based on chemiluminescence. Light is emitted every time a nucleotide is incorporated during DNA polymerization. The machine performing the analysis synchronizes light with a specific nucleotide addition (G, A, T or C) and thus reconstructs the DNA sequence. This method is rapid but allows for the analysis of only rather short DNA sequences (approximately 50 bp) and is mostly used for the detection of specific single-nucleotide polymorphisms (SNPs).

Peptide and protein sequencing

Due to significant structural differences between amino acids, peptide sequencing is a more demanding task than DNA sequencing. Mass spectrometry is a time-consuming and error-prone method of peptide sequence prediction. Today the most widely used method is called 'Edman degradation'; it was developed by P. Edman (see Ch. 5). Here the terminal residue of the targeted peptide is derivatized and cleaved from the amino-terminal end of the protein in a sequence of alkaline and acidic reactions; the cleaved residue is then dissolved in an organic solvent for analyses by chromatography or electrophoresis (Fig. A.15). Amino-acid sequence analysis can only be continued for up to approximately 50 residues in this manner due to the accumulation of imperfect digestions.

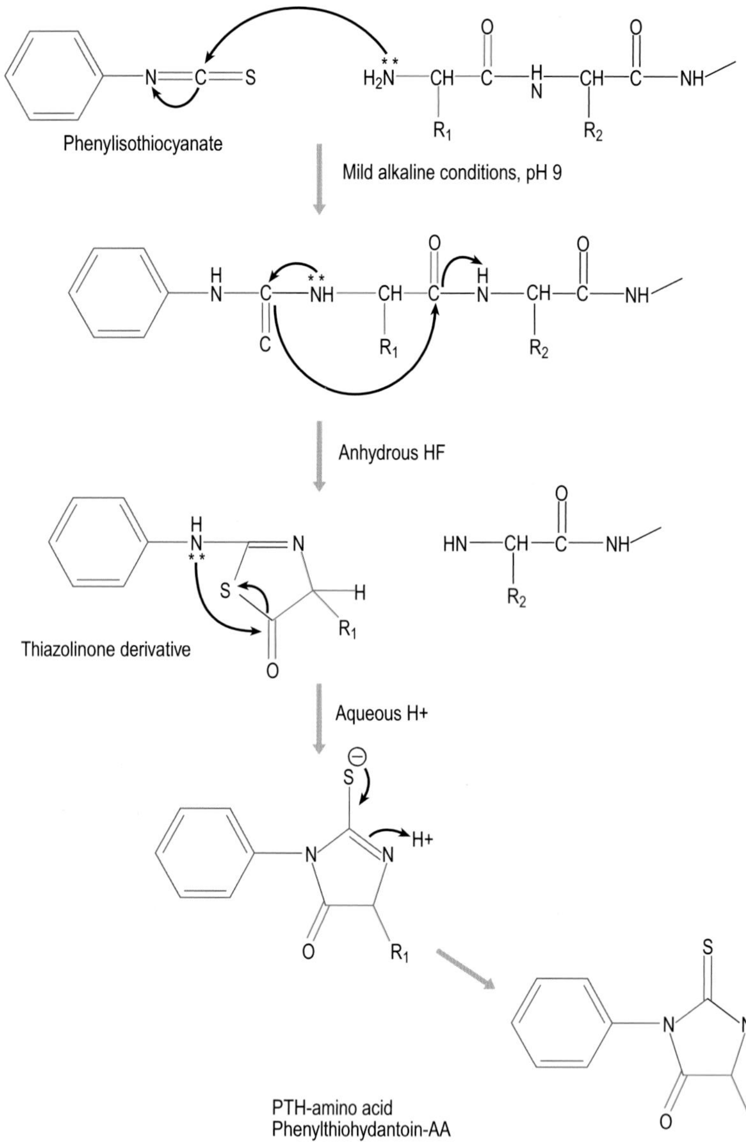

Figure A.15
Protein sequencing: the Edman method. In this technique, a protein adsorbed to a solid phase reacts with phenylisothiocyanate. An intramolecular cyclization and cleavage of the N-terminal amino acid results; the product can be washed from the adsorbed protein and detected by HPLC analysis. The method may be applied to protein sequences of a maximum of around 50 amino acids, so most proteins need endoprotease digestion prior to direct sequencing.

FURTHER READING

Meldrum D 2000 Automation for genomics, part one: preparation for sequencing. Genome Res 10(8):1081–1092. Review.

Meldrum D 2000 Automation for genomics, part two: sequencers, microarrays, and future trends. Genome Res 10(9):1288–1303. Review.

Metzker ML 2005 Emerging technologies in DNA sequencing. Genome Res 15(12):1767–1776. Review.

Two-hybrid systems

This molecular biology approach is used to study protein–protein interactions: most frequently, for the identification of novel interaction partners with a known protein.

The principle relies on the activation of a reporter gene which only occurs when the interaction of the proteins in question is present (Fig. A.16). To make this possible, the transcription factor activating the reporter gene is split into a binding domain and into an activator domain, and two fusion proteins are expressed simultaneously in yeast or bacterial cells. One of the fusion proteins contains the binding domain of the transcription factor fused to the protein for which interaction partners are searched (bait); the other one (prey) contains the activator domain of the transcription factor fused to the protein which is supposed to interact with the bait. The prey need not necessarily be a single protein, but could be a library of many proteins. If the prey protein (or a member of the prey library) interacts with the bait, the binding and activator domains of the transcription factor are brought to close physical proximity to each other and transcription of the reporter gene starts. Otherwise, the reporter gene remains inactive. The most frequently employed systems use the Gal4 transcription factor of yeast to drive transcription of reporter genes such as gal1-lacZ or β-galactosidase.

Once interaction of two proteins is demonstrated in a two-hybrid system, it needs to be verified in an independent experimental system, e.g. by co-immunoprecipitation from cells which are engineered or known to express the two interacting proteins.

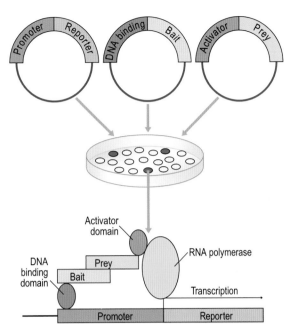

Figure A.16
Two-hybrid systems. This technique is used for identification of proteins which interact with each other. Two fusion proteins are expressed simultaneously in yeast or bacterial cells. One fusion protein contains the binding domain of a transcription factor fused to the protein for which interaction partners are searched (bait); the other one (prey) contains the activator domain of the transcription factor fused to the protein which is supposed to interact with the bait. If the prey protein interacts with the bait, transcription of the reporter gene is turned on.

FURTHER READING

Bartel PL, Fields S (eds) 1997 The yeast two-hybrid system. Advances in Molecular Biology. Oxford University Press: Oxford.

Index

Abbreviations:
PCR - polymerase chain reaction
SELDI-TOF - surface-enhanced laser desorption/ ionization with time of flight mass spectrometry